germs
are us
collaborating
FOR LIFE

ALSO BY
MELVIN A. BENARDE

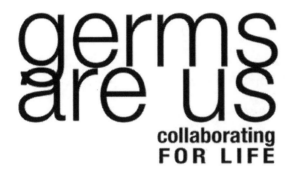

germs are us

collaborating
FOR LIFE

MELVIN A. BENARDE, Ph.D.

MADISON M PUBLISHING

Germs Are Us; collaborating FOR LIFE

Copyright © 2015 by Melvin A. Benarde, Ph.D.

All rights reserved

Printed in the United States of America

First Edition

For information about permission to reproduce selections of this book, to purchase for educational, business or sales promotional use please contact Madison Publishing at, www.germsareus@gmail.com

Library of Congress Control Number: 2014946450

Benarde, Melvin, A. 1923–

Germs Are Us; collaborating FOR LIFE/Melvin A. Benarde, Ph.D. - 1st ed.

p. cm.

Includes glossary, references and index.

ISBN 978-1500574888

1. Germs. 2.Microbes. 3. Microbiome. 4. Environmental microbiology. 5. Beneficial microbes. 6. Health. 7. Title

Cover Design: Johanna Furst

Portrait photo: Thomas Francisco

Cover photo credit: Photomicrograph of the soil mold Fusarium venenatum used to produce Quorn, a meat substitute. Courtesy of Marlow Foods, Stokesly, North Yorkshire, UK.

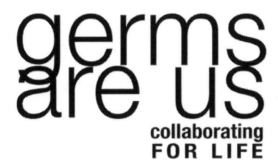

germs
are us

collaborating
FOR LIFE

Ignorance and fear are not necessary
components of human existence.

– Lucretius, On the Nature of Things, 1bce

DEDICATION

**To the microbes that make us
and our environment flourish.**

*Books are the carriers of civilization. Without books,
history is silent, literature dumb, science crippled,
thought and speculation at a standstill.*

*They are the engines of change, windows on the world,
lighthouses erected in a sea of time.*

– Barbara W. Tuchman, Guns of August, 1978

CONTENTS

PREFACE

Readers of this book are in for one surprise after another, as *Germs Are Us* reveals an incandescent paradigm: the inextricable connection between microbes and us—forever.

Germs Are Us is a game changer, expanding our horizons beyond what we've ever known, and altering our view of the way we comprehend the world. The idea may be heretical, and seemingly preposterous at first blush, but it's a'comin, and we need to know about it, and be prepared for it. Such new thinking will be eye-popping, challenging, and sometimes unsettling, but *Germs Are Us* will aid in the transition. Will we be frightened by this new knowledge? Some of us will; many more will seek information and answers, as reality comes front and center allowing us to live more informed and calmer lives.

The idea, the fact, that we humans are a composite of microbial and human cells can be downright shocking, and will be one of the 21st century's major revelations —and controversies.

While *Germs Are Us* means to be informative and revelatory, it will help us face our concerns and fears. It is a genre far removed from anything yet written on the inhabitants of the unseen world, and their tight connection to us.

The message in this bottle is huge: without our microbes there'd be no us...and little else.

In fact this book was yet another collaboration. It could not have come into being without the advice and assistance of a gaggle of family and friends. I've written a book about a raft of complex issues in a manner at once accessible yet uncompromising in its scientific accuracy. Consequently, appraisal and help are essential in a book of this nature, ranging as it does, across a panoply of rigorous issues.

My wife Anita, always my first and severest critic, could be counted on to raise questions for clarification, as would my writer/journalist son Scott, and daughter Andrea, assuring the elimination of jargon and science-speak. High praise must go to Dean Lichtman, a courageous talent who read every chapter—twice—raising salient questions, assuring accuracy and clarity. Gale Patullo, an elite grammarian, took on the unenviable chore of editing my jottings doing yeoman's work, for which my gratitude is boundless.

Gratitude must also go to Lester Levin, friend and colleague who I could bounce ideas off, secure in the knowledge that if I bounced too far, he'd reel me in. Appreciation must also go to AJ, my grandson, for the books rousing title that garnered wide applause. And what would I do without my granddaughter Erica, who took on the onerous job of indexing with her usual aplomb, stitching together myriad people, places and permitting the rapid location of all things from A to Zed.

Not to be overlooked are the reference Librarians at the West Windsor Public Library, who made scientific journal articles appear like rabbits from a top hat. I suspect they'll be relieved that his project is over. Finally, pride of place belongs to my daughter Dana, who became my general manager and guru every step of the way to the book's publication assuring that it blossomed and bore fruit. Without her uncompromising attention to details, there'd be no book. Period.

Nonetheless, with all the help rendered, and all the suggestions extended to me, *Germs Are Us*, being a complex sweeping volume, all errors, omissions, interpretations and conclusions are mine alone.

Melvin A. Benarde, Ph.D.
Princeton, NJ
2015

INTRODUCTION

As I walked into our nearby Sam's Club, a couple, husband and spouse I guessed, were blocking the way with their shopping cart. As he attempted to hold the cart handle, she laced into him shouting, "don't touch it," "don't touch it, do you want to get infected?" That poor guy, has he got trouble, and far more than germs! That's not an isolated case. Not by a long shot. So, for example, a recent article in the New York Times, typical of the many we've been treated to in the media, informed us that researchers at the University of Houston, University of South Carolina, and Purdue University, working together, found huge numbers of bacteria on TV remote control units in hotel rooms in their states, and presumably this germy condition exists in all hotel rooms. Furthermore, they tell us, these germy clickers are far more fearsome than bedbugs. However, way down at the bottom of the article, the lead researcher, Prof. Jay Neal, warns about over re-reacting. "You'd have to lick the remote control for a long time to get sick from it," he said. Nor does he suggest what kind of sick, but does that matter? Even the most famished among us surely wouldn't lick a clicker, it doesn't taste or smell like chocolate. Then there was my wife, Anita, at her physician's office. His nurse asked her to step on the scale. As she did, and was about to place her hands on the right and left bars around the scale, the nurse shouted, "Don't do that. Those bars are loaded with germs!"

The Metropolitan Transportation Authority in New York, the MTA, weighed in, announcing that it would be selling advertising space on the front of its fare cards to raise much needed revenue. Among several ads being considered is this one:

You Touched the Pole! Quick Use some...

Bacteri-Off

Handsanitizer

1-800-555-Germ

Yup. Keep the pot boiling. Do we laugh or cry? Hey, ya gotta laugh. There's real humor here. But a few tears are also being shed. After all, aren't microbes, our germs, all over the place? Aren't they on our shoes, in our hair, on our ties, shirts, chairs, tables, dresses, dishes, pencils, doorknobs, food, and everything else? There are mobs of microbes, on everything, everywhere. In fact, germs, microbes, are the most widespread living things on our planet. And, as we shall come to understand, we humans are more microbial than human! And, yes, the title of this book is a fact. No animal, plant, human or inanimate object is germ-free. If we were, we'd all be dead! We, and they, have been living together since we climbed down from the trees, and began walking upright, and more than likely they were with us in the trees. Do we share the earth with microbes, or is it that they share it with us? Not a frivolous question. And for most of our time together, it's been a comfortable and agreeable relationship. Although we haven't realized it we, and our germs, are inextricably linked, now and forever—beneficially!

Germs Are Us, lays bare this new paradigm, and wants to tell the germ's story, and what a story it is! Providing as it does, a robust understanding of the microbial universe, but perhaps as important, it reduces the fear of germs, counteracting the manifest absurdities that make us fear our world, and our germs, our microbes.

Recall, that FDR reminded us that, "The only thing to fear is fear itself." Apparently, every generation needs to be nudged, reminded of this enlightening caution, as we forget too easily.

And Marie Curie, winner of a Nobel Prize in Physics, urged us to be aware that "nothing in life is to be feared, it is only to be understood. Now is the time," she said, "to understand more, so we may fear less."

That's it; understanding is the key to unlocking our fear. We've been afraid of the wrong things far too long. Microbes, our germs, are surely one of these things; things we've been made to fear: manipulated by fear mongers, and an unhelpful communications media.

Three problems afflict us: lack of accurate, trustworthy information, conflicting information, and continuous exposure to misinformation. Result: fear and mental pollution, a media-genically induced dysfunction, the offspring of medical/scientific news dispensed by scientific illiterates unable to differentiate good science from poor. Time for keen understanding of germs is at hand.

The story of our microbiome, the totality of microbes that live agreeably among us, as well as, those which perform the many salutary and life sustaining activities, we know so little about, needs telling, convincingly and cogently. Just what *Germs Are Us* does.

Chapter ONE provides a remarkable celebration of the human mind's capacity to uncover nature's secrets; the revelation of an unseen, invisible world, and deals with the many experiments that led to the discovery of microbes.

Chapter TWO takes us on a voyage of discovery of the enormous microbiota that live comfortably on and in every inch of us. Here we ask, can we humans live in an environment free of microbes? Also asked is, what do our microbes do for us, and are they really necessary? The National Institutes of Health's Human Microbiome Project is introduced, which seeks to explain the critical roles our germs play, involved as they are, in so many of our metabolic processes, that will lead to new treatments for a number of diseases.

Chapter THREE wades through, shedding light on our dynamic and protective immune systems, and asks, is dirt good for us? We then examine the Hygiene Hypothesis, which supports our need for close contact with microbes early on, and why allergies and other autoimmune conditions appear to be rising. We continue with the critical question, would our immune system be overwhelmed without our vast number of beneficial microbes?

Chapter FOUR takes on a basket of those few delinquent germs that grab headlines, and our attention, and asks the question, how do they get to us, and how successful are they? We also tackle the nasty issue of Bioterrorism, asking, how difficult is it to mount a bioterror attack, and which of the nasties are at the top of anyone's terror list?

Chapter FIVE describes the considerable differences between food spoilage and food borne illness, and we ask, how did Napoleon's military campaign against Russia spur the quest and advancement of food preservation. It also explains why food irradiation is clearly the way to go to achieve greater safety of our food supply.

Chapter SIX brings us the Germs of Endearment, those remarkable producers, without which our food supply would be dull and boring. Here we blow wide open the umpteen benefits our microbes provide: groaning boards of scrumptious foods and bracing beverages, as well as additional microbial benefits in a variety of areas.

Chapter SEVEN deals with those microbes often referred to as our biogeochemical engineers, responsible for driving the carbon, nitrogen and sulfur cycles, without which there'd be no us. They are that important. We also ask, what could be the most important question of the 21st century: can our microbes reduce the level of carbon dioxide in the atmosphere, thereby restoring our normally stable climate? The possibility is surely intriguing. We also deal in depth with the pathways to development of biofuels, and the microbial mining of minerals to make us more competitive.

Finally, it explores the new world of biotechnology where synthetic microbes are manufactured, piece by piece, in labs and other places, to obtain the organisms we desire, for the many functions we need them to perform. Could this be a two-edged sword coming back to bite us?

This book is a game changer, expanding our horizons beyond what we've ever known, and will forever alter the way we see and comprehend our world. Such new thinking may not come easily, but *Germs Are Us* will surely aid in the transition that will allow us to live calmer, more enjoyable, less stressful lives.

We begin with an old and ancient friend, the wise Aristotle, (384-322 bce) who had among his many great ideas, a few poor ones.

ONE

The Invisible Becomes Visible

According to Aristotle, "as a general rule, all shelled animals, Testaceans, grow by spontaneous generation in mud, differing from one another according to the differences of the material: oysters growing in slime, and cockles on sandy bottoms; and in the hollows of the rocks the ascidians and the barnacles, and common sorts, such as the limpets and the nerites. Other insects are generated spontaneously: some out of dew falling on leaves, others grow in decaying mud or dung: others in timber, green or dry, some in the hair of animals: some in the flesh of animals; some in excrements: and some from excrement after it has been voided, and some from excrement yet within the living animal, like the helminths or intestinal worms."[1] For Aristotle, aphids arose from dew, fleas from putrid matter, mice from dirty hay, and barnacles on ships became geese, when broken off.

This philosopher extraordinaire, polymath, and intellect for the ages, student of Plato, and teacher of Alexander the Great, ardently believed in Spontaneous Generation; that life can spring from non-life. Worse yet, because Aristotle said it, it became so, and went unchallenged for well over two thousand years.

Annually in spring as the Nile River flooded Egypt's banks leaving behind nutrient-rich mud which brought with it bountiful food crops, common knowledge held that large numbers of frogs were generated by the rich mud and soil: frogs that weren't there during dry spells. Wasn't it obvious then, that frogs sprang alive from the muddy soil? Of course it was. Not!

In many towns animal carcasses were hung by their heels, and customers selected which chunk butchers would carve off for them. But hanging carcasses also drew armies of flies. Obviously, the decaying meat hanging in the sun created the flies. Definitely not!

In many areas of Europe, medieval farmers stored grain in barns with thatched roofs. As the roofs aged, they leaked, which led to moldy grain, and of course with stored grain, mice abounded in great numbers. Moldy grain must have produced the mice. That was the common wisdom, as was the fact that raw sewage flowed in gutters in most cities sans sewage treatment systems. Each morning, the contents of chamber pots were tossed out of windows, and after a meal, whatever was left on plates was also tossed onto the gutters. And truth to tell, rats swarmed and fattened. Wasn't it obvious that sewage and garbage turned into rats? Aristotle had it right, didn't he?

Recall the story of the Pied Piper of Hameln, Germany. Hameln, (Hamelin) a sleepy hamlet of ancient, half-timbered dwellings, half-an-hour drive southwest of Hanover, was a well-to-do town of corn traders that had a severe rat problem. As the brothers Grimm, Jacob and Wilhelm, wrote in their priceless children's story, and as Robert Browning popularized it in his witty ditty, that many of us read in elementary school, a Piper with his coat of many colors, appeared in Hameln, as if in answer to the Council's needs, offering to rid the town of all its rats for a fee of a thousand Guilders. The Mayor and Council quickly and happily agreed.

The Piper drew his Fife from his coat pocket and began to play a haunting tune that brought a flood of rats scurrying out of the buildings to his side. As he marched along heading out of town, rats continued bounding out of barns and houses following the Piper. Leading them to the Weser River, he removed his colorful clothes, walked into the river where the rats quickly followed and drowned. The Piper now requested payment, but the Mayor laughed at him, offering only fifty Guilders. Furiously angry, the Piper left. Two days later he returned wearing dark clothes and a red hat, and began playing a merry tune that had all the children chasing and dancing after him. 130 of them followed him all the way out of town and up into the nearby mountains and into a cave, and were never heard from again.

To this day, Hameln celebrates the Pied Piper and the rats, each year in May. It's off the beaten tourist track, and worth a visit.

As for spontaneous generation, the eminent 17th century Flemish (Belgium) Chemist, Johan Baptiste van Helmont, offered a recipe for the production of mice. Simply place some rags in a pot with a few grains of wheat and mice will appear in about two weeks. Both male and female will be present and they will reproduce additional mice. Eminence will do it every time.[2]

This was too much for Francesco Redi, who had to challenge Aristotle's widely accepted notion of spontaneous generation. However, challenging Aristotle was tantamount to challenging the Church at Rome, as the Church held tightly to the notion of spontaneous generation as a defense of the virgin birth of Christ. But challenge he did, and successfully, by a series of simple, yet elegant experiments that laid spontaneous generation to rest—for a time.

Who was this Redi fellow, bold enough to challenge existing authority? Redi was a Tuscan, born in Arezzo, Italy, in the heart of Tuscany, in 1626, and educated at the University of Pisa. As a doctor, he became Court Physician to Ferdinand de Medici, Grand Duke of

Tuscany. At the time it was commonly believed that maggots formed naturally from rotting meat. To test the notion of spontaneous generation, also known as Aristotelian Abiogenisis, he placed slices of meat into two jars, one of which was sealed, the other open to the air. Flies flew into the open jar and maggots, (fly eggs, larvae) appeared on the meat. The sealed jar had no flies and no maggots. In his second series, he placed slices of meat in another two jars, covering one with gauze to permit the entrance of air and the odor of decaying meat to escape, while the other was fully open. Again, the meat in the gauze-covered jars remained free of maggots, but flies hovered over the jar, and maggots developed on the gauze. The uncovered jar, as in the first test, contained flies and maggots on the rotting meat.[3]

Redi's simple experiments were a staggering blow to the notion that life could arise from non-life. The idea of controlled experiments was a totally new contribution. His experimental results were printed and distributed as: Esperienze informo alla Generazioni degl'Insetti, Experiments on the Generation of Insects. This should have laid spontaneous generation to rest—but it didn't. We humans do resist change.

Redi remains also well known as a poet for his outstanding work, the dithyramb, Bacco in Toscana, Bacchus in Tuscany. It's too humorous and witty to let it pass without a few lines. To wit:

The conqueror of the East, the God of Wine

Taking his rounds divine,

Pitc'd his blithe sojourn on the Tuscan hills;

And where the imperial seat

First feels the morning heat,

Lo, on the lawn, with May-time white and red,

He sat with Ariadne on a day,

And as he sang, and as he quaff'd away,

He kiss'd his charmer first, and thus he said:-

Dearest, if one's vital tide
Ran not with the grape's beside
What would life be (short of Cupid?)
Much too short, and far too stupid.
You see the beam here from the sky
That tips the goblet in mine eye;
Vines are netrs that catch such food,
And turn them in to sparkling blood.
Come then—in the beverage bold
Let's renew us and grow muscular:
And for those who are getting old,
Glasses get of size majuscular:
And in dancing and in feasting,
Quips, and cranks, and worlds of jesting,
Let us, with a laughing eye,
see the old boy Time go by,
who with his eternal sums
Whirls his brains and wastes his thumbs.
Away with thinking! miles with care!
Hallo, you knaves! the goblets there.
Gods—my life, what glorious claret!

Whoever said that scientists have no soul? This remarkably talented chap flourished in a region of high intelligence and creativity. Redi's Tuscany was home to Petrarch, Vasari, Dante, Boccaccio, and Michelangelo, an immensely fertile region for artists, poets, painters, and of course, scientists. But theirs was, and continues to be an uphill battle.

As damming as Redi's experiments were, spontaneous generation refused to go quietly, receiving support from an English biologist and Roman Catholic priest. In 1745, John Tuberville Needham, using "mutton gravy hot from the fire," in open glass containers, allowed the broth to cool and found the clear broths soon became cloudy and putrid. Surely this was strong proof of spontaneous generation. Discovery of microbes in air was still a long way off, ergo, and naturally, Needham was held victorious. And it does give one to wonder how it was possible that at this time, Sir Isaac Newton (law of gravity, and calculus), spoke out in praise of spontaneous generation, and Alchemy, another of his pet notions. Hey, and why not, transmuting base metal into gold had much to recommend it at the time.

Twenty years were to pass before another creative Italian, Lazzaro Spallanzani, took up the cause. In 1749, his parents sent him to Bologna to study at that ancient university where he concentrated on math and natural sciences. In addition to obtaining a philosophy degree in 1753, he was ordained a priest in 1757. Although not a physician, he made important contributions to medicine, and was the first to propose freezing sperm cells for later use. How about that for imagination? But it was his experiments suggesting and hinting that microscopic life in air was the probable cause of Needham's cloudy and putrefying broth solutions that brought him the notoriety he deserved.[4]

To demonstrate this, he placed broths in glass flasks, sealed them tightly then heated the broths to boiling. All remained clear. Whatever caused Needham's broths to cloud up, had entered from the air," he wrote. This should have driven the final nail into what had to have been the dying corpse of spontaneous generation. But myths are hard dying.

Needham would have been a better investigator had he followed Spallanzani's caution. "If I set out to prove something," he remarked, "I have to learn to follow where the facts lead me. I have to learn to whip my prejudices."[4] Needham wasn't listening, claiming that a "vital force" necessary for spontaneous generation had been destroyed by boiling the solutions in sealed flasks which prevented the "vital force" from entering the flasks. Obviously the mind can dredge up sentiments to support our most cherished flummery. Nevertheless, Needham received the support he didn't deserve from a wholly unexpected and unintended source: the discovery of oxygen and its necessity for life, by the eminent 18th century French chemist, Antoine Laurent De Lavoisier. Spallanzani's elegantly simple experiments were criticized for not having sufficient oxygen in the sealed flasks to support life. They didn't know it at the time, but it was nevertheless true. Microbes were not yet known, but they too required oxygen. Any wonder that Aristotle prevailed for two millennia!

The 17th and 18th centuries passed into the 19th, with spontaneous generation still at large and all the rage, when in 1861, Louis Pasteur in France, demolished that lingering and persistent prattle. It took that long; and then it wasn't any easier. But one of the delights of science is its capacity for showing us that the world is not as it often seems. Good examples follow, tumbling one upon the other.

In 1861, the French Academy of Sciences sponsored a contest for the best experiment either proving or disproving spontaneous generation. Louis Pasteur's winning experiments sprang from Needham's and Spallanzani's, and showed conclusively—well almost—that living things are present in air, and that they can readily grow in nutrient solutions. To settle the matter, he approached this cleverly in several ways. Using sterile, (germ-free) cotton plugs, he drew air through them, then placed these plugs in clear boiled beef broth. Two days later the broth teemed with growth. Living things were obviously in air.

Filling flasks with broth again, he sealed them shut, and brought them to boiling. Months later no growth. To top that off, he again placed clear broth in flasks, heated their necks in a flame to soften the glass, then drew them out in long S-shapes and other curves, but kept the ends open to the air. The broth in these Swan-neck flasks was brought to a boil and allowed to stand. And stand. And stand. No growth, even though air could pass into the flasks. The few airborne bacteria that might enter the long, S-shaped necks were trapped on their inner surfaces. When he tilted his flasks allowing broth to reach the lowest points in the curves, where airborne particles could have settled, the broths rapidly became cloudy—with life. Pasteur had refuted the long held notion of spontaneous generation, and conclusively demonstrated that living things were everywhere, including the air.[5] He proved decisively that Omnis Cellula e Cellula–only cells arise from cells; which harkens back to Lucretius, the 1st century Roman writer, and his De rerum natura, On the Nature of Things, in which he wrote, "de nihilo nihil," nothing comes from nothing.

In Pasteur's un-tilted swan-necked flasks there is no growth to this day! His original flasks remain on display at the Pasteur Institute. The next time you're in Paris, amble off the beaten tourist paths to the Institute and have a look. Spontaneous generation was finally laid to a much needed, rest and the existence of invisible life firmly demonstrated. Of course, some remained unconvinced. Nothing new there.

There was, however, an unaccounted for fly-in-the-ointment. Spores. Spores are a dormant condition whereby some microbes become dormant, and in that dormancy, resist normal heat treatments for extended periods. Pasteur and others assumed that these "seeds," (from the Latin, germen) these microbes, could not survive boiling water. It remained for Prof. Ferdinand Cohn of Breslau University, Breslau, Prussia, (at the time), now Wroclaw University, Poland, to discover these thermo-resistant microbial spores, and remark on their implication for spontaneous generation. Cohn explained that these heat resistant cells could readily revive after dormancy, and grow. Therefore, to fully and finally dispatch spontaneous generation, nutrient solutions had to either be boiled for at least two hours or be superheated above 212°F (100°C) the temperature of boiling water, to kill-off any loitering spores. When that was done, spontaneous generation's last legs were gone for good. It was also Prof. Cohn who showed that microbial cells divide by fission, splitting in half, indicating that they can readily multiply and grow. An enormous contribution at the time.[6] He also made a clear distinction between spoilage and pathogenic (harmful) microbes in food, which we shall meet up with in Chapter FIVE.

Microbes Revealed

Well before the spontaneous generation brouhaha was being batted back and forth, a sometimes-lens-grinder in the thriving Dutch City of Delft, near the Hague, was picking his teeth.

Delft, well known for its Delftware, decorative plates and vases of cobalt blue-white ceramic ware, was home to Antoni van Leeuwenhoek, official wine taster, Alderman, Haberdasher and amateur lens grinder.

Several lovely paintings of Delft were done by the celebrated artist Jan Vermeer, who was not only born in Delft, but in 1632 the same year as Leeuwenhoek. No doubt they knew one another. Delft was also the home of Baruch Spinoza, another grinder of lenses, and a philosopher, whose mind was percolating with contrary ideas, calling everything into question. Indeed, Delft was a city in ferment.

During the year 1674, Leeuwenhoek placed his fingernail between his teeth, scraped along the surface of his teeth, and deposited a bit of the scraping on his homemade microscope which could magnify some 300 times, just enough to be astonished to see "little things" swimming about "Animalcules" he called them. He also found them in rain and river water. Here was the first ever recorded observation of unicellular life: later to be identified and referred to as germs or microorganisms.

Much later. Nevertheless, microbiology was born.

Interestingly, Leeuwenhoek's homemade lenses were placed between silver, or brass, plates of his own design and riveted together to form the basis of his microscopes. These lenses were originally used to inspect the quality of cloth he offered for sale. Not only was he a master craftsman, he was widely respected as an honorable entrepreneur.

In the 50 years between 1674 and 1723, Leeuwenhoek sent 375 letters about observations of his "animalcules" to the Royal Society of London. In one of them he wrote, "Dear God, what marvels there are in so small a creature." In another, he noted that, "there are more animals living in the scum (plaque in our jargon) on the teeth in a man's mouth (women were no exception) than there are men (he surely meant people) in the whole kingdom." He had no idea how close to the truth he was. To fully appreciate the diversity and magnitude of life on earth, get a microscope. The very first bacteria seen by anyone were shown in Leewoenhoek's sketches that accompanied his letter of September 17th, 1683, to the Royal Society.

"I then most always saw, with great wonder, that in the said matter there were many very little living animalcules, very prettily a-moving. The biggest sort...had a very strong and swift motion, and shot through the water (or spittle) like a pike does through water. These were most always few in number. "The second...spun round like a top, and...were far more in number. To the third...seemed to be oblong, while anon they looked perfectly round. These were so small...yet therewithal they went ahead so nimbly, and hovered so together, that you might imagine them to be a swarm of gnats or flies, flying in and out among one another."

What an exciting time it must have been for this gifted amateur. Can anyone imagine what eyesight he had to have had to make his fabulous observations, bringing his petit microscope, some four inches long, directly in front of one eye! Perhaps most phenomenal was his notation that "seeing these wondrous dispensations of nature whereby 'little animals' are created so that they may live and continue their kind, our thoughts must be abashed and we ask ourselves, can there even now be people who still hang on to the ancient belief that living creatures are generated out of corruption?"[7] Obviously he was well aware of the notion of spontaneous generation and disavowed it unconditionally. That, dear reader, was 160 years prior to Pasteur's demolishing the idea with his brilliant experiments. For Leeuwenhoek, it was intuitive. Isn't this a guy you'd want to clink a glass of wine with? Surely it's for good reason microbiology textbooks refer to him as the father of microbiology.

Stirrings

Human, animal and plant disease have been an integral part of our existence since we walked the earth, and wondered why. The idea, the notion that living things, "seeds" some called them, could be the source of infection and illness, remained below the horizon, but there were stirrings.

From the 12th to the 19th centuries, bloodred spotting on starchy foods captured the imagination, especially when the red spotting appeared on sacramental bread and wafers. Dozens of blood-like sightings on bread, cake, meat, and chicken, but most often on the Host, were recorded between 1174 and 1874 in Italy, France, Germany, Belgium and Poland.

The Miracle of Bolsena, the most famous spotting, occurred in the Church of Santa Christina near Bolsena, Italy, in 1263.[8] On his way to Rome a German priest stopped at Santa Christina, to celebrate Mass. As he bent over the Host, during consecration, "the blood that Christ had sweated in Gethsemane oozed from the Host and dropped down upon the linen of the alter." He couldn't believe what he saw. The Pope had to be told. The Priest hastened on to Rome to bear witness. In memory of this miracle, Pope Urban IV issued a Bull, Transitaurus de hoc Mundo ad Patrem; For the purpose of moving the world to the Father, which established the Feast of Corpus Christi in honor of the Eucharist, celebrated to this day. But that was far from the end of it.

Blood-red spots also appeared on Polenta, (a thick corn meal porridge often called "Italian Grits", which was an essential dish among many farm families,) in a number of Italian villages, causing civil disturbances during the 18th and 19th centuries. Then, in 1879, Bartolomeo Bizio, a Pharmacist in Padua, completed a series of tests, remarkable for that era, (this guy would easily have been nominated for a Nobel prize had it been established by Alfred Bernhard Nobel, given the ingenuity of Bizio's experiments), and found that the red spots on the Polenta were produced in damp and warm environments, and noted that the corn meal and other grains carried "seeds" (from the Latin, germen, pronounced as the g, in ginger meaning, bud, sprout, seed, germ, and/or embryo) which reproduced themselves. Bizio named these living things, Serratia, in honor of Serafino Serratia, an Italian physicist. He also added a species name, marcesans, from the Latin, marcesere, to wither, or decay, because "as it decays it dissolves into a (red) fluid and viscus matter which has a mucilaginous appearance," which shook the countryside with fear and trembling.[9]

We now know that the Miracle of Bolsena and the Feast of Corpus Christi, as well as the "bloody polenta" were due to the growth of the common airborne bacterium, Serratia marcesans. We were approaching the horizon—closing in. The "seeds," the "germs" were getting names.

Raffaello Sanzino, otherwise known as Raphael, considered one of the greatest of Renaissance painters, was requested by Pope Julius II to create a work commemorating the Miracle of Bolsena. In 1512, the elaborate painting depicting a Priest offering communion with wine, and a wafer broken open to reveal a red stain was unveiled. To the faithful the red "blood" proved the wafer was transformed into the body of Christ. This appearance of blood was seen as a miracle affirming the Roman Catholic doctrine of transubstantiation, which held that the bread and wine became the body and blood of Christ at the moment of consecration during the mass. This colorful painting can be seen in the Stanza di Elidoro, the third Rafael Room, a huge Papal apartment, in the Palazzi Pontifici, at the Vatican, in Rome.

A Hungarian Obstetrician

For women about to give birth, Vienna, circa, 1840, was a nightmare. Childbed Fever deaths in hospitals was so frequent that women often preferred to give birth in back alleys, after which they would bring their infants to the hospital, a practice not limited to Vienna. At the time, Childbed Fever, puerperal sepsis, was referred to as The Doctor's Plague. Ignatz Phillip Semmelweis, a Hungarian OB, practicing at the Vienna General Hospital, wondered why maternity clinics were "houses of death." Why, he wondered, was his division having a far higher maternal mortality than the midwives division? To his shock and consternation, an answer arrived with the untimely death of his close friend and colleague, Dr. Jakob Kolletschka, who died from a wound accidentally inflicted while dissecting a cadaver. Kolletschka's symptoms were the same as those of women who died of Childbed fever. It hit him! He had his "aha" moment. He, his students and the other OB's, were the culprits! They had been doing autopsies on women who died of Childbed Fever just before examining women in labor. *They* were infecting the women with whatever it was they picked up from the cadavers. Midwives had no contact with cadavers. He knew what to do. All students and all OB's had to wash their hands with soap, followed by rinsing in chlorinated water (Chlorina liquida) *before*

13

entering the maternity wards. The death rates plummeted! Listen to him. "The cause of Prof. Kolletschka's death was known: it was the wound by the autopsy knife that had been contaminated by cadaverous particles. Not the wound, but the contamination of the wound by cadaverous particles that caused his death, as well as the death of women with Childbed Fever."[10,11] He could not know what those "particles" were, but whatever they were, chlorine solutions could remove them. It had to be something in the environment, as so many preferred to believe. He was ridiculed by the surgeons and OB's at his hospital, but in time, his seminal insight began slowly moving about the continent. Resistance continued, but the horizon was coming into view.

An Appalling Famine

Consider that Irish Catholics didn't pour out of Ireland for the US and Canada because they needed an ocean voyage. No. They packed up and departed the "old sod" because a microbe devastated their potato crops, on which they had subsisted. Their meager diet of potatoes, were eaten in place of bread. Unbelievably, potatoes were the sole source of food for 30 percent of the people, and essential for another 30 percent.

Potato blight first occurred in autumn, 1845, lasting till 1852. The editor of the Gardeners Chronicle and Horticultural Gazette trumpeted the news that "...we are visited by a great calamity which we must bear. On all sides we hear of destruction. As a cure for this distemper, there is none."[12] Today, we call this blight-er, this microbe, this fungus, *Phytophtora infestans,* one of the first microbes to be associated with a plant disease. We were getting closer.

Starvation was rampant. A wholesale exodus followed as hundreds of thousands left the country. Between 1845-1851, the population of Ireland decreased by more than 30 percent. Among the hundreds of thousands that crossed the Atlantic to America, were two impoverished families: the Kennedy's and the Fitzgerald's. JFK, John Fitzgerald Kennedy, born in 1917, became President of the United States, in 1960, because a fungus forced his great-grandfather out of Ireland.

The Broad Street Pump

Dr. John Snow (1813-1858) was a thinking man's physician. When he was a young medical apprentice he was sent to help during an outbreak of Cholera among British coal miners. His careful observations convinced him that the disease was usually spread by unwashed hands and shared food, not "bad air."

In 1854 Cholera struck London a second time. This time he was ready. He learned that the city's water supply came from two competing companies, the Southark & Vauxhall Company, and the Lambeth Company. Snow interviewed Cholera patients, or their families, and found that most of them purchased their water from the Southark & Vauxhall Company. He also learned that this company took its water from the Thames River below locations where Londoners discharged their raw sewage. By contrast, the Lambeth Company's intake pipes were in the upper reaches of the Thames well before the water reached London's raw sewage outlets. By calculating death rates for those using water from each company, something that had never been done before, his data clearly showed that those households receiving water from the Lambeth Company had a mortality rate five times less than those purchasing their water from the Southark & Vauxhall Company.[13]

Snow inferred the existence of a "Cholera poison" transmitted by polluted water. He also noted that the cause of the disease must be able to multiply in water, and he believed that consecutive cases suggested a means of transmission, more so than could be accounted for by coincidence. He tells us, "that diseases which are communicated from person to person are caused by some material which passes from the sick to the healthy." Of course, he was right, but he couldn't know why, or what that material was. But he was close, very close. As he put it, "the morbid material is ingested through the mouth, multiplies in the gut, and is excreted with feces." Wow, was he ever close! Here was a thinking, analytical physician like no other.

As cases developed, he spotted the location of each household on a map. As the days passed into weeks, the spots grew thicker. He then located the sources of water and marked the location of each community pump on his map. Spots were heavy around one pump, and extremely light around another. Snow found that a brewery near the lightly spotted pump had a deep well on its site where its workers, who lived in the area, got their water. But these brewery workers also slaked their thirst with beer. He realized that these men and their families were, in effect, protected from the community's cholera-laden water. Conversely, the heavily spotted area on the map fairly shouted out, "it's the Broad Street pump, in Golden Square," in the Soho district.

As Snow tells it, "*I had an interview with the Board of Guardians of St. James parish on the evening of Thursday, 7th September, and I represented the above circumstances to them. In consequence of what I said, the handle of the pump was removed the following day. This, of course, prevented anyone from fetching more water from this pump.*" Why, you may ask, did Snow bring his data to the Vestrymen of St. James Parish? A relevant and reasonable question. Under English Law, a sanitary code was established that vested power in local Boards of Health. St. James, an Anglican Parish, was the local Board of Health for the Soho area. Ergo, Dr. Snow was following protocol by going to them with his request. Too many microbiology textbooks, along with the media, continue to maintain that Snow himself removed the handle and stopped the epidemic in its tracks. Perhaps this statement will finally allow the dust to settle on the question of who in fact removed the handle of the Broad Street pump, and if it's removal actually stopped the epidemic in its tracks.

Donald Cameron and Ian G. Jones, of the Department of Community Medicine, Edinburgh University, Scotland, inform us that, "the pump handle was removed by or on behalf of the local Vestrymen, certainly not by John Snow, and both Snow and his contemporaries clearly state that the outbreak was declining anyway."[14] And here is Reverend Henry Whitehead, a contemporary of Snow's on the matter of a declining epidemic. "It is commonly supposed," he writes, "and sometimes asserted even at meetings of medical societies, that the Broadstreet outbreak of cholera in 1854 was arrested in mid-career by the closing of the pump on that street. That this is a mistake is clearly shown by a tabulation, which, though incomplete proves that the outbreak had already reached its climax, and had been steadily on the decline for several days before the pump handle was removed."[15] Doubt should finally give way to the numbers.

Whatever it was that was causing cholera, Snow's evidence surely indicated it was waterborne. This led to public health efforts to clean up the Thames. Although the association between water supply and cholera was strong, it was not directly causal. But cleaning up the Thames further strengthened the association, as cholera cases plummeted.

Here was a thinking physician, so far ahead of his peers, that they were leery of him. Nevertheless, in 1853, he offered a comprehensive theory for the causes of infectious and communicable illness in which he stated that for each infectious disease, there is a distinct and specific cause, and that the causal agent is a living organism. Furthermore, that the quantity of infectious material transmitted is increased by multiplication after infection, to produce the observable symptoms.[13] Mind you, this was half-a-dozen years before Louis Pasteur in France, and Robert Koch in Germany, would discover and identify microbes! How much more explicit could Snow have been?! What a remarkable piece of Sherlockian intuition and creativity!

Remarkable as it was, believe this: the powers that be, the government officials, replaced the Broadstreet pump handle after the cholera epidemic of 1854 subsided, and thoroughly rejected his theory of causation as repugnant. The idea of a fecal-oral transmission was "too unpleasant for the public to contemplate." The prevailing theory of Cholera causation at the time was that it was an airborne disease concentrated in low-lying areas where the disease settled. Additionally, offensive odors, especially breathing the odor of decomposing animals was deemed causal. That made much better sense. Didn't it?

Of course it wasn't until well after Snow died that British physicians grudgingly acquiesced to the idea that cholera was waterborne. Would you believe that the evidence that Cholera was waterborne was not generally accepted in England, Europe and the US, until 1936!

Who was John Snow? Nothing less than a legendary figure in the history of public health, epidemiology, and anesthesiology.

Prior to his concern with cholera, Snow was a pioneer in the use of anesthetics, a true experimenter who calculated accurate doses of both chloroform and ether for use on individuals who would undergo painless surgery or childbirth. Consequently Queen Victoria chose Snow and his chloroform procedure when she gave birth to her son Prince Leopold in 1853, and again in 1857, when she gave birth to Princess Beatrice. This led to wide acceptance of obstetric anesthesia.

Furthermore, Snow's agile mind was quick to realize that bread adulterated with alum, (aluminum potassium sulfate) used as a whitener, was the cause of childhood Rickets. His keen observational power found that Rickets was far more common in children of working class families, who were fed almost entirely on bread, than those children who had a greater variety of food. He was enough of a chemist to understand that alum destroyed the wheat's natural calcium phosphate that normally strengthened bones. Snow also found that those families that baked their bread at home, used no alum, but those that bought their bread at bakeries, were always heavily adulterated.[16, 17] Few, if any physicians thought this way.

John Snow died prematurely at age 45 from kidney failure due to continued experimentation with a wide variety of anesthetics. For Epidemiologists, he is considered the grandfather of that discipline, as his studies of Cholera and alum in bread were, and remain, models of scientific reasoning.

Across the Channel

Indeed, there were stirrings in England, and ferment across the Channel in France, where Louis Pasteur, Prof. of Chemistry, and Dean of the Faculty of Sciences, University of Lille, visited a brewery that had both sound and sour beer, which led him to his microscope, where, with careful examination of the beers, he saw what convinced him that he was looking at living organisms-a lá Leeuwenhoek–which he called ferments, responsible for both the sound and sour beer, as well as for the fermentation of beet sugar. Moreover, the sour wine had a different type of living thing than the sound product. Ah! From this, he went on to write that just as microbes can grow in beer, wine and milk, so too they can multiply in people and animals and produce disease. "What a fabulous assumption!" What a burst of creative imagination! Here was the genesis of the germ theory of human illness. And, by the way, the key to the development of the Germ Theory, had to be a thorough rejection of spontaneous generation. Why?

In the early years, it was anti-intellectual, which prodded thinkers to go after it. But in the later years, during Pasteur's and Koch's time, as the new science of microbiology was emerging, it was a necessity. After all, if life, a microbe, could arise in a nutrient solution by chance alone, there was no sense, no point in studying the nature of its action, or its metabolism and other characteristics, as it might never be encountered again, or there could well be a different microbe at any one time. Either way, such an event would defeat the development of a systematic means of identification and control.[18] It would be chaotic.

Being able to identify organisms, seeing the same ones, repeatedly, allowed Pasteur to identify one microbe, one ferment, as he referred to them, that could convert a sugar solution into alcohol, wine, while another readily identified, would convert the sugar solution into undrinkable acid. This could be repeated again and again, assuring the outcome would be predictable, preventable and/or controllable. In the case of pathogens, those disease inducers, each organism, each microbe, could be identified as it had its unique "fingerprint," which gave rise to the concept of *one agent, one disease*, leading directly to the Germ Theory. Spontaneous generation defied any of this.

For Pasteur, it was clear. Listen to him, "In the interior of the grape, in healthy blood, no such germs exist; crush the grape, wound the flesh, and expose them to the ordinary air, then changes, either fermentative or putrefactive, run their course. Place the crushed fruit or the wounded animal under conditions which preclude the presence or destroy the life of the germ, and again, no change takes place; the grape juice remains sweet and the wound clean." And he concluded, "The application of these facts to surgical operations, in the able hands of Joseph Lister, was productive of the most beneficent results, and has indeed revolutionized surgical practice."

And so it was, that in 1857 Pasteur published his study, "Sur la Fermentation Appeleé Lactique," On the Lactic Fermentation, which became his public manifesto and announcement of the germ theory of fermentation. In this Report, he showed that the souring of milk was due to microbes that converted milk sugar, lactose, to lactic acid, and that the acid clotted the milk protein, casein.

We call this sour, clotted milk, yogurt, sour cream, or buttermilk, depending upon which bacterium, which germ, produces the scrumptious mouthful. He also found that when wine, alcohol, was left open to air, it turned into vinegar, acetic acid, which was the conversion of alcohol by yet a different set of microbes present in air. The versatility of microbes was evident to him. They were surely phenomenal chemical factories. He dubbed these microscopic-sized organisms, microbes: a well-chosen designation.

Perhaps of utmost importance, without the presence of these ferments, no changes occur! That's pivotal! By gently heating wine and milk, he killed off the ferments that produced the alcohol and acids. Pasteurization was discovered, which we'll meet again, in Chapter FIVE.

Similarly, when human surgical wounds are kept free of ferments, these seeds, these germs, wound infections do not occur.

Joseph Lister, Prof. of Surgery at the Glasgow Royal Infirmary, Glasgow, Scotland, learning of both Semmelweis' disinfection techniques and Pasteur's heat treatments, began heating and soaking his surgical instruments and dressings in carbolic acid (phenol), which proved highly successful in reducing surgical infections, and provided further proof of the role of germs, microbes, in disease, as phenol, which killed germs, also prevented wound infections.

But the salient question that remained to be answered was how do we know an illness is infectious and microbially related?

The first demonstration of the role of microbes, germs, as agents of disease came from the discovery in 1873, of the microbe causing Leprosy, followed several years later with the isolation of the Anthrax bacillus an infectious disease of sheep and cattle, that we the people are readily susceptible to. The scores of diseases transmissible from animals to we humans are called zoonotic diseases, zoonoses, which we'll deal with a bit further on. One thing to remember, at least 75 percent of our illnesses are animal related.

Robert Koch, a young German physician practicing medicine in Wollstein, a small country town in the district of Posen, northern Germany, using criteria suggested by Jacob Henle, his former professor and friend, sought to establish a causal relationship in 1876 between an organism he called Bacillus anthracis, that he had recovered from a dying animal, and Anthrax, a fatal disease of sheep and cattle.

To do so, Koch injected healthy mice with the blood of diseased sheep. The mice sickened. Placing bits of spleen from ill mice into sterile beef serum, he obtained luxuriant growth of his Bacillus. He then inoculated these organisms into a number of healthy mice, which also became ill. From these sick mice he was able to again retrieve his Bacillus. This series of stringent tests resulted in the Koch-Henle postulates that became the gold-standard for determining causality of microbial related illnesses. These postulates, now universally accepted and used, require that:

1. The suspect organism must be present in every case of the disease, but absent in healthy animals.

2. The suspect organism must be obtained from an infected animal and grown in pure culture.

3. The disease must be reproduced when the obtained organism is inoculated into healthy animals.

4. The same organism must be obtained from the ill animals.

Koch's exacting proof of the relationship between his Bacillus anthracis and Anthrax was then independently verified by Pasteur, which effectively ushered in the Golden-age of Microbiology/Bacteriology, with its germ theory of disease, and its underlying principle of one agent, one disease; as John Snow had theorized fourteen years earlier. Now, a once invisible universe had been revealed. The realization that yeasts, a germ, played a significant role in fermentation was the spark igniting a necessary and sufficient link between the activity of microorganisms and the physical and chemical transformations they could induce in animal and plant tissue, and that these "seeds," these "germs," could also initiate human illness. The race was on: and what a race it was.

In the remarkably short span of 34 years between 1876 and 1910, not all that long ago, a baker's dozen of the most dreaded illnesses, Hydrophobia (Rabies), Tuberculosis, Tetanus, Yellow Fever, Syphilis, Gonorrhea, Anthrax, Typhoid Fever, Pneumonia, Cholera, Diphtheria, Dysentery, and Rocky Mountain Spotted Fever, were discovered and confirmed by imaginative and persevering scientists using the Koch-Henle postulates. They worked. Along the way, those seminal root-nodule, nitrogen-fixing bacteria (to be discussed shortly) responsible for giving us abundant food crops, were identified, as was hypersensitivity, the theory of Immunity, immunization, and vaccination. All revealed. What a time it was! Could it have been anything but a Golden Age?!

Time out for a clarifying diversion.

For lucidity and accuracy, here and evermore, let it be understood that microbes and germs convey two distinct ideas. Therefore, I propose we use microbes when referring to all unicellular, beneficial micorganisms, saving germs for those delinquents, related to our infectious and communicable illnesses, as they were what the early researchers were hunting for and discovered. And, as they referred to these wee beasties as seeds or germs, they came to represent the entire universe of the denizens of the unseen world, and that's what got into textbooks, dictionaries, and the communications media. Time is now for a change. As we shall see, over the past twenty years, a veritable revolution has ensued during which microbes have been shown to be much more beneficial than harmful. We'll pursue this new paradigm at length, but for the moment, let us not lose the thread.

The rapidity of the discoveries noted above, was breathtaking, and the dazzling roster of medical scientists included the most creative minds from Germany, France, England, Denmark, Japan, Russia, the Netherlands, Austria, and lastly, but hardly least, in 1910, Howard Taylor Ricketts, a University of Chicago Microbiologist, discovered the organism responsible for Rocky Mountain Spotted Fever, and joined this singular pantheon. These prestigious researchers thoroughly demolished Aristotle's other entrenched notion, that the physical environment was the cause of our illnesses. Aristotle had a long and successful run, but was undone, eventually.

But the germ theory was truly, and almost entirely a European invention. It still had to cross the Atlantic to post-civil war America, and enter the consciousness and awareness of both the medical community and the public.

How was it received? The short response, poorly. Exceedingly poorly. That an invisible thing, a living thing at that, could sicken and kill a man, a cow or a tree, was unimaginable. A more nuanced response impresses us that "looking back at this period we find that American medicine was ill equipped to deal with this problem." Few, if any of the medical schools of the time made anything more than a pretense of teaching pathology, and bacteriology, then in its infancy, was hardly thought of"[19] And, in 1875, one distinguished pathologist claimed that if what is really known of the laws of disease were told to the members of the profession, more than half of them would indignantly discredit it. At the time, America and its 38 states, was wholly uninvolved, which may well account for the attitude toward the medical revolution on its doorstep.

Objectors and dissenters to a germ theory were everywhere. Most, for example, firmly believed that TB, Tuberculosis, was due to an inherited or acquired disposition. There was an almost insurmountable obstacle to a theory of contagion. The idea of personal contact between or among individuals was just too much to bear even though discoveries were following in rapid succession. Dr. Robert Koch had predicted that it would take no more than two generations for the universal acceptance of the idea of human-to-human contagion, but that was lost on American physicians who couldn't shake the belief in inheritance of TB. Fully 50 years were to pass before the theory of contagion would become a reality in American medicine. But that had to await the Flexner Report with its rebirth of American medicine and its new medical schools. Silos of information supporting the germ theory were piling up, but few were listening-or worse, were ready to listen.

Most discouraging was the fact that in 1866, during the Cholera epidemic in Chicago, Dr. N.S. Davis, a physician there considered the infection due to "seeds, or "germs", scattered throughout the city, so many years after John Snow's work showing it to be a waterborne disease, but few, if any were aware of his work.[20] It was no different when Typhus Fever occurred in New York's lower east side in 1894; it's cause and means of transmission remained unknown. As late as 1900, many New Yorkers remained convinced of the miasmatic theory of disease: that illness was due to bad air: mal aria.

The germ theory in America was at a dead end. Until there was full understanding of that theory, rubber would never meet the road.

A formidable and intriguing question was, why did America so thoroughly lag Europe for so long, so ignominiously, given similar backgrounds and resources? The response at the time may have held more than a grain of truth. "There was little prestige to be gained in research because the commercial spirit of the Anglo-Saxon world placed the emphasis on practice-reflecting the businessman's sense of values." Furthermore, the profession opposed and rejected innovation. It was self-satisfied. There was no incentive to adopt rigorous techniques of an evolving scientific approach. Ergo, the germ theory of Pasteur and Koch, having crossed the ocean to post-civil war America, was virtually DOA- Dead on Arrival.[20]

Worse yet, major opponents of the germ theory were- believe this-supporters of spontaneous generation-years after its stubborn demise! From the paucity of articles in American medical journals, circa 1880, on Lister's antiseptic procedures, you could be forgiven if ever you thought the germ theory even existed. Ignorance of European research and results was widespread following the Civil War. And most telling, the quality of personnel in the medical profession was at a low level.[21] Additionally, optical instruments such as microscopes were rare and of poor quality until the last decade of the 19th century. As far as American Medical journals were concerned, the germ theory was not accepted, or mentioned only for ridicule. The new science of Bacteriology scarcely existed. Curiously enough, not so much for the general public, who were reading Popular Science Monthly, Scientific American, The Tribune Popular Science, and the American Journal of Science and the Arts, which were informing their readers about the germ theory and its direct relation to illness. However, and unfortunately, this popular awareness was limited to affluent families that tended to their personal needs. For the millions of families living in poor urban areas, microbes were wholly unknown.[21]

As the 1860's gave way to the 90's, the germ theory appeared to be born again as though the opposition of the previous twenty years had never occurred. It remained for the young physicians who studied in Europe to return and put into practice their new found science. And, as we shall see, President Garfield's bullet wounds got none of the benefits.

Abraham Flexner and the Carnegie Foundation for the Advancement of Teaching, had had enough of America's lagging so far behind Europe. The Foundation's

Administration urged Flexner to take on the task of evaluating the country's medical schools and medical education.

Louisville, Kentucky, born Abraham Flexner, was prepared for that responsibility. After graduating from Johns Hopkins University, and studying at the University of Berlin, he joined Carnegie's faculty. His report, *Medical Education in the United States and Canada*, published in 1910, revolutionized medical education. Half of the almost 200 so-called medical schools with their poor quality, closed down. Flexner's Report was responsible for instituting the radical reforms that elevated U.S. medical education to leading position in the world, and took the germ theory along with it. The drastic changes in medical education heralded a revolution that led inexorably to higher standards for entrance to medical schools, curriculum revisions that required strong biomedical sciences, and hands-on clinical training, safer surgery, preventive vaccinations, improvements in personal hygiene, and widespread community sanitation. Simply put, The Flexner Report was the most important event in the history of American medical education.

Flexner didn't stop there. He was the founder of the Institute for Advanced Study, in Princeton, New Jersey, and was its Director from 1930 to 1939, during which time he managed to coax Albert Einstein to come and join the faculty.

President Garfield's woefully ignorant physicians were prime examples of why the Flexner Report was so vital.

James A. Garfield, 20th President of the United States, was not your common garden-variety machine politician. Garfield came to the presidency with clean hands, which promised a new dawn in the mosh pit of Washington politics. After only four short months as head of the nation, he was shot: Brought down by Charles Guiteau, an unhinged office seeker who stalked, and put two bullets into Garfield.

In mid-June 1881, Guiteau borrowed fifteen dollars and bought a .44 caliber British Bulldog pistol.

Garfield and Secretary of State James G.Blaine, arrived at Washington's Baltimore and Potomac railroad station on the morning of July 2nd, 1881, where Garfield was to take the train to Elberon, at the New Jersey shore, where his wife Lucretia and their three children were expectantly waiting for him.

When Garfield walked into the station, Guiteau was standing directly in back of him. No more than five feet from him. Guiteau's first shot sliced through Garfield's right arm and kept on going. As he turned to see who shot him, Guiteau's second shot struck him in the back. Neither shot was fatal. They were healable wounds. Guiteau was quickly wrestled to the floor, cuffed, and taken away. Garfield was carried to an upstairs room in the station where a passle of physicians took turns sticking their dirty fingers and unsterilized instruments into his wounds, trying to locate the lead bullets. That was just the beginning of what would become Garfield's trial by fire.

The Philadelphia World's Fair, The Centennial, held from May 10th to November 17th, 1876, celebrated the 100th anniversary of the Declaration of Independence, and ushered in the modern machine age. The vast crowds, which included James A. Garfield, Alexander Graham Bell, and Dr. Joseph Lister, were fascinated by working models of the typewriter, telephone, airbrake, and self-binder reaper. Also of note, were Dr. Lister's talks to American physicians, trying to persuade them to use his antiseptic techniques. Unfortunately for Garfield, most of them simply shrugged off Pasteur, Koch and Lister's widely established discoveries. Five years before Garfield's unnecessary and ghastly death, Dr. Samuel Gross, President of the Centennial's Medical Congress, and one of the most respected surgeons in the country, had this to say to his peers: "Little if any faith is placed by any enlightened or experienced surgeon on this side of the Atlantic in the so-called Carbolic Acid (phenol) treatments of Prof. Lister." President Garfield would pay dearly—with his life—for that sentiment.

By the time Garfield was shot, Dr. Doctor (believing he would be a physician, his mother named him Doctor) Willard Bliss had been a practicing surgeon for thirty years. But he had little to no respect for Lister's use of Carbolic Acid spray to disinfect and remove microbes and their potential for infection. Dr. Bliss took charge of his patient at the railroad station and later at the White House.

What follows, is Candice Miller's description of Garfield's treatment by Bliss, and my attempts at paraphrasing. Ms. Miller is the recent author of that highly lauded book, and rightly so, Destiny of the Republic: A tale of Madness, Medicine and Murder of a President, published in 2011.

Miller tells us that, "As soon as Bliss arrived at the station, he assumed immediate and complete control of the President's medical care." And, she continues: "Opening his bag, Bliss selected a long probe that had a white porcelain tip...doctors used these probes to determine the location of bullets. If the tip came up against bone, it would remain white, but a lead bullet would leave a dark mark." She also writes that pressing the unsterilized probe downward and forward into the wound, Bliss did not stop until he reached a cavity three inches deep in Garfield's back. At this point he decided to remove the probe, but found he could not. "In attempting to withdraw the probe, it became engaged between the fractured fragments and the end of the rib," Bliss later wrote. He finally had to press down on Garfield's fractured rib so that it would lift and release the probe. Of course all this without an anesthetic.

After it was out, he began to explore the wound again, this time with the little finger of his left hand. He inserted his finger so deeply into the wound that he could feel the broken rib. Bliss removed his finger and calmly selected another probe. Bending the probe into a curve, he passed it into Garfield's back, downward, forward and backward in several directions. After enduring Bliss's excruciating examinations, and listening to ten different doctors discuss his fate, Garfield asked to be taken back to the White House—anything was better than this room. The horror and murder was to begin in earnest.

In the United States, circa 1880, the most experienced physicians continued to refuse to use Lister's antiseptic procedures, complaining that it was too time consuming, and dismissing it as unnecessary, even ridiculous. "Had Garfield been shot just 15 years later, the bullet in his back would have quickly been found by X-ray images, and the wound treated with antiseptic surgery. He might have been back on his feet within weeks. Even had Garfield been left alone, he almost certainly would have survived." Yes, resistance to change is difficult, but to think that in the U.S. we would have to wait to the beginning of the 20th century, to achieve these benefits is beyond imagination.

"In order to successfully practice Mr. Lister's antiseptic method," one doctor scoffed, "it is necessary that we should believe, or act as if we believed the atmosphere to be loaded with germs." And loaded it was.

When Garfield's wound was dressed one morning, "a large quantity of pus escaped, carrying with it fragments of cloth that the bullet had dragged into his back and a piece of bone that was about an eighth of an inch long. Dr. Bliss was not concerned about the pus. On the contrary, he considered it a good sign, as did many like-minded surgeons at the time." Just two years earlier, William Savory, a well-regarded British surgeon and prominent critic of Joseph Lister, had proclaimed in a speech to the British Medical Association, that he was, "neither ashamed nor afraid to see well formed pus." And he declared, "a wound was satisfactory under a layer of laudable pus." Bliss could not have agreed more heartily.

Garfield's wound, the medical bulletin announced one night, "was looking very well," having, "discharged several ounces of healthy pus." But Garfield was deteriorating. Each time they inserted an unsterilized finger or instrument into Garfield's back, something that happened several times every day, they introduced bacteria, which not only caused infection at the site of the wound, but entered Garfield's blood stream.

"Unbeknownst to his doctors, cavities of pus had begun to ravage the president's body. One cavity in particular, which began at the site of the wound, would eventually burrow a tunnel that stretched past Garfield's right kidney, along the outer lining of his stomach, and down nearly to his groin! An enormous cavity, six inches by four inches, would form under his liver filling with a greenish-yellow mixture of pus and bile." He was literally rotting to death. So toxic was the infection that it was a danger even to those who were treating him. One morning, while dressing the president's wounds, Bliss reached for a knife that was partially hidden under some sheets. Unable to see the blade, he accidently sliced open the middle finger of his right hand. "It is thought that some pus from the President's wound penetrated the cut," the New York Times reported the next day, "and produced what is known as pus fever." The resulting infection caused Bliss's hand to become so painfully swollen that he had to carry it in a sling. Recall Ignaz Semmelweis's experience with Childbed Fever and the death of Dr. Kolletschka! But Bliss still refused to admit that he could not save the President's life.

On the evening of September 19th, at 10:30 PM, and after a day of a bulletin announcing how well he was doing, President Garfield died-murdered-by a gang of physicians totally resistant to the germ theory and Lister's antiseptic procedures. The poor man was tortured for ten long, miserable weeks. Ignorance was, disastrously, Bliss.

As the 20th century wandered into the 21st, remarkably new discoveries about microbes, immensely beneficial microbes, began emerging. And, as the following chapter reveals, we and our microbes, are inextricably linked, now and forever.

TWO

Our Microbiota: Our Beneficial Microbiomes

As we move down our mother's birth canal, and immediately upon emerging into the world, we acquire and become part of a life-long acquisition of microbes that inhabit every inch of us. By our teen-age years we support one of the most diverse and complex microbial ecosystems on planet earth. But that's only the beginning.

Microbes are the oldest living things on earth and far and away its predominant population. We live on a planet dominated by microbes. Every grain of soil, every drop of water, on this vale of tears is rich with microbial life. "Ten billion bacteria live in a gram of ordinary soil, a mere pinch held between thumb and fore finger."

We now know that we humans owe much of our individuality to the microbes that dwell comfortably on and in us. Getting to know and understand this, may alter the onerous name and bad press that has dogged microbes since Pasteur, Koch and the other giants of microbiology who discovered the pathogens they were desperately seeking. Between 1850 and 1950, microbiologists were quite rightly chasing infectious disease and the organisms responsible. Microbiology could easily have been called the study of pathogens and their diseases. Nevertheless, their exalted accomplishments are universally apparent. All credit to them!

Since the 1970's however, the preoccupation has been with the immense universe of beneficial microbes, and the vast microbial world inhabiting our bodies, the air, soil, and oceans, making human, animal and plant life possible and productive.

Yet another post-modern idea that is gaining wide currency is the reality of co-evolution between our non-pathogenic, beneficial microbes and our immune system. It has also been demonstrated that our common intestinal bacterium, the ever present E.coli, separated from its closest relative Salmonella typhimurium (a prominent agent of Salmonellosis) about 120 million years ago when mammals first appeared. More than likely, E.coli evolved with mammals and is well adapted to grow in the intestine of warm-blooded animals, including us humans. With this co-evolution E.coli is resistant to the normally pestiferous effects of bile acids, and can also use lactose, milk sugar, as a source of carbon, which most other bacteria cannot use. The huge and beneficial microbial universe, unknown to most of us, works diligently for us 24/7, sub-rosa, forever. Our microbes, yes, our microbes are nothing less than inseparable and indispensable. This is the big new story currently unfolding.

It's not the birds nor bees. Neither is it creepy crawlers of any description. It surely isn't mammals, our four-legged co-inhabitants. No, it isn't any of these. It's the microbes that rule the earth. They were here at the beginning and have been preparing the earth for us for over three billion years. We are their descendants.

Microbes exist literally in every nook and cranny of our bodies; on the highest mountains, in the deepest oceans, and everywhere in between, including the food we eat and the air we breath. Moreover, we live within a virtual sea of microbes. Globally, microbial cells are a billion times more abundant than the stars in the heavens. Take a breath of air and you sample the microbial world.

Despite decades of war against microbes, we've been calling them germs; it is now evident that we are more microbial than human. That's got to be a bit of a shocker, and a paradigm shift of robust proportions.

The message in this bottle is huge: without our microbes on and in us, there'd be no us! *Germs Are Us* redefines our world, revealing the legion of unimaginable benefits microbes render. We and our microbes, our microbiome, are inseparable and indispensable. Together, our ten trillion cells, their hundred trillion cells, our 22-thousand genes, their eight million genes, co-mingled, yes, you read that right, create a supra-organism-us/them. To banish them, is to banish ourselves. They can live without us, as they have for billions of years, we cannot live without them! That's the pivotal issue, the essence.

Do we share the earth with microbes, or do they share it with us? No longer a frivolous question: one we consider throughout this book.

It's the numbers: immense numbers that reveal a remarkable story. And non-fiction at that. We are simply outnumbered by our microbes. We, our bodies, head to toes, every inch of us, eyes, ears, nose, skin, hair, teeth, tongue, arms, legs, guts, consist of ten trillion human cells, numbers as large as our national debt. But that number pales in comparison to the thriving communities, yes indeed, plural, of over a hundred trillion microbial cells–bacteria, fungi, yeasts, and protozoans that have taken up agreeable and comfortable residence on and in us. That hundred trillion doesn't include viruses, which can add another 30 to 40 billion. These humongous numbers constitute the newly discovered microbiome.

By studying this new population, scientists have learned a startling truth: our microbes not only allow us to live, but keep us healthy. We are partners *for* life;

forever. That for is profound, capturing as it does the double truth.

This then is the new paradigm, which we've got to come to grips with, understand and become comfortable with because, for the most part, microbes are beneficial, not withstanding the few nasties that can and do cause trouble from time to time.

Would it be too much of a stretch to assume that you will come away believing that our microbes rule? *Germs Are Us* may just change the way we think about who, or what we actually are. It's time to end the "Manichaean view of microbes as we good; they evil": a mentality that has stoked the war on microbes.[1] Their story and our togetherness needs to gain traction. After all, who would believe that healthy people are swamped with microbes, germs.

Consider our bodies as a collection of microbial ecosystems-microbial habitats. Our teeth, gums, and tongue, each with its own select types, and each side of each tooth with a different set of microbes. Imagine! Some 500 to 1,000 different species have thus far been identified in our mouths, and it's only the beginning, the early stages.

Our saliva is home to another 600-plus types, harmlessly enjoying its warmth, moisture and nutrients. Hard to pass up. And each square centimeter of our lungs is home to thousands of microbes; a shockingly new finding as our lungs were long thought to be sterile; microbe-free. They're not.

Is it too hard to believe there are different types of microbes on our right and left hands? Whoever said the right hand doesn't know what the left hand is up to, had it about right.

Our gut, our intestines, large and small, harbor over a 100 trillion microbes;a number that may go to a quadrillion:that perform significant metabolic functions including metabolizing complex dietary polysaccharides, starches and cellulose,as well as producing Vitamin K, so necessary for blood clotting, not otherwise accessible to us. They also harvest energy for us from our foods by digesting dietary fiber, and other chemicals our human cells cannot. That's a key: bear that in mind. Our microbes are doing the vital work, our human cells cannot do.

My stash of microbes, my microbiome, though different than yours, as each of us are a bit different from one another, suppress the growth of the delinquents, those nasties that attempt to come aboard to work their wiles on us. Needing all the help we can get, our microbes are there for us.

Furthermore, their presence helps mature our unimaginably complex immune systems, educating the plethora of specialized cells to recall past events that could come back to haunt us. Our microbes school our immune cells to differentiate foreign organisms, protein, from our human protein, which translates to protection from risk of infections, bowel diseases, allergies, asthma, diabetes, and much more. We'll pick up on that in Chapter THREE.

The newly accumulated evidence suggests that over the past half-century, we've become far too clean, having been incessantly bombarded with messages to scour, and scrub the dirt away: clean, clean, clean. Kill those bugs. Sanitize everything! Result:our immune systems may lack adequate contact with foreign microbes and may be unable to differentiate friend from foe.

Consider this recent disclosure. Every gram of our fecal matter contains some 10 billion viruses. And we expel some 350 billion every day. And that's only viruses. Bacteria contribute yet another ten billion cells, and we haven't gotten beyond a small fecal mass. Moreover, a recent study checked stool samples of 124 healthy people, finding an average of 536,122 genes in each sample; 99.1 percent were bacterial! Hey, just counting their genes and cells makes us more microbial than human. Is that a hellofa jarring thought? Nevertheless, we are entwined forever-for life.

This vital partnership is the story this book reveals. That's the new evocative idea, the model that holds that there is no human life sans microbes. We are inseparable, and they are indispensable. As a Boa Constrictor swallowing a Capybara, that idea requires time for digestion.

With that as prelude, we now take a more detailed look at our various microbial menageries, our microbiome, a term Joshua Lederberg, a Nobel Laureate, coined as descriptive of the internal microbial ecosystem and its connectedness to our genome, that would signify the community of symbiotic and pathogenic organ isms that literally share our body space."[1] He was also prescient enough to note that "any comprehensive view of human genetics and physiology is a composite of human and microbial genetics," placing him way ahead of scientific understanding at the time.[2]

Digging into our co-inhabitants microbiome conjures questions of our individual identity. So, for example, what do we think we are, may be more to the point then who do we think we are? Why? Because we now know that we are not quite what we thought we are. We've thought of our selves as nothing less than totally human; a hundred percent human, and apart from any other form of life. That's no longer possible, as uncomfortable and threatening as it may be. The idea or fact of our being a supraorganism composed of microbial and human cells, and microbial and human genes, is gaining substantial traction as a consequence of the Human Microbiome Project, HMP, that takes us to the cusp of a totally new understanding of what it means to be human: a paradigm shift of sci-fi-like proportions.

To deal with this, the National Institutes of Health, NIH, launched a five-year investigation to determine the totality of microbes on and in us. "The ultimate objective of the HMP (was) to demonstrate that there are opportunities to improve human health through monitoring or manipulation of the human microbiome."[3]

Launched in December 2007, this five-year project funded at a level of 150 million dollars over that period, was kicked off with four major centers: The Baylor College of Medicine, Houston; The Broad Institute, Cambridge; The J. Craig Ventor Institute, San Diego, and Washington University School of Medicine, St. Louis; four institutions considered world class in genetic sequencing and microbe detection and identification. Two hundred fifty volunteers were to be sampled, divided equally between men and women, to provide a data base of information that would serve as a reference for future studies.[4] And as Prof. Julian Davies of the University of British Columbia, Vancouver reminded us a decade or more ago, "our existence is dependent on bacterial species living in and on us."[5]

The five years were up in 2012, and in a series of momentous reports published on June 14, 2012, some 200 members of the HMP, from some eighty universities and scientific institutions discussed their five years of research. They had obtained samples from 242 healthy volunteers, 129 men, and 113 women, collecting microbial samples from fifteen body sites in men and eighteen from the women. Some three samples from each volunteer were secured from their mouths, nose, skin (two behind each ear and inner elbow) lower intestine (stool-self collected) and three vaginal sites in women, for a total of 11, 174 samples, of which 4,788 specimens were available for study.

"Like 15th century explorer's describing the outline of a new continent, HMP researchers employed a new technological strategy to define for the first time, the normal microbial make up of the human body," remarked Dr. Francis S. Collins, Director of the NIH, who went on to say that "the HMP created a remarkable reference data base by using genome sequencing techniques -which will be described shortly, to detect microbes in healthy volunteers."

This sequencing technique can detect and identify microbes that refuse to grow in laboratory cultures. It is now believed that over 10,000 microbial species occupy our human systems. The researchers could not even name all the newly found types of microbes sequencing revealed; they were so new. But they are believed to play a critical role in human health and illness. Of utmost importance however, the primary goal of the HMP is understanding what sickness is, but to do this, it is necessary to define a healthy microbiome. That's essential.

We know we are loaded with microbes. But they too have their preferred environments. Microbes view us as "prime real estate." Some prefer high humidity. For them, our belly button and armpits beckon. Others prefer warm, moist habitats like that provided between our toes. Still others prefer our buttocks and forearms that offer dry, open environments, or the oily crannies of the side of our noses. They are a picky lot, but they know what they want and what's good for them. Furthermore, they defend themselves by secreting antimicrobial chemicals that kill-off foreign intruders. By protecting themselves, they protect us. A win/win affair if ever there was one.

Of course our mouths are warm and friendly places; warm, moist, loaded with nutrients and with highly variable environments. So open up, and let's have a look. With so compelling a habitat, it's no wonder that as many as a thousand different types have taken up residence there. In addition to the extraordinary diversity of organisms, HMP scientists found an average of twenty billion microbes crowding out harmful bacteria. Although the dominant organisms are *Streptococcus mitis*, *Strep. salivarus*, *Stre.p mutans*, and *Strep. viridans*, there are Staphylococci, Neisseria, Candida and Diphtheroids among many others.

Interestingly the numbers and types vary from person to person. Apparently at any given time each of us has

100-200 different types in common, but we also vary with two hundred different types. Strep mutans, found primarily on our teeth, is one of the most studied. Obtaining its energy from sugars in our foods, it converts the sugar to lactic acid that can corrode dental enamel, which can lead to dental caries—cavities.

The formation of biofilms on the surface of our teeth, dentists refer to as plaque. These films consist primarily of the quartet of streptococci noted. The new data also suggests that changes in the microbiota of the plaque can predispose susceptible people to dental caries. Changes in the microbiota from a healthy state can shift the oral environment in ways that lead to decay. Unquestionably, the mouth is a complex ecosystem where some microbes produce proteins that beckon others to come and join the community.

Our saliva is a natural habitat for over six hundred different species of microbes, peaceably enjoying the neighborhood. Curiously enough, saliva appears to be a constant around the world with similar sets of organisms in both western and eastern countries. As you might well imagine, this came as a surprise, given the widely varied diets around the world.

Our throats appear to harbor hundreds of millions of virus particles in the mucus bathing the area. For the most part, these have yet to be identified. However, it does look as though these particles not only don't sicken us, but tend to infect unwanted bacteria, helping to maintain our microbiome in a healthy condition.

And microbal lore held that our lungs were sterile territory. They're not. Streptococci, Prevotella and Veillionella are comfortably ensconsed. No, they are not contaminants from our mouths and our throats.

As we speak, billions of bacteria, fungi and yeasts are crawling and creeping over our skin, our body's largest organ. From our forehead, with its oily habitat, where Propionibacterium reside, and moving along the scalp and sides of our noses, to our legs, which are normally dry, open swaths, a great diversity of bacteria and fungi preside. Every square inch of skin swarms with a billion microbial cells. Between our toes the Firmacutes, coccoid, and rod-shaped organisms, have found an accommodating home.

Our armpits with its warmth and moisture are home to a diverse collection of bacteria that release those sweaty sock and locker room aromas. Brevibacterium is one of them, which we'll catch up on when we attend to a number of the expensive cheeses we crave. Yes, you read that right.

And what of our belly buttons, where that moist, indented cranny is far too safe from soap and water. Researchers at North Carolina State University, Raleigh, found on swabbing the umbilicus of 100 volunteers, in their Belly Button Biodiversity Project, a surprising and unexpected, 1,400 different types of microbes in that convoluted depression known as the umbilicus, which they believe is an underestimate! We and they, have yet to learn the function, or functions, these many organisms attend to. You can bet that whatever emerges will be headline grabbing.[6] And, recent research suggests that our eating habits are controlled, that's not a misprint, by our gut microbes. Apparently they manipulate us, yes, you read that right, to eat when they desire—when they need nutrients. Imagine! Our desire for pickles or ice-cream at midnight may not be our craving, but theirs! We may have to re-think what "our' really means.

Huge numbers of *Staphylococcus epidermidis* have found a comfortable playground on our skin, preventing the potentially harmful Staph. aureus from gaining a toehold, or some such thing. We've got to applaud that type of teamwork, or at least offer an "Amen".

Actually our skin is teeming with bacteria. In that exclusive crease between our buttocks three major types of germs dominate, but on the buttocks themselves, a half-dozen species are prominent; including proteobacteria and bacteroidetes. There isn't a nook or a cranny without its resident flora.

At birth, infants delivered vaginally become smeared with their mothers' microbes as they pass through the birth canal: lactobacilli–at least a half-dozen species–prevotella and atopobium become bound to them. Babies delivered via cesarian section obtain a microbiota similar to that of their mother's skin, along with those of the Obstetrician, Nurses and the immediate hospital delivery room. In that environment they become inhabited with *Staph. epidermidis, Enterococcus feacalis*, and *E.coli*: an entirely different set of microbes-a collection that does not appear (as we shall see) to be as prorective as the vaginal cohort.

Let's now have a look inside. Obviously our diet plays a role in shaping the microbial composition of our gut: stomach, small and large intestine. As we peer into the gastrointestinal system, the gut, with the greatest preponderance of both numbers and types of microbes, one in particular flags our attention: *Bacteroides thetaiotaomicron, a t*ongue-twisting monicker if ever there was one. It enjoys the acidic, oxygen-depleted, rough and tumble darkness of the stomach, obtaining its energy by consuming polysaccharides, the complex carbohydrates found in veggies, fruits and grains. By digesting this long chain molecule, we are provided with glucose and other small molecule sugars we sorely need. Our genome lacks the genes needed to code for enzymes that metabolize complex carbohydrates. Thankfully, this bacterium not only has the gene for degrading complex molecules but also has genes for hundreds of enzymes that can split crop fibers providing the nutrients we need but cannot otherwise get. Not to be outdone, other species of bacteroidetes breakdown fats, and proteins, and the prevotella chomp nicely on fiber and carbohydrates. To do without our microbial zoo is unimaginable. We need them. Can't live without them!

Hundreds of species of microbes prefer our stomachs where they graze on mucus lining our stomach walls. But it's the colon, the large intestine that is the microbial metropolis with literally thousands of different types and trillions of cells. It's here in the colon that our microbes have the final touch, breaking down starches and other difficult molecules, toxins among them, and also provide vitamins we need.

This microbial community is remarkably stable. Once these microbes are established, and mature along with us, they remain in our gut for decades contributing to our individual uniqueness. And, as we shall see, autoimmune diseases in which our immune cells are unable to differentiate self from non-self (self being us, and non-self being foreign protein) are now correlated with dramatic changes in gut microbiota.

As for obesity, it appears that the mix of gut microbes may determine whether we gain or lose weight! Overweight individuals appear to harbor greater numbers of firmacutes, of which there are a number of types, while the leaner among us favor the bacteroidetes, with their numerous types. Similar sets of microbes have been observed in hospitalized patients. As the heavier folks lost weight, their gut microbes shifted from firmacutes to bacteroidetes. *Methanobacter smithii* is prevalent in large numbers of our overweight individuals and may be at least partly responsible for pushing people to over eat.

This firmacute/bacteroidetes seesaw relationship was also found in mice, which may suggest why our neighbor seems to eat everything in sight without gaining an ounce. This remains to become a medical regime, but not too far from becoming one. It may just become a procedure for safely shifting our gut flora one way or another. At the moment, it's a wait and see.

And then there is the penis, upon and within which, researchers have found streptococci, lactobacilli, chlamydia, prevotella, and fusobacteria. However, widely different microbial communities exist on circumcised and uncircumcised men. The uncircumcised, shelter far greater numbers and types of microbes on their penis. Circumcision reduces the number and types of bacteria on the glans, or head of the penis, while the uncircumcised penis has a collection resembling the microbial types associated with female vaginosis: lactobacilli. What this means has yet to be determined.

New research informs us that the vaginal microbiota changes during pregnancy. Microbes that digest milk begin to multiply (which, curiously enough, suggests their presence is waiting to be called upon) and will be swallowed by infants during the birthing period.

Breast milk feeds both the infant and the microbes he/she carries, which assures a growing and competent gut microbial ecosystem that helpfully crowds out unwanted bacteria and helps maintain a healthy baby.

Clearly, we and our microbes have evolved a mutually satisfactory and beneficial relationship that has contributed to our health, and fitness. The questions that surely follow are: how were we able to learn all this, and what was the impetus for the Human Microbiome Project?

It began with the discovery of DNA, Deoxyribosenucleic acid: the remarkable molecule of heredity, and the ability to decipher its code. Let's talk about that.

For the longest time geneticists believed that genes, the elements, the units of inheritance, were proteins. That suddenly changed in 1944.

Oswald Avery, Maclyn McCarty and Colin MacCleod, of Rockefeller University, New York, demonstrated unequivocally in a tantalizing series of microbial experiments that DNA was the chemical of inheritance. Their experiments proved that the heritable condition of virulence from one infectious type of pneumococcus could be transferred to another non-infectious bacterium using only DNA devoid of any contaminating protein. They also showed that this transformation could be prevented by an enzyme,

DNAase, that chewed-up the DNA.[7, 8]

This then, connected genetic information with DNA for the first time and set modern genetics in motion. Although that was surely the stuff of a Nobel Prize, which bafflingly didn't materialize, there was a germane piece of work that preceded theirs, that motivated their splendid set of experiments.

Frederick Griffith, a physician/microbiologist working in Liverpool, England, in the late 1920's devised an experiment that opened a crack in thinking about transmission of hereditary chemicals, although DNA was not yet on anyone's radar. However, it was well known that strains of Streptococcus pneumoniae could be both benign and virulent. On culture media streptococci could grow as rough-looking "R" colonies, or smooth, glistening, virulent, "S" colonies. Furthermore, Griffith, had seen the possible reversion to virulence in the throats of convalescent patients as well as healthy individuals, which prompted his mouse experiments.

Concisely stated, Griffith's experiments on the transfer of virulence in the pathogen Strep.pneumoniae began by inoculating subcutaneously live, harmless "R" pneumococcal organisms into mice, which had no ill effect.

In the following experiment, he inoculated live "R" streptococci along with dead "S" streptococci. Low and behold, the mice died. On autopsy, he recovered live virulent "S" streptococci. He was shocked and amazed. Who wouldn't be! Something was wrong. He had to repeat this experiment. However many times he repeated it, the results were the same. The only interpretation possible was that the harmless "R" forms had been transformed to the virulent "S" forms. In 1928 Griffith referred to this change from "R" to "S", as transformation.[9, 10] That was where it was left until Avery, McCartney and MacCleod picked up on Griffith's experiments sixteen years later, with the goal of determining what it was that produced that transformation. Here, then, was evidence that Griffith's transforming material was DNA, and that DNA had to be the source of genetic information.

Genetics was about to explode. The race was on to understand how genetic instructions were stored in the DNA molecule, and what was the structure of this epochal chemical?

Unfortunately Griffith did not live to see DNA detected. He perished far too early. The result of a direct hit on his house by a German bomb during an air raid in February 1941.

At this point, no one had a clue about what DNA looked like. Efforts turned to X-rays to obtain the molecule's photograph. Enter Rosalind Elsie Franklin, a British biophysicist, and X-ray crystallographer. Working at King's College, London, Franklin was out front discovering diffraction structures that led to DNA's physical framework.

Although James Dewey Watson, an American Zoologist collaborating with Francis H.C. Crick, a physicist at Cambridge's Cavendish Laboratory, were also trying to determine the shape of DNA, they had seen a photograph of Franklin's original high resolution X-ray diffraction pattern that revealed DNA's physical structure. Now they could correctly deduce that the genetic information was encoded as the sequence, succession, order, of nucleotides in the DNA molecule, and rushed to publish their double helical formulations. For this, they were awarded a Nobel Prize in Physiology or Medicine, in 1962. Rosalind Franklin did not share in the award as she died at the tender age of thirty-seven, taken away by an ovarian cancer.[11]

The structure of DNA provided fundamental information about genetics: two connected spiral staircase-shaped double stranded helices winding together like parallel handrails, were complementary to one another, furnishing the key to how genetic information is stored, transferred and copied. Complementary means that knowing the sequence of nucleotide building blocks in one strand, you know the exact sequence of building blocks on the other strand.

A nucleotide is a building block of DNA, and each nucleotide contains one base, one phosphate molecule, and the sugar molecule deoxyribose. The bases in DNA nucleotides are adenine, thymine, cytosine and guanine. Adenine always matches up with thymine, and cytosine always matches up with guanine. Long strings of nucleotides form genes, and groups of genes are packaged tightly into units called chromosomes.

Although Gregor Mendel didn't use the term gene, he was well aware that "discrete factors" carried and transferred hereditary traits. Who was this Mendel fellow who is considered the Father of Modern Genetics?

The Abbot, Johann Gregor Mendel, conducted his famous experiments on pea plants in the gardens of the Augustinian Abbey in Brno, the Czech Reublic. Working alone and without any biological background, this solitary gardener, but a stickler for details, stood the old world on its head. By 1865, his years of breeding and cross breeding of his pea plants unraveled the basics of heredity. But his fundamental work was not recognized until the early years of the twentieth century. Of course his "discrete factors", were today's genes and their DNA.[12]

Today we know that genes do not do the heavy lifting. They contain the codes, the instructions, for making the many proteins we need to function. But proteins cannot copy themselves. To make more protein our cells use the instructions coded in DNA.

That we inherit traits from our parents has a long history. That common sense observation led to agriculture and the breeding and cultivation of animals and crops for the more desirable qualities we wanted.

Cells need protein. When cells need more protein they use the instructions coded in nucleotides, the sequence of its four-letter alphabet, a, c, g, and t, which as noted above, represent the four nitrogenous bases, adenine, cytosine, guanine, and tyrosine in various arrangements, sequences, repeated over and over, is the astonishing alphabet, the genes a-b-c's, in which the genetic code is "written." Millions of these four bases ocurr in all of us, as well as all animals and plants. The order or sequence of these bases makes us and all animals and plants unique.

This code is our Rosetta Stone, which enables scientists to decipher proteins: the proteins of all living things, as all have the same alphabet. The words of the code, the instructions, govern and direct how and when the literally hundreds of thousands of proteins, depending upon the human, plant, animal or microbe involved, will be made. The "words" are determined by the order of the four bases along a strand of DNA.

The four bases always occur in pairs: as noted, a always pairs with t, and c with g. "a", on one strand of the double helix pairs with t on the opposite strand, as c does with g. This is crucially important, as their arrangement along the DNA strands is the means by which information is stored and "read."

Each sequence of bases actually spells out an amino acid, the building blocks of proteins. Consequently, the code specifying an amino acid must consist of at least three bases. These three-letter "words" are called codons, 64 in all, and can spell out any of the twenty essential amino acids. So, for example, ttt codes for lysine; cat codes for methionine; gcc for alanine, and acc for tryptophane. Along a strand of DNA, the triplet codons could look this way: atgacggagcgg. The words are read in groups of three bases that spell out all amino acid sequences. These amino acids then join to form chains of peptides, which link-up to form chains of polypeptides, which join to form proteins. The various combinations of the twenty amino acids can literally produce millions of proteins.

The take away message in all this is, that a chemical is a chemical, is a chemical, or, a protein is a protein, is a protein, no matter in what living thing it occurs. All species of living things have the same four letter genetic alphabet, a,t,c, and g. The cells of flowers, frogs, flies and finches make the proteins required for whatever their singular needs are. But lysine and alanine, or any of the essential amino acid in frogs, flowers or my neighbor Francine, are identical. Never forget that.

Furthermore, each of us has the same number of 'words" but, and this is a substantial but, some of the words have different spellings. These different spellings mean different proteins. And yes, these different proteins can be the difference between health and illness. These different proteins are the mutations.

Mutations can cause a gene to encode a protein that fails to work, or work incorrectly. At times an error can fail to make a protein. Mutations may sound like trouble, but not all are harmful. Some have no effect; others may produce new versions of proteins that confer survival advantages. And yes, some do cause illness and disfigurement.

Abraham Lincoln had exceedingly long arms and legs, a thin body and deep-set eyes. Lincoln had Marfan's syndrome. Today we know that Marfan is a genetic disorder of connective tissue, due to a mutation. The protein TGF-B, transforming growth factor-beta, normally instructs the cells about what to do during the body's development.

TGF-B's function is altered in Marfan syndrome. In those of us free of Marfan, a protein, fibrillin-1 attaches TGF-B to connective tissue. In Marfan's, fibrillin-1 is defective, a wrong spelling in a stretch of code. Rather than attaching to connective tissue, TGF-B remains unanchored. During this lack of attachment, it allows cells to function abnormally, often resulting in the signs of Marfan syndrome.

Antoine Marfan, a French pediatrician first described this condition in 1896. The gene linked to it was first identified by Dr. Harry C. Dietz, of Johns Hopkins Medical School, Baltimore, and Dr. Francesco Ramirez, of Mt. Sinai Medical School, New York City, in 1991. Come to think of it, Charles de Gaulle, and Nicolo Paganini, the Italian composer and violinist were also believed to have had Marfan's syndrome.[13]

Little to nothing could be done for the unfortunate folks, with conditions due to gene malfunctions, until recently.

In January 2014, we learned that those one in 50,000 men with the inherited, degenerative and incurable vision condition, Choroideremia, could regain sight by replacing a defective gene with a healthy one!

Choroideremia is a progressive, degeneration of the light sensitive cells of the rods and cones at the back of the eye, caused by the loss of RAB Escort Protein–REP-1; a defect in a single gene on the X chromosome, that affects mainly boys.

A team of researchers at the University of Oxford, England, led by Dr. Robert E. McLaren, assembled a deactivated, harmless virus to shuttle billions of healthy, synthetic versions of the gene, tailor-made in his lab, under the retina of blind individuals: restoring function of their light sensitive cells. Each injection of this retinal gene therapy sends ten billion viral particles, each carrying a copy of the healthy gene into the eye, replacing the faulty protein.

Dr. McLaren believes this procedure can be used to restore vision in those with age-related macular degeneration as well as those with retinitis pigmentosa.[14] Isn't that worth a ten on anyone's hit parade?

With the above as a primer, we now turn to a specific gene 16SrRNA, found in all microbes. This is the gene that researchers search for to help identify known and unknown microbes, as each type of microbe has the 16SrRNA gene along with its unique nucleotide sequence that permits its identification. As we shall see, it is the pattern of nucleotides that provides the ultimate identification: the species-specific signature, which is currently the "gold standard" for identification and classification. DNA sequencing determines the order of nucleotides in fragments of DNA. The bases may be attached in any order that, as you can imagine, offers a vast number of possible arrangements. Each protein is made according to its specific pattern of nucleotides, and the order of bases also dictates DNA's structure and function. Ergo, this serves as a bar code of life, informing us of the types of microbes residing on and in us that will not grow on laboratory culture media, and it does so rapidly. Of additional importance, microbes bivouacking in hospitals can be rapidly identified and dealt with. In the discussion that follows, we will see that microbes are being discovered where they were never known to exist, nor the role they play in our lives.

With sequencing we have entered a new land where our scientists are the new pioneers, and whose discoveries will be modifying our lives beneficially.

Without sequencing the National Institutes of Health, NIH, would not, could not have embarked on its ambitious and thus far highly productive Human Microbiome Project that cracked open a new era of scientific studies to comprehend the complex interaction between our microbiota and us. Its importance cannot be overstated.

In his book, The Language of Life, Dr. Francis S. Collins, Director, of the National Institutes of Health, tells us that "your body is made up of approximately 400 trillion cells," ... "But if you add up the number of microbial cells on your skin, in your mouth, and nose, and in your intestinal tract, the total comes up to a quadrillion-a thousand trillion or 1,followed by 15 zeros" He further maintains that "Not only are there far more microbial cells than human cells, but they are enormously diverse contributing millions of their genes to our modest 21-22 thousand genes. So it it not far fetched to think of us, together, as a supraorganism." That's not only a new paradigm, it's a head spinner.

Here we launch into an explanation of the polymerase chain reaction, sequencing, and fingerprinting, followed by an account of NIH's Human Microbiome Project, and conclude with notable examples of the successes the HMP and sequencing has wrought for us.

Polymerase Chain Reaction

Kary Mullis won the 1993 Nobel Prize in chemistry. Frederick Sanger, a British biochemist, won two Nobel prizes: one in 1958, for helping to unravel the chemical structure of protein molecules, and again in 1980, for developing techniques for reading stretches of DNA.

Sanger's first Nobel was granted for determining the exact sequence in which the fifty-one amino acids of the Insulin molecule were linked together. These fifty-one, are a medley of the twenty essential amino acids repeated as the code instructs.

Back to the American, Kary Baker Mullis, and his polymerase chain reaction, PCR, which he developed while a chemist at the Cetus Corporation, Emeryville, California.[15] PCR can selectively amplify a single molecule of template DNA producing millions of copies from miniscule amounts of DNA. That's the key that unlocks it all. PCR is at the core of DNA sequencing as it is almost a verity of identifying unknown microbes, that DNA is always in short supply, requiring amplification. PCR is the remedy, and is nothing short of revolutionary: one of the most important biologic tools ever invented. Consequently, DNA sequencing owes its existence to Kary Mullis and Frederick Sanger, who by the way, is often referred to as The Father of Genomics. Unfortunately for humankind, Sanger departed this world at age 96, on Tuesday, November 19th, 2013. He made a difference.[16]

A genome, as noted, is the totality of our genes. Our human genome differs from that of Apes, which differs from that of a fly's or a corn plant. But all use the same genetic alphabet.

Although each of us has a genome, it differs from person to person. Sequence variation within our genes makes our DNA different from that of our parents, and our brothers and sisters; surely different from my neighbor Diana and her husband Josh.

Our genomes are relatively long accounts that consist of some 22 thousand 'word" genes: the bases, repeated over and over.

One further point, ribosomes are also found in all living cells and function in protein synthesis. Ribosomes are similar to DNA, but unlike DNA ribosomes are single-stranded and consist of two subunits, each of which is composed of a protein and a type of RNA referred to as ribosomal RNA-rRNA. Most importantly, ribosomes contain a 16S subunit which, through millions of years of evolution has been extraordinarily preserved; scientists use the word, conserved, for this sub unit that has barely changed in most types of microbes.

The extraordinary conservation of rRNA can be seen in the 16SrRNA gene sequences of human fragments, corn and the microbe *Thermatoga maratima*. Thermatoga is a heat-loving thermophile (discussed in detail in Chapter SEVEN) living and growing comfortably at temperatures approaching that of boiling water.

Human:

gtg/cca/gca/gccgcggtaattccagctccaatagcgtatattaaagttgctgcagtta aaaag

Corn:

gtg/cca/gcagccgcggtaattccagctccaatagcgtatatttaagttgttgcagttaa aaag

Thermatoga:

gtg/cca/gccgcggtaatacgtaggggggcaagcgttacccggatttactgggcgtaa aggg

Notice the close similarity between the human and corn fragments and the differences in the Thermatoga fragments, but also many of the same sequences.

Therefore, it is the 16SrRNA that is hunted for among other genes in the sequencing process as it provides a specific signature sequence tremendously useful for microbial identification and classification. This 16SrRNA is not just the standard for gene sequencing, it is the gold standard for classification of microbial species, as it is the least variable DNA in all microbial cells, which translates to the fact that portions of DNA sequences from distantly related organisms are remarkably similar. That's the key![17]

Before sequencing, less than one percent of the microbial universe were known, and could be grown in lab culture media. Others couldn't be identified at all, or were not even known to exit. Sequencing has opened an Aladdin's cave of microbial riches, providing a more complete picture of the totality of microbes on and in us, as well as their other habitats and environments.

Until recently the study of unknown microbes had been problematic; if a microbe couldn't be grown on a solid or in a liquid media, it couldn't be identified. And it was soon learned that most microbes just didn't take to life in a lab. Clever people thought about this conundrum and solved the problem. No longer would it be necessary to try to grow organisms on nutrient media.

Over the past two decades genetic techniques were developed allowing entire communities of microbes to be characterized and identified by their DNA, providing a far more complete picture of the totality of microbes on and in us.

The operative term is sequencing, and is the key. My Collins dictionary informs me that a sequence is an arrangement of two or more things in successive order. For us, it is the unique order of amino acids in a protein or in nucleotides of DNA or RNA. DNA is found primarily in a cell's nucleus; RNA, ribose nucleic acid, is common in the cell's cytoplasm. RNA copies the DNA message in the nucleus, carrying it into the cytoplasm where proteins are synthesized.

To extract and compare bits of a specific type of RNA from known and unknown microbial samples to determine if they are present in a particular environment, and if they've never been known before, molecular tools are used. The technique is now widely used as a biomarker and for microbial ecologic studies. The specific type of RNA used is the 16SrRNA, which, as noted earlier, has changed little over millions of years as microbes have evolved, the slight changes that have occurred, provide clues about how various microbes are related.

Because the 16SrRNA gene is short, less than two-thousand bases, it can be quickly and cheaply copied, and then sequenced.

When a researcher has a test tube containing a sample of saliva, intestinal contents, or water from a deep-sea hydrothermal vent, and would like to know just what microbes are in his/her sample, the cells in the sample can be split open to isolate the 16s gene among the other genes.

To identify these otherwise unculturable organisms, the Polymerase Chain Reaction, PCR, along with nucleotide sequencing are the current procedures of choice.

PCR and DNA Sequencing

PCR is an enzymatic process that amplifies,

replicates, the amount of target DNA in a sample. Kary Mullis isolated his DNA polymerase from the thermophile, *Thermus aquaticus*, thriving in a hot spring, at Yellowstone National Park, Wyoming. Interestingly, although DNA polymerase is a protein, as all enzymes are, it is curious that a protein can tolerate temperatures of 95° (203° F) without coagulating a lá fried or hard boiled eggs. For his polymerase to be effective at this near boiling temperature, Mullis fished out the Taq polymerase gene from Thermus that allows this protein to remain functional. Not only is it heat tolerable, but it is incredibly accurate, making less than one error in 20 thousand base pairs.

With the availability of this gene it was no longer necessary to add fresh enzyme after each cycle: the entire process could now be automated and billions of copies of DNA fragments provided within hours. Surely worth a Nobel.

More often than not there is never enough microbial DNA in a sample to obtain an adequate sequencing of nucleotides. PCR assures an adequate supply rapidly and cheaply. For those interested in the details, read on. Otherwise, skip down to the Human Microbiome Project.

PCR involves three steps; denaturation of the sample, annealing, and extension.

First, the unknown microbial sample is heated to 95° (203° F) to cleve the hydrogen bonds binding the double-stranded helical molecule together, yielding two single-strands of DNA.

Primers are then added to the mix. These primers, tailor-made nucleotides, are added to prepare the strands for annealing–the attachment of the enzyme DNA polymerase to the complementary region of the single-stranded molecule. A primer is a strand of nucleic acid that serves as a starting point for DNA synthesis. It's required for DNA amplification because the DNA polymerase that catalyzes the process can only add new nucleotides to an existing strand of DNA. These primers are usually short, chemically synthesized nucleotides.

In the final extension step, the strands are extended by the polymerase, providing the necessary amount of DNA for sequencing, or as it is being referred to, fingerprinting, to begin.

The contents of the reaction tube is then transferred to an Agarose, polyacrylamide gel. Drops of the "unknown" DNA mixture are placed in wells or lanes on the Agarose sheet. Sample fragments of known microbial DNA are placed in wells or on other lanes. Samples of the unknown can be spotted on 3,4, or more lanes, forming a series.

Each of the primer bases, a, t, c, and g, are tagged with a fluorescent dye; either red, yellow, blue or green. The gel plate is then placed in an automatic sequencer for electrophoresis and analysis. Electrophoresis is a technique that sends an electric current through the gel causing the DNA fragments to move down the gel. The gel plate is hooked up to a high voltage electric source. When current is switched on, DNA fragments, with their negative charge, move down the gel toward the anode, the positive pole. Currently PCR is done in an automated instrument, a thermocycler.

The smaller, lighter fragments move faster and further then the larger, heavier fragments. After a set time, the current is switched off. The DNA nucleotides are separated into colored bands along the gel, in their various lanes. These bands are scanned by a laser beam as it passes a specific point on the gel, producing a profile of each nucleotide. Each base emits its colored light of a characteristic wavelength, and is recorded as a colored band forming a chromatogram. Additionally, after moving down the gel, strands only one nucleotide longer than another become separated. A sequence of these results can be displayed on a computer screen and the base sequence of the original DNA determined. A computer program determines the DNA sequence resembling the triplet shown earlier for human, corn and microbe. It's the closest thing to a fingerprint: a bar code of life.

Sequencing a genome may seem easy, given its automation; actually its a formidable task, requiring finding the nucleotide sequence of small fragments of a genomes DNA, but getting these small fragments together into an entire genome, is much like assembling a jigsaw puzzle from a pile of scattered pieces. Nevertheless, currently an automated DNA sequencer can specify more than 100,000 bases of DNA per day, while a large facility can produce over ten million per day.

This explosion of sequencing and the use of automated procedures with their ever-increasing speeds motivated the National Institutes of Health to embark on its Human Microbiome Project.

Although it has long been known that microbes, germs, in our abdominal cavity, our stomachs, small and large intestine, have been, and are responsible, for certain human illnesses, it is only recently that we have come to understand that gut microbes also play a major role in keeping us healthy.

The Human Microbiome Project

To discover their roles, the microbes involved, and their and our interactions, the NIH launched its HMP in 2007, in which the sequence of genes in the microbiome of healthy volunteers would be determined: a mighty undertaking.

With the worldwide explosion of sequencing, it was now possible to pursue what had been elusive and unknowable: an understanding of the immense microbial universe residing on and in us.

The HMP was launched in 2007, as a two hundred million dollar, five-year project, tasked with the mission to comprehensively characterize our human microbiota and determine its role in both health and illness.[18]

In the beginning, 242 healthy volunteers were sampled one to three times at 15 (male) and 18 (female) body sites, including mouth, tongue, teeth, behind the ear, inner elbow, nose, vagina and stools, generating 5,177 microbial profiles from 16SrRNA genes. In addition, some 890 human reference strains were obtained for sequencing. "Collectively these data represent the largest resource describing the abundance and variety of the human microbiome, providing a framework for current and future studies."[19]

This project also brought together over two hundred scientists from eighty institutions around the country to aggregate their findings into a comprehensive census of the microbial endowment of healthy people. It was becoming evident that we humans co-evolved with our microbial communities and that they play a substantive and beneficial role in our lives. But when the normal composition of our microbiome becomes unbalanced, we can get into serious trouble especially as the five to eight million different microbial genes nestling within us, vastly dwarf our meager twenty-two thousand. Recent studies have solidly associated microbiome imbalances in illnesses such as cancer, obesity, inflammatory bowel disease, asthma, and nutritional conditions, and as we shall see, a clutch of others.

The following study fetches this relationship into sharp focus.

The Columbian Connection

For over a thousand years peptic ulcers have tormented us, but no one considered it a microbial problem. The mantra was, "no acid, no ulcer." All that changed in 1984, when two physicians, Drs. Barry J. Marshall and J.Robert Warren of Perth, Australia, found these ulcers were the work of the bacterium Helicobacter pylori. This microbe produces the characteristic inflammation, acidity, chronic gastritis, and is the second leading cause of gastric cancer worldwide.

Drs. Pelayo Correa and Barbara Schneider of Vanderbilt University's Ingram Cancer Center, together with researchers at Dartmouth University's Geisel School of Medicine, were interested in learning if co-evolution between people and the Helicobacter influences risk of illness.[20]

Dr. Correa, a gastroenterologist/pathologist, and a native Columbian, had long wondered about the different gastric cancer rates between the Andean mountain dwellers and the people living along the coastal areas.

Pursuing such a relationship, they studied two distinct communities in Columbia, South America, to determine if co-evolution between Helicobacter and these populations affected their risk of cancer.

They discovered that the risk of developing gastric cancer depended heavily on both the ancestry of the individual along with the ancestry of the bacterium with which that person is infected. The team of scientists tested 233 individuals from two populations, one located in the high mountains of Columbia, and the other in a coastal village.

Sampling and sequencing the organism in both groups, they found that the rate of gastric cancer was 25 times higher among the mountain people. Among those living along the coast, the population was primarily of African descent; their dominant type of H.pylori was closely related to Africa.

The mountain people were predominantly Amerindian, with little to no African ancestry. Their H.pylori was closely related to Europe.

Drs. Correa and Schneider also showed that the European Amerindian descendants were at far greater risk of developing more severe gastric cancer then those of African descent. Moreover, the mountain dwellers had worse outcomes then those with the African microbial strains. Additionally, they found that people from either the mountains or coastal areas who had the lowest percentage of African ancestry had more severe cancers if they also had a greater percentage of H.pylori of African ancestry.

The researchers concluded that co-evolution among people and H.pylori reduced gastric cancer risk in those of African ancestry. The Amerindian people would have been exposed to H.pylori more recently, which indicates that they would not have had sufficient time for coevolution to occur, which would explain the far higher incidence of cancer among them.[20]

This revealing study clearly highlights how our microbiome affects our risk of disease. It also demonstrates the clear benefit of sequencing for DNA nucleotides.

As if to dot the i's and cross the t's, a more recent study adds strength to the microbiome-risk of cancer relationship.

Researchers at Mt. Sinai's Icahn School of Medicine, New York City, led by Dr. Sergio Lira, found that changes in the gut's microbial composition can sharply alter the development of bowel tumors, irrespective of genetics. It appears that if their mouse model can be transferable to us humans, that bacteria are needed, more likely, required, for tumor development. Listen to them: "In the presence of antibiotics, or of a slightly different set of cecum microbiota, (the cecum is the cul-de-sac forming the beginning of the large intestine) tumors did not develop." Clearly specific microbes within the microbiome are linked to chronic inflammation and the development of cancer. These researchers also informed us that, "after finding that antibiotics prevented polyp formation, they fed feces from antibiotic-free mice, to germ-free mice and found that the once germ-free mice developed tumors. When they sampled the intestines of their tumor-bearing mice they found heavy concentrations of Clostridial organisms, along with increased levels of inflammatory-causing immune cells. Yet another piece of the puzzle nicely in place.[21]

With the passing of 2012, the Human Microbiome Project had run its course. Currently the question is how to establish cause and effect between the microbiome and health, and the lack of it. Unfortunately, exaggerated claims by probiotic producers that their products can restore or alter the microbiome can discredit the field as their marketing is far out in front of the science.

At the International Human Microbiome Congress in Paris, in March 2012, participants raised the idea of an HMP2. Dr. David A. Relman, a physician/microbiologist at Stanford University's School of Medicine, offered a substantive proposal; that an HMP2 could mount a microbiome version of the famous and productive Framingham Heart study, by following thousands of people from birth for at least twenty years to see how their microbiomes fluctuate overtime and correlate with disease states.[22] I'd vote twice for that, as the HMP is providing a roadmap of the totality of microbes dwelling on and in healthy adults, which should be a game changer of popular opinion.

Interestingly, a powerful new tool has become available for dedicated researchers seeking to make fundamental discoveries. These investigators can now ask questions of the masses of data in public data banks such as NIH's Genebank, which, at the end of August 2013, held 167 million gene sequences along with 154 million bases. Digging into this can lead to notable discoveries without ever going into a lab, or mounting a population survey. They need only computer power, laptops or super computers.

Researchers who never conducted an experiment of any kind can take advantage of the public data bases to excise information that can lead to an advance, by culling out the DNA of large numbers of ill individuals, comparing them with healthy controls, seeking genetic fingerprints, sequences, linked to diseases. To do this, huge amounts of data are required, which are available, but it will not be easy. Mathematical rigor is needed. So, for example, a team of computer whizzes at Microsoft Research, Los Angeles, using Microsoft's Azure cloud-based super computer, compared the genomes of thousands of people in the United Kingdom's (England) Welcome Trust's data base, analyzing some 64 billion pairs of genetic markers, found new associations which may serve as markers for bipolar disorders, coronary heart disease, hypertension, inflammatory bowel disease, rheumatoid arthritis, and types 1 and 2 diabetes. Of course these are not cause-effect relationships, but they are a beginning to be followed up. As these databases are freely available, anyone can mine them for whatever nuggets may be lurking in the vicinity. Research that took years, can now occurr in hours, or days.

To take advantage of the opportunities hidden in the many data banks, NIH launched a new project called Big Data to Knowledge-BD2K, funded to the tune of ninety-six million dollars over four years. This project sets up a number of Centers to encourage development of novel approaches aiding discovery by data miners of new relationships tucked away within the billions of sequences. The opportunities and potential benefits are huge: for all of us.[22]

We Now Consider a Sampling of our Microbiomes and Their Human Interactions

Human breast milk contains a diversity of bacteria. Prof. Katherine Hunt and her team of researchers at the University of Idaho, Moscow, and Washington State University, Pullman, studied the microbial communities in human breast milk to determine its long-term stability. Using current sequencing procedures, they found after sampling three times over a month, that milk from sixteen healthy women, the optimal nutrition source for healthy infants, contains a great diversity of bacteria; far greater than previously reported.

Microbes such as staphylococci, corynebacteria, and propionibacteria, typically present on adult skin, were found in milk of all sixteen women, suggesting that skin may be the origin of these organisms. Consequently, to avoid the possibility of inadvertent contamination, the women's breasts were disinfected with an iodine-based solution before sampling.

Re-sampling found the most abundant genera were streptococci, staphylococci, serratia, corynebacteria, and propionibacteria; eight additional genera representing less than one percent of the total were also found. They learned too, that the stability of these microbial communities varied among the sixteen women. Stability also varied within individuals.

Streptococci were found to be the most abundant inx others. Several women had no clear dominant genera. The use of sequencing increased the capacity to obtain the less abundant genera, thereby generating a greater diversity than previously reported. Interestingly, lactobacilli and bifidobacteria previously reported in milk were found only rarely in any of the sixteen women. Because previous studies on breast milk had been done in Europe, dietary, genetic and/or environmental factors could account for the differences.

Nevertheless, a core microbiome was definitely present in these women. They noted too, that "the genus found in greatest abundance in the milk samples (streptococcus) is only a minor component of sebaceous skin microbiota." Similarly, propionibacteria are reported to be the most abundant on skin, but was not among the top five in their milk samples.

Clearly then, human breast milk introduces infants early on to a wide diversity of microbes that go directly to their gastrointestinal tracts. However, protective effects of breast feeding against diarrheal and respiratory illness, and the reduced risk of developing obesity cannot be inferred at this time, from the substantial difference in fecal microbiota between breast fed and formula-fed infants. Further studies are in progress to determine if other factors such as race, number of children, and type of delivery contribute to maintaining child and mammary health.[23]

The results of this study support the conclusion that human breast milk contains a far more diverse microbiota than previously known. It also found that the stability of individual core microbial communities is transient. It doesn't contribute solid information about the role the breast milk's microbial community plays in colonization of babies' gastrointestinal tracts or maintaining mammary health.

Prof. Kjersti Aagaard and her team of thirteen investigators at Baylor College of Medicine, Harvard University's School of Public Health, and the Massachusetts Institute of Technology, set out to determine the catalogue of vaginal microbiota in healthy adult females during pregnancy, compared to the non-pregnant vaginal community, and its meaning for new born infants.

But they make the point that for the longest time the overarching popular and medical belief held that microbes were foreign and had to be removed, banished, if health was to be achieved. This view is wholly at odds with the fact that microbes are present on and in us from the time of our birth. We are not sterile as we enter the world. The HMP with its totality of microbes residing on and in us should be a game changer of popular and medical opinion.

By the time of delivery, the infant has been exposed to the maternal vaginal microbial community as well as that of the delivery personnel. Exposure arrives via a richly microbial vaginal canal, feces, swallowing and breathing, skin to skin contact, along with maternal breast milk, as well as physician and nurses involved in delivery, among others.

Prof. Aagaard's team found that "although human adults have highly differentiated bacterial communities that are relatively stable," in pregnancy the vaginal microbiota shifts to a reduced diversity and numbers, but with the emergence of protective lactobacilli. They reported that compared to a non-pregnant cohort, four lactobacilli strains, L.iners, L.crispatus, L.jensenii, and L.johnsonii become dominant, and suggest that these organisms have biologic significance by producing enzymes and other protective chemicals limiting the growth of other organisms. Additionally, they found that pregnant vaginal microbial communities appear to return to the richer more diverse microbial types found in the non-pregnant vagina, in the last weeks of gestation.

In concluding, they comment on the remarkable distinction between the pregnant and non-pregnant microbiota, suggesting that these findings show the dynamic nature of our combined genomes, and "its role in vertical transmission of microbes through subsequent generations."[24]

Evident and well documented are the discoveries that a galaxy of microbes, both in numbers and types, call the uterus home. Tissues once thought to be sterile are now known to be rife with microbial life. The microbiome project has shown that no area or body tissue is microbe-free. That's a salient take-away message.

Microbes and Anti-tumor Agents

Two recent publications, one by a team of thirty-two French scientists representing a half-dozen institutions found that gut microbes reinforce, boost, the effects of anti-tumor agents. They demonstrated in mouse models that with the absence or lack of Lactobacillus johnsonii and Enterococcus lirae, the anti-tumor treatments of the normally effective platinum compounds were far less effective. Apparently these normally present gut organisms stimulate the generation of immune T-cells (detailed in Chapter THREE) that destroy tumor cells. Moreover, the researchers were shocked to find that antibiotic therapy increased the risk of tumor development by reducing the populations of L.johnsnii, and E. lirae.[25]

If that wasn't powerful enough, a team of twenty-one investigators from various labs of the National Cancer Institute, Frederick, Maryland, obtained similar results. They reported that disruption of the gut microbiota by antibiotic use substantially impaired the response of tumors to the antitumor compound, Cyclophosphamide. Their data clearly showed that Lactobacilli control the tumors response to therapy by affecting the immune system positively or negatively, depending upon the presence or lack of these microbes. This surely "highlights the potential to improve cancer treatment by manipulating human gut microbiota."[26]

The fact that two research groups working independently of one another with two different protocols, obtained similar results, provides strong support for their conclusions. Should their findings prove out in human trials, it would surely change current medical practice, as quite obviously, these studies demonstrate the complex interplay between microbes, the immune system and type of therapy. Clearly, gut microbes are essential for activating the immune cells that battle cancer cells.

For years it has been evident that antibiotics markedly reduce a diversity of beneficial intestinal organisms. With the new knowledge that antibiotics wipe out these specific, beneficial microbes, thereby increasing tumor activity, limiting antibiotic use in individuals braving chemotherapy, seems a no-brainer. Furthermore, cancer patients with the additional insult of a microbial infection, the consequence of an impaired immune system, are recipients of a double whammy, as they take antibiotics to defeat the infection, which reduces the effectiveness of their anticancer therapy as the antibiotic kills off the microbes normally enhancing the antitumor agents. At least this is the scenario expected to play out in us humans, if the mouse results prove transferable to us. Again, it's another wait and see. But sucking up probiotics at this time, is exactly what is not called for.

Kwashiorkor and Malnutrition

Malnutrition is a major contributor to childhood illness and death. Kwashiorkor has long been a puzzling and elusive form of malnutrition. Kwashiorkor is a Ghanian word meaning, the sickness the child gets when the new baby comes. That is, the older child no longer gets the proteins and amino acids in breast milk that now goes to the new infant.

Although rare in the U.S., far too many elderly in nursing homes exhibit protein deficiency as protein is more expensive than fat or carbohydrate. And too often, the elderly are unable to chew protein-containing beans, and may also avoid beans for their gas production. When Kwashiorkor does occur in the U.S., it is a sign of child abuse or severe neglect. However, it is widespread in African countries where the food supply is limited. In these circumstances, children manifest enlarged livers, bloated stomachs, decreased muscle mass, changes in skin pigmentation, loss of weight, diarrhea and much more.

Led by Drs.Michelle F. Smith, and Jeffrey Gordon, along with a team of scientists from Washington University, School of Medicine, St. Louis, and the University of Malawi, College of Medicine, Balantyre, Malawi, they set out to investigate the role of the gut microbiome, as a means of solving the underlying and perplexing problem.

To do this, they studied 317 pairs of Malawian twins from birth to age three. Over the three years, half of the twin pairs remained well nourished, while 136 had a poor response, and 23 exhibited severe malnutrition.

During the years of the investigation, the undernourished and malnourished twins were fed a peanut-butter-based ready-to-use therapeutic food, (this paste contained milk powder, oil, sugar, and a micronutrient supplement) and their fecal microbiome were sequenced to ascertain the types and numbers of their microbial load. This was compared to the fecal microbiomes of the healthy twins. Additionally, one group of germ-free mice received fecal transplants from healthy Malawian children. Another group of mice received transplants from children with Kwashiorkor. Both groups were then fed the typical Malawian diet.

The researchers found that feeding the peanut-butter ready -to-use therapeutic diet produced beneficial gut microbiota that relieved the Kwashiorkor. When that diet was stopped, the Kwashiorkor returned. The mice receiving the fecal transplants from malnourished twins had marked weight loss, as well as substantial changes in their amino acids, carbohydrates and metabolic pathways that were only temporarily improved with, the peanut-butter paste diet. Metabolic analysis indicated that the microbes in Kwashiorkor produce products inhibiting enzymes that compromise effective energy metabolism.

The investigators concluded that, "these findings implicate the gut microbiome as a causal factor in Kwashiorkor." They go on to say that "these results may be useful for developing new and more effective approaches for treatment and prevention."[27, 28]

Undeniably, the human gut consists of a complex and diverse microbial community that varies from person to person. Apparently as our microbes play a major role in our daily functioning, it has been suggested seriously, that as our microbes have had billions of years to enhance their ability to exploit their environments, and that over a million years of our co-evolution, microbes have evolved an uncanny ability within our internal environment, to manipulate us for our mutual benefit. To put an even sharper point on this, Bacteroides ovatus, a gut microbe has now been isolated and shown to digest complex carbohydrates, polysaccharides, called xyloglucans, fibrous material, found in fruits and veggies. More than ninety percent of us have at least one of these xyloglucan-digesting organisms in our gut.

Researchers at the University of Michigan's medical school, tell us that their findings underscore the importance of these bacteria for our diet, health, and nutrition. I don't find that too hard to believe. Do you?

As we shall see, in the following chapter, microbes play a significant role in meshing with our immune system.

This extensive sampling of the human microbiome provided a first characterization of the normal microbiota of healthy adults. The large sample size and the many sites sampled allows an understanding of the relationships among our microbes, and provides support for individual variation, that may well lead to understanding and dealing with microbiome-based illnesses. However, it remains for future studies to learn why our site-specific microbial communities vary so extensively. Moreover, similar studies will be needed for populations around the world to see how they compare: how different, or how similar.

The excitement among the HMP scientists is palpable; as it should be. We should be cheering them on, as they are providing us with the spankingly new knowledge about ourselves, which can only be beneficial. We can now think of our microbiome as another genome. Ergo, with two genomes, each working for us, we can surley be thought of as a supraorganism. Dwell on that message for a spell. With that in our grasp, we now consider our immune systems internal defense forces, and their tight connection to our microbes.

THREE

The Internal Defense Forces:
Our Dazzling Immune System

The battle is joined. At the moment of birth, and unabated until our arrival at the happy hunting grounds, our astonishing immune system is our muscular defense against legions of nasties-microbes, germs, intent on using us for their pleasure, and sickening us if they can.

However, microbes that we encounter daily seldom cause illness. Something to keep in mind. Most are destroyed rapidly by our internal defense forces. One thing is certain, this internal defense force, our immune system, is not just immensely complex, it is truly mind-numbing in its complexity. Nonetheless, we can get a grip on it firm enough to appreciate its complexity and understand its functions as well as its tight connectedness to our microbiome. By the way, immunity comes via the Latin, immunis, meaning free of burden, referring to our ability to resist microbial disease.

With all the complexity, it is essential to remember that a cardinal function of the immune system is to assure the ability to distinguish self from non-self. That is, to be able to discriminate us from them; them being foreign proteins; not to attack our proteins. Errors, though rare, can occur, and on those rare occasions when our immune cells do attack us, autoimmune diseases arise. Consequently, the question that arises is, how can the immune system recognize the huge number of microbes and other foreign proteins that threaten us? Surely the system cannot know or anticipate which foreign antigens lurk in its neighborhood at any moment. No, anticipation isn't involved. It's the antibodies of the adaptive system that enter the fray differentiating them from our cellular proteins.

Two major fighting forces forever alert and on standby, are ready for the never-ending battle. On the front line, with its set of defenses is the innate brigade: natural, and non-specific, existing since birth, inherited from parent to child. Being non-specific, these innate troops can respond and pursue any foreign protein, any microbe. Furthermore, the innate system can respond immediately to invaders, taking them on and holding them in check until the adaptive system produces its specific antibodies.

Skin, the innate's major barrier, is abetted by the flushing action of tears and saliva, containing enzymes capable of destroying foreign proteins. Additional backup comes from mucus that traps microbes in nose, throat and the respiratory tract; spitting, coughing and sneezing expels them.

Our muco-ciliary elevator (broncho-pulmonary cilia) carries trapped organisms up and out of the trachea, the windpipe that channels air to the lungs. This works just fine if you don't smoke. Smoking paralyzes the cilia stalling the elevator.

Hydrochloric acid in our stomachs is deadly for those few pathogens that make it passed the innate's first line of defense. The heavy weapons involved in much of the above are chemicals: fatty acids in sweat that inhibits bacterial growth, and lysozyme and phospholipase in tears, saliva and nasal secretions. Histidine peptides, known as histatins, also play a major microbe-inhibiting role in saliva.

Defensins, appropriately named, are peptides in the lungs and gastrointestinal tract that have antimicrobial activity. Surfactants and Opsonins in lungs that bind to microbes signal phagocytic cells of the presence of foreign proteins. The beauty of these innate cells is their ability to function within minutes to hours. Moreover, this initial defensive position can also prompt supporting troops, if there is need.

Awaiting calls to action are the humoral and cell-mediated militia: with their neutrophils, macrophages, natural killer cells, dendritic cells, along with B and T cells. We'll meet up with each of these a bit further along.

A second line of defense, call it the "big guns," are cells of the adaptive immune system that is antigen-specific. Here we deal with the antigen-antibody duality. An antigen, most often a protein, induces a specific immune response, as it is foreign to our body, which our body does not sanction. Antibody is a specific protein produced in response to an antigen and which reacts with the antigen. Our antibody molecules are Y-shaped, and attach their forked end, the tail of the Y, to an antigen, neutralizing it. Visualize two antibody molecules catching a microbe between them. Rod-shaped, spherical, or spiral microbial forms fit nicely into the Y's and are firmly trapped. Additionally, by chemically removing the tail, making the Y into a V, the risk of side effects can be greatly reduced when dealing with the vicious venom of black widow spider bites, as well as scorpion and snake bites.[1] For the most part only foreign proteins elicit an antigen-antibody reaction, but polysaccharides and lipopolysaccharides can also set off that response.

When needed, immunoglobulins can be called into the fray. They go by the name Ig. Each of the five of them,

IgG;IgM;IgA;IgD and IgE, are produced in response to an antigen and function as an antibody, and as we shall see, each has its specific function.

To summarize, the innate system is non-specific, natural, and native, and is in place prior to exposure to antigens, and can respond to antigens immediately. The adaptive system is specific, and acquired. It is induced by an antigen and remembers scrimmaging with them. Subsequent encounters stimulate increasingly effective defense mechanisms. With its collection of specialized cells it amplifies the protective mechanisms of the non-specific system, making them better able to eliminate foreign invaders. However, the adaptive system can take days or weeks to join the struggle.

So, the task of our immune system is to recognize danger signs involving foreign proteins, antigens, and then, with exquisite precision mobilize antibodies: other proteins that bind to and neutralize, or kill the offending microbial antigens. But our immune system has to be cognizant of the difference between our self-proteins, and non-self, foreign proteins. Therein hangs a tale, a tale of on-going combat between the forces of light and darkness, between our immune system cells and those miscreant microbial cells.

Consider that if the nasties, those delinquents never met with opposition, we'd either be chronically ill, or dead; suggesting that even these germs do not want to lose their comfortable abode. After all, they had the world to themselves for thousands of millennia, and had to keep evolving to maintain themselves in the face of dreadfully harsh environments.

With the rise of mammals, and especially we hominids, they found much more agreeable surroundings. And we humans, also evolving, co-evolving along with them, were able to adequately defend ourselves. Neither epidemic nor pandemic, however onerous—the Black Plague, waves of cholera, typhoid, typhus, smallpox, or the Spanish Flu, smiting tens of millions of us, could never wipe us out. Why? Because our formidable immune defenses spread widely about our bodies, were ever vigilant.

This immune system, a network of mind-bending complexity, and so specialized in its various functions deserves not only recognition, but accolades for a job well done. Therefore, it is altogether fitting and proper to bring it front and center for your elucidation, comfort and applause.

We begin with the irresistible fact that our bodies provide ideal quarters for both beneficial microbes and potentially harmful germs. For them, nothing can match our body's warm, moist, highly nutritious habitat. Consequently loads of them try to gain admission. Our ability to repel them is referred to as immunity. Germs attempting to slide under the radar and gain a foothold, must get passed our first line of defense: our skin, tears, saliva and mucus.

Without cuts or abrasions, germs (microbes) cannot get through the skin, our body's largest organ. Tears constantly wash out foreign particles from eye surfaces, and saliva does the same for our mouths. Germs entering the nose cause nasal surfaces to secrete protective mucus, and attempts to enter our lungs can trigger a sneeze or cough forcing invaders out of the respiratory tract.

Mucus membranes line the entire gastrointestinal, respiratory, urinary and reproductive tracts. This membrane constantly secretes mucus that traps and inhibits entrance of germs to tissues and cells. But it's not perfect. As we know, the Treponema of Syphilis, Mycobacteria of Tuberculosis, and Streptococci of Pneumonia, for example, can and do slip under our defenses, with our help.

The mucus membranes of the respiratory tract along with the fine hairs, the cilia, also there, move synchronously propelling inhaled germs trapped in the mucus, upward toward the throat to be spit out. This constant movement, known as the mucociliary elevator, works well in those of us that do not smoke. Cigarette smoke paralyzes the cilia that then lie back, impairing the elevators forward motion, and of course making those individuals susceptible to a range of potential illnesses.

The stomach's hydrochloric acid-like environment readily kills organisms ingested with food. And urinary flow is yet another mechanical means of preventing microbial colonization of the urinary system.

Should a nasty get passed these gatekeepers, they meet and must contend with an incomparably specific immune system that stockpiles a huge arsenal of exceptional cells.

Our highly sophisticated adaptive immune system, unlike any other, is not in one place. It's far flung. The various and diverse organs of the immune system are collectively known as lymphoid organs–lymph–from the Greek, meaning a pure, clean stream: an appropriate description considering its appearance and purpose.

Here's how it works. Cells that will grow and become the many types of specialized cells that circulate throughout the lymphatic vessels and lymph nodes are born in bone marrow: a nutrient-rich gelatinous tissue found in the center of the long, flat bones of our pelvis and legs. The cells of greatest concern are lymphocytes- a trillion of them. All white cells, leucocytes, are of two main types: B-cells, which grow to maturity in bone marrow, hence the designation B, and T-cells, which mature in the Thymus gland, just above the heart, behind the breast bone, from whence cometh the T.

B-cells produce millions of specific antibodies belonging to a family of large protein molecules called immunoglobulins: five in all, designated Ig's: IgG, IgM, A, D, and E. IgG, as you are probably well aware is also known as gamma globulin, and is the most prominent. IgG may just be the elixir patients and physicians have been waiting for to mitigate their Alzheimer's disease, obsessive-compulsive disorders and schizophrenia, which appear to have autoimmune causes. Should this prove to be true, in tests currently in progress, it would banish all manner of pills, as IgG antibodies are an unlimited resource. Here again, it is stand by for further devlopments.[2] IgM, usually found in star-shaped clusters in our blood streams, is the first to arrive on a battle site, and is the most effective killer. IgA guards the entrance to our body and as such is concentrated in tears, saliva as well as secretions of the respiratory and gastrointestinal tract. IgD, helps B-cells initiate the immune response, the battle, and E, is responsible for the watery eyes and runny nose of allergy symptoms is generally present only in small amounts, but during an allergic turmoil, it's level increases dramatically.

The first time an allergy-prone person is exposed to an allergen (an antigen) such as grass or weed pollen, that person's B-cells make huge amounts of the grass or weed IgE antibody which bind to specific cells in the lungs, skin, tongue and mucosal linings of the nose and gastrointestinal tract. The next time that person contacts either pollen, the IgE-primed cells in the lungs, skin and tongue, release powerful chemicals that induce wheezing, sneezing, itching and other allergic symptoms.

These protective antibodies arise explicitly for the specific foreign protein it is attacking, which must be mind-boggling in its complexity and specificity. As you can imagine, there are literally millions of antibodies, each with a specific "memory" of a protein encountered once before, years ago. And when there is a second occurrence, the antibody is mobilized to halt potential invaders doing their nasty business. Amazing is an under statement for the exquisite chemical signaling going on here, along with the warriors called into combat.

It is estimated that the healthy folks among us, which means most of us, have 10 million different antibodies stored away in immune cell memory: a mind-bending number considering that anyone of these millions could be called up to do battle with a specific antigen: a germ. Any wonder that Immunologists have long wondered how these ten million different proteins could be stored– fit onto a limited number of genes. They are not alone in asking that question. The type of fitting system has to be yet another mind-bending creation.

Let's be clear. Any microbe or foreign protein, animal or plant that can trigger an immune response is referred to as an antigen-from *anti*body *gen*erator. Tissues and cells from another individual except an identical twin also carry non-self markers and are seen as foreign antigens, which explains why tissue transplants are often rejected. These antigens can also be toxins, or any proteinaceous substance capable of triggering an immune response. Recall too, that antibodies are the reason specific germs can make us ill only once in our lifetime. Although this memory doesn't apply to all viruses, we shall see, a bit further on, how that is being dealt with.

T-cells also patrol the blood and lymph for foreign invaders, attacking and destroying them along with diseased cells they now recognize as foreign protein. These T-cells orchestrate, regulate and coordinate the overall immune response. But they depend on special cell surface molecules-proteins- to help them recognize self from non-self. That is, not to mistake the proteins of our muscles, nerves, skin and all our other organs from foreign non-self protein. To make so horrendous a mistake, can and does happen, with the crisis of an immune meltdown that can sicken and/or kill us. The bad, bad consequences go by the name autoimmune diseases.

So, how do our immune cells distinguish self from non-self? An essential question, as this is at the heart, the core of the immune response.

All cells in our body are covered with major histocompatibility complex proteins—MHC's—whose function is to bind peptide fragments from pathogens and display them on cell surfaces for recognition by T-cells that can digest them. Disease proteins in a cell are split, broken into pieces by the cell's proteolytic enzymes. These broken pieces become attached to the MHC's which transport them to the cell's surface where the surface MHC's flag down killer T-cells to get rid of these foreign antigens.[3] These passing T-cells recognize all surface protein complexes as self, as the surface MHC's distinctive peptides, collections of amino acids, direct them not to attack. Without this distinguishing ability, the immune response cannot occur. Again, perfection is not of this world. Sometimes the immune systems recognition apparatus breaks down and the body begins to manufacture antibodies and T-cells directed against our body's own cells and organs. So, for example, T-cells that attack pancreas cells contribute to Diabetes, while an antibody known as rheumatoid factor is commonly found in individuals with rheumatoid arthritis.

When our immune system lacks one or more of its components, an immunodeficiency disorder can occur. These can be inherited or acquired via an infection. AIDS (acquired immune deficiency syndrome) is an immunodeficiency disorder provoked by the HIV virus that destroys T-helper (Th) cells. After gaining entry to a cell, the offensive virus takes over the cells machinery and copies itself incessantly, then invades helper T-cells and macrophages-large scavenger white cells-both normally needed to organize an immune defense. The AIDS virus splices its DNA into the DNA of the cell it infects: the cell is then under the control of the virus. This process is repeated interminably until the infected individual is hellishly ill with AIDS.

Our protective antibodies are made explicitly for the specific foreign protein it is attacking, each with a specific memory of a protein it encountered once before. Decades more often, than not. Haven't we learned over the years that with most infectious diseases, once we become ill, and recover, we are protected for life from a reinfection. Well, mostly. But it took sharp minds to work out the condition of resistance and susceptibility to infectious disease.

History informs us that a natural experiment demonstrating the fact of immune memory occurred in the Faroe Islands, a remote speck of land between Iceland and Norway. In 1781, a devastating measles outbreak drastically reduced the Islands population. During the ensuing 65 years, the population rebuilt, and the Islands remained measles-free. In 1846, with the arrival of a ship from Denmark, measles struck again, infecting some 80 percent of the population with a grievous death rate. Ludwig Panum, a Danish physician investigating the outbreak, astutely observed that, "of the many aged people still living on the Faroe's, who had measles in 1781, not one was attacked a second time." He also found that "all the old people who had not gone through with measles in earlier life, were attacked when they were exposed to infection."[4] Panum learned that immunity to measles was long-lived and that re-exposure was not essential for maintaining long-term protective immunity. After 65 years measles antibodies were still available and protective, indicating the long-term memory of immune cells, especially the lymphoid memory T-cells that retained memory of the virus. Interestingly, Thucydides, the Greek historian, in describing the plague of Athens in 430 bce, wrote that, "the same man was never attacked twice."

The intriguing cast of immune system players cannot be considered complete without brief attention to the central role of dendritic cells, a class of phagocytic cells with long, thread-like fingers that come in several types.

Dendritic cells functions in our immune system was discovered by Dr. Ralph Steinman, of New York City's Rockefeller University, for which he was awarded a Nobel prize in Medicine or Physiology in 2011. He died at age 68, of pancreatic cancer, three days before the award was announced; not knowing he was to be awarded.[5]

Dendritic cells are long, thin, branched, tree-like cells, (referred to as dendrites-from the Greek, meaning, tree) found in lymphoid organs and at the interfaces between our bodies and the environment. The epidermal layer of our skin has a rich network of dendritic cells; they also line the surfaces of our airways where they function as sentinels, checking and inspecting proteins and other environmental particles.

They, in fact, are the sentinels patrolling the body seeking out foreign invaders. When they come upon one, they bind it, and break it up into smaller pieces, and present them to T-cells. They then travel to lymph nodes or spleen where they signal B-cells to make huge numbers of antibodies that neutralize the invaders; they also stimulate production of killer T-cells that launch attacks to destroy and dispose them.

Nevertheless, their work is not done. Dendritic cells also have a major role in preventing dangerous immune cells from attacking our body's tissues—attacking, itself. New evidence now shows that dendritic cells provide the vital link between antigens and all types of lymphocytes, the many and diverse white cells. These cells have recently been shown to have MHC receptors on their surfaces that enhance uptake of antigens making them recognizable to cytotoxic T-cells. Furthermore, and this is mind -boggling, these astonishing cells are able to specify which type of T-cell is needed for the specific type of antigen present: virus, bacteria, or other parasite. Different T-cells for different antigens! Remarkable, is a world of understatement. Obviously there is good and sufficient reason why dendritic cells are looked upon as "conductors of the immune orchestra." Surely, its sweet silent music is our continued good health. Dr. Steinman should have been awarded a Nobel twice over for his momentous discovery.

As noted earlier, we are earthlings, which means perfection is elusive. When our immune cells fail to recognize us, an immune firestorm can occur. You will of course recognize these autoimmune conditions:

Grave's disease; Multiple Sclerosis; Juvenile Onset Type1 Diabetes; Rheumatoid Arthritis; Inflammatory Bowel Diseases (Crohn's and Colitis), and Systemic Lupus Erythematosus, are among the 70-80 others for which one in five of us suffers. We also know that some 24 million men, women and children around the country are host to the many and diverse conditions, with women leading in the number of diseases that attack us humans. Some are rare, some more common.

Uncertainty abounds: why autoimmunity is not triggered more often, or even why it occurs when it does remains an open question. So, what do we know and what remains to be discovered? Would one cause fit all? A reasonable question and one in which the jury remains out. Nevertheless, important discoveries are being made.

There is strong suspicion that a foreign protein bears great familiarity to one or more of our self antigens, which is termed "molecular mimicry," and that our T and B cells cross-react with our tissue antigens causing an immune meltdown, and an autoimmune disease.

Recently the discovery of a protein fragment capable of causing Diabetes in mice spurred researchers at National Jewish Health and the University of Colorado (Denver) to propose a new hypothesis about the cause of Diabetes and autoimmunity generally.[6] They propose "that the unusual and rare presentation of protein fragments (peptides-groups of amino acids) to the immune system allows highly reactive T cells to escape the Thymus gland, and never having "seen" these fragments before, but, as they have encountered these peptides elsewhere in the body, trigger an autoimmune attack." This appears to have much to recommend it, but as science requires, before it can be accepted as fact, others will have to obtain the same or similar results. Ergo, it's a wait and see.

On the other hand, another interpretation maintains that autoantibodies are nothing more than antibodies generated in response to pathogenic bacterial cells that were destroyed as a result of an active immune response; in effect, collateral damage. Yet another wait-and-see.

The most recent findings to be published come from Harvard Medical School where Dr. Julia Wang and her team offer a new "unifying theory." They have turned away from proteins, pursuing carbohydrates, telling us that "the abundance of a carbohydrate in skin and connective tissue called Dermatan Sulfate turns traitorous," and the resulting disease may be systemic as in Lupus, or rheumatoid arthritis, or localized as in Type1 Diabetes or Grave's disease. Dr.Wang believes "dermatan sulfate plays a pivotal role in regulating a type of B cell she refers to as B-1a. Levels of both dermatan sulfate and B-1a cells are elevated when cell turnover is high, as in wound healing." She also indicates that, "when dead cells pile up, dermatan sulfate may help speed the clearing of these cells by the immune system." She goes on to say that when cells with a high affinity for the molecule die, the resulting complexes can become unrecognizable as self.[7]

These complexes stimulate the proliferation of B-1a cells and the production of autoantibodies, which in turn mark healthy tissues for destruction. When these antibodies bind to our antigens on healthy cells, other autoimmune B cells infiltrate the tissue. Change follows. This idea, this interpretation, also has much to recommend it. The idea of a unifying theory has a nice ring to it, suggesting a pulling together of the various published interpretations. This could do it, as her data appears to include a number of different organ systems.

Another recent study, taking a different tack, found that gnotobiotic, germ-free animals, have defective T-helper (Th) cell development, with a reciprocal increase in T-regular (Treg) cells. When these mice are given a diverse mixture of microbes, but one lacking such organisms as Bacteriodetes fragilis, there is no restoration of a proper immune balance, suggesting that specific organisms may have the capacity to restore pro and anti-inflammatory responses in the gut.[8] These diverse studies do point in a similar direction: microbes and the immune system must function together to maintain our health. Now, there is a startling new idea that will be pursued.

Important new information relating microbes and our body's immune system comes from studies of germ-free (sterile) animals: born with extensive defects in the development of gut-associated lymphoid tissues, and in antibody production. They also have fewer and smaller lymph nodes, all integral to immune system maturity and protective functions.

These structures form normally following the introduction of gut bacteria, suggesting a dynamic relationship between the immune system and microbes. The nagging question is, has the progress that has lowered infant mortality on the one end, and prolonged life on the other, also responsible for the major shifts in our microbiota, and with it, given rise to a clutch of autoimmune diseases and allergies. Over the past 40 years, the prevalence of Asthma among children has doubled; current epidemiologically based thinking faults urban and suburban living environments that are far too clean. Early contact with a range of microbes is sorely lacking. Dirt is good!

Enter David Strachen, and his Hygiene Hypothesis, that started the feverish rush to explore and uncover this relationship, if in fact it should exist.

Prof. Strachen, initially at the University of London's School of Hygiene and Tropical Medicine, informed us that hay fever has been described as a "postindustrial revolution epidemic." In his National Child Development Study,[9] he followed 17,444 British children from birth in March 1958, to their 23rd birthdays in 1981. From his mountain of data, he found that hay fever was strikingly related to family size, and position in the household in childhood.

Eczema during the child's first year was (also) directly related to the number of children in the household. Protection from these illnesses could readily be explained by prevention of infection in early childhood transmitted by unhygienic contact with older siblings, or acquired prenatally from a mother infected by contact with her older children. Later infection or reinfection by younger siblings might confer additional protection against hay fever.

Strachen concluded, saying, "that over the past century declining family size, improvements in household amenities, and higher standards of personal cleanliness have reduced the opportunity for cross infection in young families." He further remarked that, "this may have resulted in more widespread clinical expression of atopic disease, emerging earlier in wealthier people as seems to have occurred for hay fever.

We Take a Brief Digression for Atopy

Hypersensitivity or allergy, are interchangeable terms and occur following a persons second contact with the provoking antigen, an allergen. Localized hypersensitivity is often referred to as atopy-"out-of-place"-allergy. The developing symptoms depend on the route by which the allergens enter the body. Hay fever, allergic rhinitis, is a common example of an atopic allergy involving the upper respiratory tract. Air borne allergens, plant pollen, fungal spores, animal dander and house-dust mites, sensitize certain cells within the mucus lining of the nose, throat and lungs. Repeat exposure to any one of these antigens, cause the all too well known hypersensitive responses: itching, tearing eyes, conjested nasal passages, coughing and sneezing-the bodies attempt to rid itself of the allergens any way it can.

The hypersensitivity can also show up as asthma, dermatitis and food allergy.

Back to Professor Strachen

Several years later, Strachen followed his pioneering

work by determining if increased numbers of sibling's infection's in early life protected them against allergic sensitization.

He found that an environmental influence was operating and that it impacted allergic sensitization, and that influence was directly due to the number of siblings, birth order, and infant feeding. These were protective influences against infection. In fact, the number of older brothers and sisters, not younger, were more protective, and infants solely breast fed were also of higher risk of later hay fever.[10,11]

Strachen's studies were the engines that propelled researchers in Germany, Austria, Australia and the US to determine if his findings were universal truths, or simply a local phenomenon.

What did these other researchers discover?

Dr. Erika von Mutius, of University Children's Hospital, Munich, Germany, was one of the first to pull a team together. Her team began with the idea that children growing up in the poorer, dirtier, polluted and generally less healthful cities of (former) East Germany, would suffer more from allergy and asthma than children in (the former) and cleaner West Germany. She also knew that the East German government would never allow a comparison study. Luck was on her side. The Berlin Wall came crashing down, uniting the two Germany's in 1999. She had her comparative study, and was shocked by the results. When her team of physicians studied the East German children they found that they had far fewer allergic reactions and fewer asthma cases than the children in the cleaner west. She also found lifestyle differences between the two, including family size and more frequent use of day care for young children in the east. As she wrote, "she now ascribes to the Hygiene Hypothesis," which maintains that children around numerous other children or animals early in life are exposed to more microbes and consequently their immune systems develop greater tolerance for the triggers that set off an asthma attack.[12] Dr. Mutius also found that the largest reduction in risk was among those who were exposed prenatally and continuously thereafter.

More recently, she and Dr. Donata Vercelli of the Arizona Respiratory Center, University of Arizona, found that children who grew up on traditional farms are protected from asthma, hay fever and allergic sensitization. Early contact with livestock and their fodder, they found, along with consumption of unprocessed cow's milk were the most effective exposures. Again, early contact with a diversity of microbes matures the immune system.[12] Dirt is essential.

Numerous epidemiological studies of farm living point to activation and modification of both innate and adaptive immune responses by intense microbial exposures and possibly signals from different organ systems delivered before or soon after birth. [14]

A recently published study done in Finland shows that infants there are not exempt from respiratory tract illnesses. A group of Pediatricians led by Dr. Eija Bergroth of the Department of Pediatrics, Kuopio University Hospital, Kuopio, Finland, investigated the effect of early contact with dogs and cats on the frequency of respiratory symptoms and infections during an infants first year of life.

Following 397 infants from middle and eastern Finland, from their mother's pregnancy onward, they found that children having dogs at home had far fewer respiratory symptoms than children without dogs. Those children with dogs also had fewer middle ear infections and consequently needed less antibiotic treatments. They concluded that "our findings support the theory that during the first year of life, animal contacts are important, possibly leading to better resistance to infectious respiratory illness during childhood."[15]

That study was part of the larger PASTURE study—*P*rotection *A*gainst *A*llergy in *R*ural *E*nvironments, an

on-going investigation in five European countries-
Austria, France, Finland, Switzerland and Germany. In
this PASTURE study, mothers were followed-up from
their third trimester of pregnancy to birth of their infants
and on to a full year. Furthermore, contact with dogs and
cats were grouped by daily hours of contact: from none,
to more than 16 hours. Interestingly, it was learned that
dog contact was more protective than cat. Of utmost and
surprising interest, was the finding in those homes where
dogs spent less than six hours per day indoors, that time
period was most protective. The investigators believe
that this seeming counter intuitive fact may be due to the
dogs being out more often, then bringing in more dirt,
and microbes from their extended outdoor activities.

Is cleanliness next to godliness: or shall we offer a
prayer to give us this day our daily germs? Something
to dwell upon.

With the many studies now in hand, what can be
drawn from them? That is indeed, the question. Clearly it
is consistency. That responsible researchers around the
world, studying different populations, using varying
protocols, obtain the same or similar results bolsters the
relationship-beneficial microbes equals reduced
hypersensitivity in children and adults. Such consistency
also suggests universality of the problem: that we are
more alike than not. And, that the findings are reliable.
Moreover, the combined evidence announces that we are
all in bed, as it were, with our microbes, and that they are
protecting us; will continue protecting us, if we let them.
Stop trying to rid ourselves of them. Our collections of
microbes, germs, play a major role in who becomes ill
and who doesn't. Ergo, beneficial microbes can no
longer be seen as oxymoronic.

So, yes, several relatively small studies found that
farm family children are at far less risk of allergies, hay
fever, asthma and other autoimmune disorders. To finally
pin down and settle the question, a larger study was
needed.

Dr. Markus J. Ege, of Children's Hospital, University

of Munich, assembled a team of 150 experienced Pediatricians, Microbiologists and Epidemiologists from 14 European countries including France, England, The Netherlands, Poland and Switzerland, to provide optimum inputs and assessments, as they sought to uncover the environmental causes of asthma.

They compared children living on farms with those living elsewhere for the number of asthma and allergy cases in each group. In fact, two large studies were designed: The Parsifal (Prevention of Allergy-Risk Factors for Sensitization Related to Farming and Arthroscopic Lifestyle) enrolled 6,843 children ages 6-13 of farm families and children attending Ralph Steiner, Arthroscopic schools, while the Gabriella study, (Genetic and Environmental Causes of Asthma in the European Community) enrolled 9,668 elementary school children ages 6-12, for a total of 16,511 children.[16]

Of course it is not difficult to believe that the children raised on farms, living in the open, unpolluted air, away from the smoke and grime of city life, pitching in with farm work, feeding animals, keeping fit, would be healthy. But as so many others have found, it wasn't simply the clean air, sunshine and hard work that did it, it was their close contact with microbes-bacteria and fungi-in the farm environment.

Dr.Ege's team scrutinized microbial exposure in house dust collected in both the Parsifal and Gabriella studies; obtaining results confirming previous studies that the risk of asthma in farm-family children, was as much as fifty-percent less than those children not living on farms. Also evident was the finding that farmhouse dust, especially mattress dust, a hot spot of microbial exposure, contained a far more diverse group of bacteria and fungi than urban homes. The dust was loaded with *Listeria monocytogenes, Bacillus licheniformis, Corynebacterium, Xanthomonas, Enterobacter* and others: all gram-negative rods. It was also evident that these microbes, these germs, from and around farms, animal sheds, barns and pastures, were readily brought indoors,"and even when indoors, children living on farms were exposed to a greater variety of microbes than children who did not live on farms."

From the Gabriella study, investigators were surprised to find that fungi were prominent anti-asthma protection. Penicillium was one of the more protective. This appears to run counter to observations that molds account for increased risk of asthma due to dampness. Nevertheless, it needs to be noted that there are many different species among all types of molds that exert diverse effects. Of greatest importance they found that, newborn, farm infants became colonized by both bacteria and fungi as soon as they emerged into the physical environment, which parallels the period of development of the lungs and immune system.

Unfortunately, since 1980, the number of children developing asthma has more than doubled, and preventive measures are nowhere in sight. With the results of both Parsifal and Gabriella, along with David Strachen's Hygiene Hypothesis, and the consistent results of other European studies, it seems a no brainer that some form of microbial exposure be made available to non-farm families, sooner than later.

Evidently a rich microbial environment in childhood is protective. Microbes do matter.

It is now also clear that infants born by cesarian section, who arrive via a more sterile delivery than infants delivered vaginally, are far more likely to get asthma as they age. Along with the many studies noted, these findings indicate that our collections of microbes do guide the maturation of our immune system. Most importantly, when our immune system fails to get the microbes it needs, disease does follow. Consequently, with their C-section deliveries, some few Obstetricians are now rubbing birth canal fluid over the infants to compensate for the lack of microbes lost by not moving through their mother's birth canal. That's a bright spot.

All of us host a veritable microbial zoo, but children who develop hypersensitivities, allergies, hay fever, asthma, inflammatory bowel disease, among others, not only have a different collection of microbes, but a much less diverse one. That appears to be a key. That lack of diversity is important but even more important are the types of bacteria in the lungs of asthmatics, who were found to be harboring typical respiratory pathogens, but without symptoms of infection. Here was a significant clue. Finding pathogenic organisms in the lung was itself shocking as all microbiology textbooks inform us that the lungs are sterile: microbe-free. Nevertheless, Proteobacteria, such as Moraxella, Klebsiella, and Neisseria were in there, while normal, healthy infants and children were hosts to the Bacteriodetes, such as Bacillus fragilis and B.thetaiotaomicron, commonly found in soil, seawater, skin and intestines. Clues began to congeal.

Our "old friends" as Prof. Gordon Rook of University College, London, has dubbed them, his fine-tuning of the Hygiene Hypothesis, are microorganisms associated with farms, and farm animals, untreated water supplies, pets, and fermented foods that have been part of our microbial environment for thousands of years. These domestic companions have been significantly depleted in our inexorable push for cleanliness. The reduced numbers of "old friends" is likely associated with defects in immunoregulatory pathways that may well explain the remarkable increase in immunological disorders in our over-hygienic communities. Simply stated, our immune systems are being deprived of the "information" it requires to mature and protect us.[17]

Education of the immune system appears to require not only exposure to microbes, but, the right combination of them. It may be that the absence or changes in beneficial intestinal microbiota that contribute to development of the immune system may be operative in suburban and city-living children that explains the induction of inflammatory responses and autoimmune diseases in these children, compared to those living near and/or animals that contribute to their store of commensal microbes. Yes, dirt is good: a little soiling can go a long way for children's health, and subsequent protection against immune irregularities into their adult years.

What is it about dirt that is protective, and so fascinating for researchers studying the ever-increasing numbers of childhood allergy and asthma? Of course dirt, in our hyper-clean society is a two-edged sword for companies selling all manner of soaps, liquids and powders to sanitize us, and everything around us. Allowing kids to be a little soiled, dirty, smacks of fewer sales on one hand, and the need for a stronger marketing pitch on the other. They want us clean, no matter the cost to our health. Just how clean do we need our lives to be?

One afternoon, while in Moscow attending an International Microbiology Congress, a friend and I wandered about the city. We were getting thirsty, but there was no place to slake our thirst, until we came upon a vendor, an elderly woman purveying a brownish liquid she was dispensing from a huge glass jug that looked as if it hadn't been introduced to soap and water since the Flood. Nonetheless, Muscovites were quickly lining up waiting their turn. We joined them. As we waited, the woman filled the glass, the only glass that also appeared not to have experienced soap in its lifetime, with Kvass; a homemade, nonalcoholic brew of fermented stale rye or pumpernickel bread, which they've been drinking for centuries. She handed the glass to the next in line, received a few kopeks, waited until it was drained, refilled it, then handed it to the next unquestioning soul. No washing, no wiping, well, only on her long, unlaundered, stained coat sleeve. We were next. We looked at each other, rolled our eyes, handed over the money, downed the thirst quenching Kvass, and hung around to watch the grubby glass make its communal rounds, mouth to sleeve, to mouth.

Over the next few days we made sure we were within

hailing distance of local chamber pots. However, our Moscow sojourn proved gastronomically uneventful. Could it be that exchanging "germs" with other folks provides our immune system with experiences enabling them to protect us? Or, did we bring to Moscow a well functioning immune system that would protect us no matter what? Or, was it a bit of both?

Which brings us to George. Costanza did it! George dipped twice! Sank his chip into a dip, took a bite and dipped again! Caught in the act, he was verbally flayed for so heinous a transgression. Was it? All that has gone before about our microbiota and our dazzling immune system suggests that if George was not coughing and sneezing over the dip, releasing virulent virus particles, as he dipped, there is little to be concerned about. Most of the germs in the air, on our hands, in our mouths, on our chips, are friendlies, and help mature our immune systems by adding to their experiencing different microbial populations. So, keep on dipping, hurrah for Seinfeld, and have a Kvass the next time your in Moscow. And you may want to think about those vendors, those food mobiles in many of our major cities, and especially around many of our universities. Do they help or hinder?

Dr. Graham W.W. Rooks, Emeritus Professor of Medical Microbiology, University College, London, stated it squarely. "The bottom line," he said, "is organisms that were present in mud, untreated water, and feces were with us from the start. What has happened over the course of evolution, because these bugs had to be tolerated, they came to activate the tolerance of the immune system." and he added, "they are the police force that keeps the immune system from becoming trigger-happy. Basically, the immune system is now attacking things it shouldn't be attacking." He's telling us we've left dirt behind, and need to get it back to avoid those mounting hypersensitivities.[18]

We have also learned that bacteria on our skin play an important role in combating inflammation when injury to the skin occurs. Staphylococci on our skin works by dampening down overactive immune responses, which can lead to rashes, or cause cuts and bruises to become swollen and painful.

A recent published study found that *Mycobacterium vaccae*, a bacterium naturally present in soil, can accelerate learning and brighten moods by stimulating neuron growth and raising serotonin levels. Prof. Dorothy Matthews who led the research, noted that, "we found that mice that were fed live Mycobacterium vaccae navigated the maze twice as fast and with less demonstrated anxiety behaviors as control mice."[19]

Mycobacterium vaccae are being used in other studies as a possible treatment for depression. Lung cancer patients injected with killed M.vaccae reported better quality of life and less nausea and pain. The reason may be that this bacterium activates the same set of neurons in the brain as Prozac, which buoys moods.

Gnotobiosis

In-utero we fetal embryos are microbe-free, but as we descend through our mother's birth canal, we pick up our first collection of microbes; beneficial microbes. However, and nevertheless, from that initial contact we've been subjected to frequent and on-going cleansing: keeping microbes at arms length. Sanitize, wash, wash, sanitize, has been the steady mantra. That, it turns out, has been a two-edged sword, with consequences that have come back to bite us.

We have become a germaphobic people; abetted by the communications media-newspapers, magazines, radio and TV, all purveying antisepsis, beauty, and odor-free lives, paid for by the soap and detergent giants. Consequently, we've been short-circuiting our immune systems, preventing them from distinguishing friendly proteins, from foreign, unwanted invaders. Interestingly, supporting evidence for this comes from two significant sources: caesarian births, and gnotobiotic, germ-free animal studies.

In Caesarian births, infants arrive without having contacted a diversity of microbes along their mother's birth canal, and are immediately thrust into contact with physicians, nurses, surrounding medical devices and physical environment which provides them with a clashing cluster of foreign microbes that do not work in tandem with the specialized cells of our dazzling immune system. As is now well documented, germ-free mice suffer a similar set of hypersensitivities that are seen in allergic children and adults. Moreover, when germ-free animals are exposed to friendly microbes, they thrive.

Curiously enough, our common load of childhood viral diseases, measles, mumps, rubella, chickenpox, herpes simplex, and cytomegaloviruses, do not protect against allergic disorders. Why not? The consensus view appears to be that these half-dozen viral conditions only emerged after the ice age, 12 thousand or so years ago, as animals were being domesticated, and we picked up these viruses from them. In geologic time, that is not long enough for us, and the viruses, to have co-evolved. Not having co-evolved long enough together, means that our immune systems are not in sync, not working together with these common viruses that could otherwise be harmless. Ergo, the fundamental question that now jumps up is, why are microbes essential for the appropriate functioning of our immune systems?

The lack of protection against the childhood viral diseases is seen regularly among kids in nursery schools and day-care centers even as they wash more often. It is also evident that exposure to bacterial infectious diseases transmitted via the fecal/oral route does provide protection. Apparently there is an increasing failure of immunoregulatory mechanisms that would have reduced or prevented various inflammatory responses while allowing the normal and essential responses to function.

Clearly, immunoregulation has been shown to be faulty in both children and adults suffering allergic, autoimmune illnesses as well as inflammatory bowel disease. The hygiene hypothesis indicates that a number of co-evolving organisms such as the Lactobacilli, Mycobacteria, and Bifidobacteria were needed to be tolerated by our immune systems because they were harmless, but ever present in large numbers. Rather than cause harm, these organisms help mature our immune systems by driving dendritic cells to produce more protective T-reg cells which leads to reduced inflammatory responses.

The hunter/gatherer way of life, which lasted for ten to twelve thousand plus years, shaped us, and appears antithetical to our modern environment that precludes frequent and continuing contact with a wide diversity of harmless microbes–that we've been vigorously executing. This exclusionary way of our current lives has been coming back to bite us via dysfunctional immune systems that sorely miss, and long for, their old familiar friends. Susceptibility to chronic, hypersensitive disorders has been a nasty consequence.

To demonstrate this, using mammalian animal models, Dr. Richard S. Blumberg's team of researchers at Harvard Medical School, studied the autoimmune diseases asthma and colitis.

Their germ-free-gnotobiotic-mice live in sterile cages and eat sterile food. Microbes are unknown to them. Consequently, their bodies, especially their gut harbor nothing like that of normal microbe-loaded animals. Accordingly they are highly susceptible to colitis, intestinal inflammation and asthma.

When, in Blumberg's studies, newly born mice are exposed to microbes, there were significant decreases in the number of inflammatory immune cells in their lungs and colon, compared to mice unexposed to microbes. The exposed mice had decreased susceptibility to asthma and, inflammatory bowel disease, as they grew older.

Undeniably, appropriate immune conditioning by microbes early in life is essential to avoid allergic and autoimmune disease in later life. What was going on here? The researchers found that at the cellular level, normal mice had far lower levels of killer T cells (NKT's) in their blood stream compared to the germ-free animals. This suggested that the high NKT numbers are at the core of their high susceptibility, and that the presence of bacteria in the normal mice, block the production of NKT cells in young animals. These natural killer cells trigger inflammation after sensing foreign protein-microbial antigens.

Continuing on this path, the researchers placed germ-free mice in among normal, healthy mice, in cages teeming with microbes. Although germ-free no longer, these transferred animals still had a large number of NKT cells in their guts. That was yet another piece of terrific information. To their credit, the team took the next step: placing pregnant, germ-free females in among healthy mice which would ensure their off-spring, their pups, would contact a diversity of microbes immediately on birth. The pups blood samples revealed far fewer NKT cells in their intestines, which prevailed as they aged.[20] The conclusion was evident: NKT cells can sense the collection and diversity of microbes in the neighborhood and respond to it, and the presence of microbes is essential for a balanced immune system. A splendid piece of work. Here then, is firm data from an animal model, supporting human studies. Lovely.

Obviously we need to mix-up, tangle with microbes when we are young; very young. Think dirt. Dirt is good. Dirt means microbes, and microbes are necessary and beneficial for our health.

Gnotobiosis Continued

Studies done at both the Universities of Michigan and Pennsylvania found that we are hard-wired to live in the natural world. For tens of thousands of years our ancestors lived, worked, and played in natural settings exposed to myriad microbes. For the past 50 years we've been joined at the hip to our TV's, computers and smart phones. We've become indoor bound, house bound and solitary. The evidence fairly jumps up at us. We've been short circuiting our immune systems by preventing them from contacting the "friendlies" and "necessaries" early on by being closed away and far too clean.[21, 22]

The studies that follow reveal and exemplify the tight relationship between our immune system and our microbiota.

Over the past several years a new development has come upon the immunological/microbiological scene. Consider that medical researchers at the University of British Columbia, Vancouver, indicate that it is now well known that specific types of microbes in our gut, our large bowel, organisms never before known, and as yet unnamed, directly affect mucosal immunity. They found that segmented, filamentous bacteria, SFB's, long, hair-like organisms, newly discovered in the small intestine, promote the arrival and functioning of T-helper cells, which send chemical signals telling the gut's epithelial cells lining the small intestine, to increase output of molecules that kill-off selected invaders. Additionally, they also note that Clostridium species can promote regulatory T-cell (T-reg) development (normally originating in the thymus gland) that play a major role in inhibiting inflammation.[23]

Furthermore, rapid progress in this area has demonstrated that the gut microbiota play an essential role in immune functions generally. That our gut microbes can no longer be ignored was highlighted by yet another study showing that placing mouse pups with genetically different mothers established a microbial gut flora in the pups resembling the foster mother's rather than the birth mothers, and which was linked to changes in disease susceptibility.

Profs. Yun Kyung Lee, and Sarkis K. Mazmanian, of the California Institute of Technology's Department of

Biology, find that it is from germ-free animals that we derive salient insights about how our microbes affect our immune system. They maintain that germ-free mice have fewer and smaller Peyer's Patches, and smaller and less cellular mesenteric lymph nodes. Besides these deficiencies in tissue function, the intestinal cells lining the gut of these mice have fewer Toll-like receptors which are needed to sense the presence of pathogens. T-cells are also greatly reduced, and their cytotoxicity is extremely weak. Clearly, for the development of appropriately functioning intestinal immune cells, a large and mixed population of microbes is essential. But that's not the end of it. The absence of a formidable microbiota leads to reduced systemic antibody levels, which suggests that our microbes shape systemic immunity.

Of course, germ-free animals are highly susceptible to infectious agents just as cancer and HIV/AIDS patients are. Consequently, the need for a balanced microbiota is necessary for a fully functioning immune system: a healthy environment for our host of beneficial commensals. Hopefully, they are correct in believing that "harnessing the immunomodulatory capabilities of the microbiota may offer novel avenues for the development of antimicrobial therapies for infectious disease."[24]

And from down-under, the Australian researchers, Kendle M. Maslowski, and Charles R. Mackay, inform us that "it has been clearly demonstrated that diet has a considerable effect on the composition of the gut microbiota, and that the composition and products of the gut microbiota have unexpected effects on immune and inflammatory responses. These, they tell us, are increasingly likely explanations for the increases in inflammatory diseases such as Asthma, and Type 1 diabetes, in developed countries. For them it is evident that the gut microbiota "can be considered an extension of the self," and along with an individuals genetic make up, determines an individuals physiological functioning. They go on to note that there are striking differences between children from rural Africa and those from urban Europe in the composition of their gut microbiota.[25]

As noted earlier, this has intimations of the differences found in farm and rural children, compared to city-born children in Germany, Austria, and Switzerland and western Europe generally. Children from Burkino Faso, on a high fiber diet have an elevated proportion of Bacteroides bacteria-B.fragilis, and B. succinogenes, and low levels of Firmicutes, such as bacilli, and clostridia;just the reverse of their European cohorts. Indeed, the Burkino Faso children had gut microbes containing two genera, Prevotella and Xylanibacter, completely lacking in the gut of European children. These organisms have the enzymes necessary for the digestion of cellulose and Xylan. We western world humans rely completely on our collection of bowel microbes to digest these otherwise indigestible plant polysaccharides. Something to consider the next time you munch around, raw broccoli and cauliflower.

The fermentation of fiber in our gut produces large amounts of small chain fatty acids such as acetate, propionate and butyrate, which these Australian scientists report, are critically important for immunoregulation. Here we appear to get down to the nitty gritty of the role of microbes in affecting immune balance. Apparently European children on westernized diets have far lower levels of the small chain fatty acids, and interestingly, allergies and asthma are all but non-existent in many rural African communities.[26] More than coincidence seems to be at work. Our diets and our microbes may just turn out to be the moderators of our immune systems. However, that remains to be resolved.

Coming at it from yet another angle, Dr. Veena Taneja, a Mayo Clinic Immunologist, lead a team that found that bacterial changes in the gut microbiota may well trigger disease leading to the destruction of joints: elbows, knees, hips.

Dr. Taneja's team developed a new mouse type: transgenic, humanized mice. Indeed, these are mice that received a set of human genes and lost a set of classical murine genes: one group of their mice now have a gene for resistance to rheumatoid arthritis-RA-while another group have a human gene for susceptibility to RA. Cool! A very cool piece of work.

When the now susceptible mice received a RA inducing chemical, they responded astonishingly; revealing a sexual bias-a ratio of three females to one male with RA, as well as an antibody response similar to humans!

These researchers also found that in these humanized mice, that genetic factors along with disruption of the gut microbiota, appears to have influenced susceptibility and/or resistance to developing arthritis. Moreover, their humanized RA resistant mice had gut organisms consistent with the fecal microbiomes of healthy humans! A remarkable observation and a dandy piece of research.

Dr. Taneja now has a splendid "tool" to "understand the role of gut microbes in the pathogenesis of rheumatoid arthritis. We have shown, she also reported, "that mice with the human RA-susceptible gene harbor altered patterns of gut microbiome characterized by an abundance and/or lack of specific commensals as compared to mice with the RA resistant gene whose gut microbiomes are shaped by age and sex." In addition, the RA susceptible mice also had reduced T-helper cells.[27]

To the question, does the immune system dictate the aggregation of an individuals microbes, or is it the other way around–the microbiota supplying marching orders to the immune system, remains the fundamental and open question, remaining to be deciphered. With the Tajeda study, the way is now fairly well marked for a run up to an answer.

The arthritis-microbiome relationship was a concern of Dr. Dan R. Littman and his team of researchers at New York University's School of Medicine. They collected stool samples from people with arthritis.

Sequencing of gut bacteria in those samples found that individuals with recently diagnosed arthritis were more likely to have Prevotella copri bacteria than people free of arthritis. Large numbers of Prevotella copri were associated with low levels of beneficial microbes that normally suppress inflammatory responses. When inoculated with Prevotella, mice become more sensitive to colitis, and their levels of beneficial gut microbes drop. Dr. Littman's research outcome is the first to demonstrate a correlation of disease onset with a specific microbial species.[28]

However, it is also clear that the relationship between our microbes and our immune system is both crucial and dynamically tied to health and illness, no matter which is responsible for hitting the reset button.

It is also becoming clear, or clearer, that regulation of immune responses by the microbiota opens up an entirely new approach to understanding and treatment of human inflammatory diseases, which must surely be seen as progress, as the diverse studies noted here, all point in the same direction: microbes and the immune system must function smoothly together to maintain our optimum health.

Finally, these new and manifold investigations have raised the provocative question, "have societal advances paradoxically and adversely affected human health by reducing our exposure to health-promoting bacteria?"

Truth to tell, this is not a totally new question, although it sounds as though it were. It does harken back to David Strachan's Hygiene Hypothesis, grounded on the idea that we, and our commensal microbes, co-evolved over eons of time, and that these organisms kept our immune system running smoothly. But it lacked the current and detailed particulars inherent in our immune system.

The current wave of immunological studies have demonstrated a powerful relationship between our symbiont microbes, those beneficial ones, and their intimate performance with the great diversity of immune system cells. The evidence emanating from both animal model and human studies shows that deficiencies in Treg cells underlie asthma, IBD, RA, type1 diabetes, multiple sclerosis, and others, and that Treg cells may just prevent, and in some cases treat these disorders in laboratory animals.[25]

Without pushing this envelope too far, it is well within the realm of possibility that we're on the cusp of a major breakthrough that could finally bring relief to millions of sufferers of autoimmune diseases.

What elevates this belief? Solid evidence. If our microbiota calls the immune systems tune, loss of early and normal development of our collection of microbes, via caesarean section births, (C-sections) heightened hygienic practices, formula-based infant diets, vaccinations, and the overwhelming use of antibiotics in early infancy, appear culpable. The absence of beneficial microbes promoting the early maturation of our immune cells, seems to lead directly to immune-related illnesses. These new immunological studies may just have provided the bedrock upon which the Hygiene Hypothesis now firmly rests: that early and frequent contact with dirt, contact with animals and other children, provides the mix of microbes that prevents autoimmune illness.

That it takes two to Tango is a fitting postscript to the story of our dazzling immune system with its internal defense forces. Together we are surely a supraorganism capable of optimum health.

Vaccination

"Immunity to pathogens relies on the ability of the immune system to "remember" past infections. This property (Is) known as immunological memory...and the success of vaccination

regimens depends on it. – Charles R.Mackay & Ulrich H. von
Andrian, 2001

We turn now to our immune system before it was recognized as our invisible defense force, as the backstory holds the drama that led to one of the greatest, if not the greatest medical advances of the 20th century.

Our ability to ward off infection is referred to as, resistance, while its opposite, vulnerability, is susceptibility. Both deal directly with immunity: the ability to repel a potential pathogenic organism. And, as frequently noted, our immune system has the sublime quality of memory. That dear reader is the secret, the blueprint of our preservation.

At this point, we recall Ludwig Panum and his singular observations on the Faroe Islands. From another direction, Lady Mary Whortley Montague, a glamourous aristocrat, a woman of independent mind, an acclaimed beauty and scholar, was the wife of Edward Wortley Montague, the British Ambassador to Turkey.

In 1716, she left London to be with him in Constantinople, today's Istanbul. While there, she saw how women protected themselves from Smallpox. The more venturesome among them, gathered for Smallpox parties, where an elderly woman swiftly and skillfully opened a vein and inserted a fine needle containing a drop of fluid obtained from a fresh Smallpox pustule. A mild case of Smallpox occurred on the eighth day. Immunity to Smallpox was their's evermore.

For Lady Montague, it was evident that her children had to be inoculated. She had it done "to her dear little son Edward," and while in London in 1721, had her daughter Mary inoculated. [29]

On her return to London in 1718, she tried to educate the public and the physicians about the procedure and its benefits. All rejected her entreaties. For the physicians, this inoculation was too simple and would be a money-losing proposition.

By the way, Lady Mary had contracted Smallpox in 1715, just before going off to Turkey. It left her without eyelashes and deeply pitted skin. A beauty no more. Furthermore, the pus-filled scabs could bend noses, as it smelled like rotting fish.

Toward the latter part of the 16th century Queen Elizabeth was hit with smallpox. One of the ladies of her inner circle, Mary Sydney, nursed her through the illness, but was her self a victim, ending up hideously scarred. According to her husband Sir Henry Sydney, she was "as foul a lady as smallpox could make her."[30]

The year was 1777, and George Washington, Commander of the Continental Army, was in possession of a report indicating that the British planned to infect his troops with Smallpox. Taking a bold step at Morristown and later at Valley Forge, against what was widely decried as ungodly, he had his troops variolated-blowing dried Smallpox scabs into their noses to produce a mild illness, followed by life-long immunity, thereby thwarting deliberate dissemination of the disease by the British. Thereafter, recruits were variolated before joining a militia going into battle.

Edward Jenner was yet to be heard from. While speaking to Sarah Nelms, a young milkmaid, Sarah said to Jenner, a young apprentice to a country doctor at the time, "I cannot take the Smallpox sir, as I have had the Cowpox." Cowpox infected the teats of cows and the hands of milkers, usually young girls, producing sores and fever that was rapidly transient with subsequent immunity to Smallpox.

Edward Jenner became a physician in Berkeley, a small town 15 miles north of Bristol in the southwest of England. In May 1796, well after the revolutionary war, Jenner scarified (a slight incision on the skin surface), vaccinated, his gardener's eight-year-old son James Phipps, with Cowpox fluid from a pustule he obtained from the hand of Sarah Nelms. Young James contracted Cowpox, but recovered in six days. Weeks later, allowing time for the boy's body to build immunity, Jenner made several punctures on James's arm, inserting freshly obtained Smallpox fluid into the punctures: a fierce challenge, but young James remained disease-free. Today, that type of experiment would be totally unacceptable, unethical and immoral. Over the next year, Jenner vaccinated another 23 people with similar success. Good thing for all of us that he did this. The results of his work were published in 1798 with the ponderous title, "An inquiry into the causes and effects of the variolea vaccinea (smallpox of the cow) a disease in some of the western counties of England particularly Gloucestershire and known by the name cowpox." A title and a half, by any stretch. Still, the medical community would have none of it: not until another experiment with cowpox and smallpox in London proved him right.[31]

Jenner derived the term vaccination from the Latin Vacca, for cow. Makes sense. His vaccination procedure must rank as one of the most important medical advances of all time. In his day, it was estimated that as many as ten percent of the European population died of Smallpox annually. Those that survived suffered permanent facial pocking, a la′Lady Montague, the size of dimes, along with scarring and blindness. Finally, in 1830, Jenner was awarded £30,000 by Parliament, a tidy sum in current dollars, which he definitely deserved. Surely most would agree it was an unnecessarily long time in coming. Furthermore, Jenner's vaccine led, two hundred years later, to the eradication of smallpox from planet earth.

In 1930's America, there were over 43 thousand cases a year. Until its eradication in 1977, several million Smallpox deaths occurred yearly around the world. Little wonder then that Smallpox is currently on most lists of the top bioterror agents, even though the virus only exits in two secure laboratories: at the CDC in Atlanta, Georgia, and in Russia, at the State Research Center of Virology and Biotechnology, in Koltsovo, Novosibirsk, some 900 miles southeast of Moscow. Koltsovo, has the designation, Naukograd, or science town, and was named for the Russian scientist, Nicolai Koltsovo. Of course, the idea that the virus exits only in these two Centers presupposes that all remaining virus stocks were either turned in or destroyed. We'll pick up on that supposition in Chapter FOUR.

Fowl Cholera and Rabies

Fast forward to Paris, circa 1879, as we join Prof. Louis Pasteur, and his crucial experiments on Fowl Cholera.

Returning from a summer vacation away from his lab where he had left a flask of live Cholera organisms, he injected these "old" organisms into freshly purchased chickens. To his everlasting surprise, these chickens remained unaffected. This had to be some strange aberration. How could chickens survive a dose of cholera bacteria? From a local Cholera outbreak, he obtained fresh Cholera organisms, grew them up in his lab and injected them into another batch of newly purchased chickens. They became ill and quickly died. He was shrewd enough to inject this new batch of Cholera organisms into a number of chickens that had remained cholera-free. Not one became ill. Pasteur was shocked. Astonished! After a moment of silence, he exclaimed, to his assistants, "Don't you see, these animals have been vaccinated." He had recalled Jenner's work on Cowpox. Jenner had so modified the human immune system (not yet known) that it was no longer receptive to the Smallpox virus. And here, Pasteur's "old" Cholera culture had become "attenuated," and had affected some transformation in the chickens system making them unresponsive to the normally lethal Cholera bacteria. Here was the dawn of a universal principle: vaccination could be a means for specifically enhancing resistance to a potentially harmful germ. Pasteur believed this resistance should be called vaccination.

Clearly, both we humans and animals are "tagged" for life by contact with microbes, whether directly or indirectly: frank illness or vaccination. A new science of immunization was born. But wait: Pasteur was about to shift uncertainty to certainty.

Rabies in Europe, and post-civil war America was terrorizing. It had to be confronted and stopped.

In his early work with rabies Pasteur demonstrated that the spinal cord of rabbits dead of the disease could become attenuated, non-virulent, by keeping the cords in sterile, dry air for several weeks. Then, by inoculating dogs with increasing doses of these attenuated cords, the dogs remained immune to highly virulent rabies tissue extracts: the virus was not yet known.

The decision to try his rabies vaccine on people was problematic, but was forced on him when young Joseph Meister was brought to his Paris laboratory from Alsace. Young Meister had been badly bitten on his arms, legs and thighs. Pasteur conferred with physicians who were certain the boy would die of his wounds.

At 8:00 PM on July 6, 1885, Joseph received his first injection; the first rabies injection any human had ever received. Over the following eleven days he received eleven additional injections with an attenuated rabbit spinal cord solution. Each injection contained a stronger dose. Joseph not only survived, but remained healthy. In his 20's he became gatekeeper at the Paris Institute, and at age 64, in 1940, we are told, he committed suicide rather than divulge the location of Pasteur's burial crypt to German soldiers occupying Paris. This notion of his death does not appear to pass muster. Rather, the more realistic account indicates he was depressed, overwhelmed by guilt, having sent his family out of Paris ahead of the on-rushing German army, and believing they had killed his family. In tragic irony, his family returned to Paris on the day he committed suicide by placing his head in a stove.[32]

On your next trip to Paris, wander over to the Institute to see the statue of Joseph trying to fend off a rabid dog.

By 1886, some 2,500 people had received the Rabies vaccine, which established this practice worldwide. Pasteur had demonstrated conclusively that a solid immunity was certainly possible.

Von Behring and Antiserum

In the late 1880's researchers at the Pasteur Institute found that microbe-free Diphtheria solutions when injected into test animals produced all the symptoms of Diphtheria. They called this liquid toxin. Following this, in 1890, Emil von Behring, a German physician found that graduated doses of heat sterilized broth cultures of Diphtheria or Tetanus bacilli injected into test animals caused the animals to produce a chemical substance in their blood that protected them from acquiring Diphtheria or Tetanus, when the animals were challenged with virulent Diphtheria or pathogenic Clostridial organisms. Von Behring called this newly formed protective chemical, antitoxin. As if that wasn't good enough, he went on to show that this antitoxin could be injected into other animals, protecting them as well. They too, had become immune: indirectly; passively.

Furthermore, when animals with symptoms of Diphtheria were inoculated with this antiserum, they were cured! But that wasn't the end of it. Von Behring found that mixtures of Diphtheria toxin neutralized by Diphtheria antiserum, could be injected in people, producing life-long immunity. He was singularly responsible for developing the means of banishing Diphtheria as a scourge of humankind. Consequently, in 1901, he was awarded the first ever Nobel prize in Physiology or Medicine.[33] His is not a name people remember. And far too many people still avoid vaccines and vaccinations. We'll pick up on that shortly.

Ehrlich and Immunoglobulins

Paul Ehrlich was another highly imaginative German physician/scientist. He is the Ehrlich of "magic bullet", fame. His grand idea was that an ideal therapeutic agent could be created that killed selectively: only the organism targeted. This followed directly from his discovery of Compound 606, Arsphenamine, which effectively destroyed the Spirillium microbe responsible for Syphilis. But that's yet another tale.

At the moment our concern is with his brilliant work on immunity. It had been known that after Smallpox infections, specific immunity was transmitted from parent to offspring. However, Ehrlich rejected the idea of genetic inheritance. After tests with mice, he deduced that a fetus was supplied with what he called antibodies from the mother's circulating blood. In one experiment, he exchanged the offspring of treated and untreated female mice. Those that were nursed by the poison-treated females were protected from the affects of the poison, providing proof that antibodies could be conveyed in breast milk.

Ehrlich then teamed-up with Von Behring in Dr. Robert Koch's newly formed Institute of Infectious Diseases, in Berlin. It was Koch who suggested that the two work together to improve the antiserum for treating Diphtheria. With his strong chemical background, unusual for physicians at the time, Ehrlich was able to rapidly increase its potency, boosting its level of immunity.

Shortly thereafter, Ehrlich developed his famous "side-chain theory." As he saw it, the reaction between toxin and components of a serum, as well as the effect of the toxin itself, was a chemical reaction. He explained the toxic effect using the example of Tetanus toxin. Cell protoplasm, he said, contains special side chains (currently we refer to them as macromolecules, large protein molecules, immunoglobulins) to which the toxin binds, affecting its function. If an animal survives the effect of the toxin, the blocked side-chains are replaced by new ones. This regeneration, he maintained, can be trained: the name for this was immunization.

If there is a surplus of side chains they can be released

into the blood as antibodies. He was in fact telling us that antibodies bind to antigens, tagging them, and that these "tags" trigger the immune response that mobilizes B and T cells that kill off the invaders.

Of course he couldn't know the many details of the immune response at the time, nevertheless he had provided the theoretical basis for immunology for which he was awarded the Nobel prize in Physiology or Medicine in 1908; sharing it with Ilya Metchnikoff, who was awarded it for his discovery of Phagocytes, and Phagocytosis, those microbe devouring cells of the innate immune system. What a fabulous period of creativity and discovery, and not all that long ago.[34]

Poliomyelitis

1955, is a year well worth remembering. Although Dr. Jonas Salk developed the first successful vaccine against that awful affliction, Poliomyelitis, Polio, in 1950, it was in 1955 that he announced to the world that his new vaccine was safe and effective. This not only changed medical history but also medical practice by preventing thousands of otherwise crippling cases.

Salk received his undergraduate education at The City College of New York, and his medical degree at New York University School of Medicine. In 1947 he was asked to take the Directorship of the Virus Research Laboratory, University of Pittsburgh School of Medicine. While working there, he joined forces with the National Foundation for Infantile Paralysis and had an idea for the development of a vaccine that he worked on for eight years.

His genius was to move from the traditional vaccines using living organisms that produced mild infections, to a vaccine that protected but did not cause an infection. As his animal studies showed benefits, he, his wife and children were early volunteers testing his killed vaccine. When their infections proved harmless, a nationwide testing program was begun in 1954. One million children ages 6-9, the "polio Pioneers," were enrolled. Half received his new vaccine; the other half received a placebo. On April 12, 1955, the results were announced. Safe and effective!

For his epoch making accomplishment, Dr. Salk was awarded the Congressional Gold Medal of Honor; the Presidential Medal of Freedom, and the Albert Lasker Award for Clinical Medical Research. Dr. Salk never patented his vaccine, nor did he ever receive a dime from it. He was committed to end the suffering Polio produced.[35]

This vaccine, using killed virus ended the annual threat of Polio epidemics with its toll of paralysis and death. Millions of children received three injections for the three types of Polio viruses. Although booster shots had to be given periodically, Salk's vaccine conferred IgG immunity that prevents the virus from multiplying. Recall that viruses, unlike bacteria and fungi, can only multiply inside human, animal and plant cells, where they take over the cells machinery multiplying ad nauseum.

Dr.Albert Sabin, another gifted physician/researcher, working at Cincinnati's Children's Hospital, took a different approach to Polio prevention. Sabin developed an antipolio vaccine based on an attenuated live virus taken orally in pill form that gave longer lasting immunity.[36]

Nevertheless, both vaccines were used around the world, eliminating Polio from most developed countries. In 1988, the number of new cases worldwide was about 350 thousand. By 2007, it was less than two thousand.

These vaccines blocked person to person contact, thereby protecting the entire community; a grand example of Herd Immunity at work. Currently, the rate of vaccine-associated illness appears to be a single case in 750 thousand vaccine recipients. About as close to zero as any medical procedure can get.

Because Polio is similar to Smallpox in not having an

114

animal reservoir, it should be just as eradicable. Should be, but it won't, unless and until ignorance is vanquished first. WHO, the World Health Organization, informs us in a new report that Polio will be difficult to eradicate in both Pakistan and Afghanistan until the Pashtuns stop rejecting the vaccine. According to WHO, Karachi, Pakistan's largest city, is the only major city in the world where Polio persists. The Pashtuns account for less than fifteen percent of the population, but have 75 per cent of the cases.

In Afghanistan, where the Pashtun hold sway, they refuse to be vaccinated believing that vaccination is a plot to sterilize Muslims. Until prominent religious leaders speak out in favor of Polio vaccination, their people will continue to be disabled by the virus, and the virus will continue to be carried around with great risk to others.

In December 2012, news flashed around the world that nine female Polio workers in Pakistan had been killed. The Polio eradication program is in turmoil and door-to-door vaccination has been suspended. Obviously the number of cases will begin to rise. How bad this will be for other countries remains unclear. Let us hope that history does not repeat. After Nigeria's rejection of Polio vaccinations in 2003, the Polio virus spread to 20 other countries. Unfortunately a copycat killing occurred in Nigeria in February 2013, where gunmen killed another nine Polio workers in Kano, Northern Nigeria. Here too, most of the dead were women, shot in the back of the head. Where this will end is anybody's guess. What is known for certain is that Polio remains endemic in Nigeria, Pakistan and Afghanistan, and will be a threat to others.[37]

March 2013 began with a financial blockbuster. Mayor Michael Bloomberg, of New York, announced that he had joined with the Bill & Melinda Gates Foundation, providing a donation of a hundred million dollars to try to eradicate Polio. His donation will be given to the Global Polio Eradication Initiative which has had a credible track record on narrowing the number of countries with Polio from 125 to three–Nigeria, Pakistan and Afghanistan.

The Mayor is resolute: "The loss of life of those who were trying to give out the vaccine is tragic, but I think it should commit us to making sure that we don't walk away, and we get the job done."

Eradicating Polio is not only difficult because of the opposition of radical Muslim leaders, but the illness spreads unseen as those infected never show symptoms. What other illness is so silent?

Bill Gates, speaking along side Mr. Bloomberg, wants the full $5.5 billion dollars needed for eradication donated this year, rather than keep operating "hand to mouth." If it is obtained, he predicts an end to Polio by 2018. I'm betting on it.[38]

Influenza

Vaccines against Influenza, the Flu, must be re-created yearly as the virus has the uncanny ability to change—mutate—and with its frequent mutations, last year's vaccine is no longer protective. This means a new vaccine must be assembled yearly to protect against the viruses currently circulating.

Three different types of influenza virus are recognized: A, B, and C. Type A infects humans, birds, pigs and horses. Type B, only humans and Type C, infects primarily humans, but at times, animals.

For the virus to cause an infection, it must attach to specific proteins, called receptors, on the surface of cells high in our respiratory tracts, before they can gain entry to these cells.

These flu viruses usually have a rounded shape with a layer of projections on their surfaces. Two types of projections, each made of a different protein readily identify them: the sharp, spiky hemagglutinin, designated HA, some five hundred dot the surface; the other is the mushroom-shaped neuraminidase, NA, some hundred of them are scattered about the virus surface. As we shall see, both the HA and NA projections are antigenic; provoking the immune system.

Along with the three major types of virus, there are numerous subtypes that make defending against the flu a tricky business as the virus has disguises; a constantly changing set of camouflages resembling HA and NA antigens. Nevertheless, the many subtypes are identified by the numbers: H's from 1-16, as H1, H2, H3, and on up, along with the N 's from 1-9. These numbers only designate the order of discovery. The first antigenic type was isolated in 1933 and received the designation H0N1.

Together the H's and N's control the viruses infectivity. Hemagglutinin is the prominent player as it binds to polysaccharide chains on the cell surface, then injects the viral genome into the cell where replication and proliferation begin. Neuraminidase plays a securing function. After the virus leaves an infected cell it ensures that the virus particle doesn't get stuck on the cell surface by clipping off the ends of the polysaccharide chains. A neat trick. For the two, it's as good a one-two punch as ever existed.

Furthermore, H's and N's have no trouble mixing and matching their subtypes constructing new combinations, which is another of their sly ways of beating antiviral agents, and at times coming up with a particularly lethal H and N combination.

It is the H spike that attaches to cells forming the linings of our nose and throat. And it's also the H's that activate B cells to be ready to repulse the invading virus.

Each number represents a major shift in proteins of the viruses makeup. Hence each change requires a new vaccine. That's the riddle and problem, which needs a seasonal solution. So for example, the flu pandemic (that swept around the world) in 1957, was given the notation,

H2N2. In1968, we were attacked by H3N2, coming at us from Hong Kong. The Spanish Flu of 1918-1919, aka "La Grippe" lives in infamy, having taken the lives of as many as 50 million around the world. In contrast to the others that normally deal death blows to the very old and very young, this one hit on teenagers and twenty somethings, and went by the designation H1N1, and is still considered the most devastating epidemic in recorded world history. During those fateful two years, children skipped rope to the rhyme:

I had a little bird

Its name was Enza

I opened the window

and in-flu-enza

Most of those deaths were due to secondary infections, such as Staphylococcal pneumonia. The possibility of that happening today is small as we have medications to effectively combat these infections, and we also can rapidly diagnose respiratory infections.

H5N1 was the bird flu that hit on us in 2004. H9N2 identifies domestic duck flu, and H7N2, is the flu in turkey's and chickens, while H1N2 is the flu endemic in us humans, pigs and most birds. These viruses are a crafty lot. The avian virus H7N9 has never before infected humans, nevertheless, as of April 2013, 108 people in China have been infected, with 22 deaths. This is only an estimate as mild cases usually go unreported as most people don't seek medical care. Although this virus does not yet appear to move readily from person to person, the CDC is warning all state public health departments to be on the lookout for it.

It is this frequent shifting of H and N antigens that continues to produce worldwide pandemics as none of us have antibodies to the new H's and N's appearing each season. The antibodies we built up last season simply dwindle away from one December to the next. Last year's antibodies simply do not produce a lasting memory in our immune systems.

So, how is a vaccine against flu developed each year? This is one of WHO's arresting conundrums. Each April and May they search the world for information about the virus subtypes circulating, and pass this information to pharmaceutical companies certified to produce the millions of doses required for injection in October and November, prior to the viruses arrival in December, January and February.

After injection of the polyvalent vaccine, usually a combination of three of the most dangerous subtypes circulating, the vaccine prompts the immune system to produce antibodies to this new set of H's and N's. Four to six weeks will be needed for our antibodies to attain peak levels.

To the question, can I get the Flu even though I was vaccinated on time? The answer is, yes. No current vaccine can include the many types of Flu circulating in any season. Consequently we can be vaccinated against 3 or 4 of the major types, but contact a fifth, and become ill. And there are those rare individuals whose immune systems are either unresponsive or only partially responsive to the antigens. None of this includes individuals with compromised systems such as those with HIV/AIDS who may be vulnerable to any microbe in the neighborhood.

As children are far more vulnerable than adults, it is the children that need to be vaccinated early on, yearly, for utmost protection of the community, the herd.

Flu viruses spread via infected respiratory droplets that travel only short distances, about a meter, three feet, 36 inches–in circumference around the expelling individual. The insidious problem is that infected individuals start producing and expelling virus by sneezing and coughing, before they start feeling feverish. This means they become stealth spreaders, going about their business, their daily activities, contacting others, possibly infecting many. Cunning is the only word for this virus, and there is no way to protect against that. Furthermore, after the initial infection, we remain infectious for about a week.

This yearly attack and riposte, has many researchers thinking hard about a universal vaccine, one that would be protective against any virus type, no matter the H and N combination that comes along, and remain protective for years. This means saying goodbye and good riddance to yearly Flu shots.

Current research suggests a goal of two flu shots in our pre-teen years, followed by a booster shot as adults. Such a universal vaccine would be a T-cell vaccine as T-cells can attack the protein of any type of virus.

If you're 50 or 60, even 70 years old, you'll live to not only learn about this new vaccine, but obtain it, and become flu-free for the rest of your life. So, hang in there.

Acambis, a British Company, now in Cambridge, Massachusetts, appears to be working seriously on animal studies for eventual development of a human universal flu vaccine. This type of vaccine would be produced constantly as its formulation remains the same over time. No shortages, no wondering if the most appropriate collection of viruses has been assembled. Sure seems worthy of a Nobel or other grand prize.

By the way, all vaccinations, whether made of killed microbes, live, attenuated microbes, or a universal vaccine consisting of a solution aimed at activating T-cells, are examples of artificially acquired active immunity. This is far and away different from artificially acquired passive immunity that injects antibodies directly into our bodies. These preformed antibodies come from animals or humans who have had the illness and are now immune, or in the case of horses, vessels for antibody production. These antibodies are circulating in the serum of these immune animals and humans, and as it's the serum (portion of the blood) that is used, the liquid is referred to as antiserum.

Down the road, several years along, passive immunity will be considered quaint. Nevertheless, and however, vaccines of all types have to be seen as the greatest medical advance of the 20th century, for all the lives saved and illnesses prevented.

Furthermore, it was recently learned that pregnant women who received flu vaccine during the 2009 influenza pandemic lowered their risk of delivering preterm babies. Typically flu vaccine rates among pregnant women bounced between 13 to 18 percent. Because of an aggressive vaccination program against the H1N1 strain, the vaccination rate jumped all the way to 45 percent, where it has stayed over the past three years.

This new study showed that not only was flu vaccine safe for both mother and fetus, but it was also protective. Researchers at the Rollins School of Public Health, Emory University, Atlanta, examined records of 3,327 pregnant women and found that infants born to vaccinated mothers had a 37 percent lower likelihood of being born premature, as well as weighing more at birth than babies born to unvaccinated mothers.

Dr. Saad Omer, the leader of the investigation was quoted as saying "Our thinking is that by preventing flu infection, we are reducing the likelihood of inflammation in pregnant women and therefore having a protective effect against preterm birth." That has got to be motivation to push flu vaccination to even higher rates over the next few years.[39]

Then there is depression. Can depression affect a vaccine's effectiveness? So curious a relationship would seem hardly tenable. Until a team of researchers at the Cousins Center for Psychoneuroimmunology, UCLA, published their remarkable findings in February 2013. They showed that a relationship exists.

Although their study was concerned with depression and effectiveness of the Shingles vaccine, they discovered that depression among their enrollees did lower the vaccines effectiveness. That must have been quite a surprise. They also found that those individuals who took antidepressants had normal responses to the vaccine even when their depression persisted. And those being treated for depression showed a boost in immunity. Why that should occur remains to be solved.

The study's team then speculated that treatment of older people with depression could well increase the effectiveness of the flu vaccine as well.[40]

Given the statistical fact that the elderly are at greater risk of severe illness and/or death from flu than any other age group, it sure seems worthwhile to provide flu vaccine to those elderly with depression.

The deeper we dig, the more gold there seems to be.

Until the new universal flu vaccines come on line, we've got to protect ourselves with what we've got.

We've got Flublok. Flublok, the newest advance in flu vaccines is the brain child of Protein Sciences of Meridan, Connecticut.They've developed a vaccine that is not, repeat, not grown in chicken eggs, which, means egg protein allergy is a thing of the past for those susceptible to egg protein allergy, and have avoided flu vaccines.

Flublok, the world's first recombinant protein-based flu vaccine is a highly purified egg-free vaccine made without the use of a live virus. Only a small piece of the virus needed for immunity is used. In this instance it's the hemagglutinin, H, protein antigen of the viruses surface spike.

Each dose of Flublok contains H proteins that match the three most prominent strains circulating in a given season. Nevertheless, Flublok will need to change its vaccine configuration yearly to match the major strains in circulation. Flublok is currently available, and has been approved by the FDA for adults 18-49 years old. Because of the newness of this vaccine, the FDA is moving slowly on it to be sure it is safe which is why it is currently limited to those ages 18-49.

You have only to check with your local health department to find out where Flublok is being dispensed.[41]

Scamming

Given our countries long and inglorious history of snake oil purveyors, snake oil tonics, potions, elixirs and brews, it was only a matter of time or a crisis, for scammers to market fraudulent flu remedies. When there is a specific health issue in the news, fraudulent products spike. Nothing new there. Obviously you've got to be cautious.

In late January 2013, the FDA and the FTC, the Federal Trade Commission, sent a warning letter to Flu and Cold Defense, of Boca Raton, Florida, for making misleading and unproven claims about its Germ Bullet Nasal Spray, a proprietary blend of eleven organic botanicals, and the company's website claimed that an FDA recognized virology lab had tested the formula and "confirmed that it had potential capability to kill cold and flu viruses."[42]

Of course, Germ Bullet had not been reviewed by the FDA for safety and efficacy, but why bother about such details? Say anything you can get away with on the Internet, where Green Bullet was being sold through such retailers as CVS.com, as well as pharmacies and natural food stores.

The FDA wants us to be on guard, wary of dietary supplements, foods such as herbal teas, and products such as air filters and light therapies that claim to:

• *Boost your immunity naturally without a flu shot.*

• *Be a safe and effective alternative to a flu vaccine.*

• *Prevent you from catching the flu.*

• *Support your body's natural immune defenses to fight the flu.*

Let's be clear about it: the only way to prevent the flu is with an FDA approved vaccine. Stay tuned. The next flu season is only months away.

HIV/AIDS

With the close of the 20th century, and the arrival of the 21st, vaccinations took on new directions, and included diseases never before considered vaccine candidates. For the longest time the therapy was directed at smashing the microbes with powerful drugs:to no avail. Enter vaccines, and we begin with Human Immunodeficiency virus and its illness, Acquired Immunodeficiency Syndrome. HIV/AIDS is not only a disagreeable infection, we'll have more to say about that shortly, but the virus is one of the slyest, perhaps the slyest. Its ability to evade every drug and drug-cocktail sent against it is legendary. Let's have a look.

This virus is different; it attacks and destroys Th-cells, T-helper (lymphocytes) cells that would normally prevent infection. But its onslaught doesn't stop there: it enters B-cells, macrophages and endothelial cells that line blood and brain cells. With this type of penetration, many things happen; all bad. Immunosuppression is bad enough, but entering brain cells can bring with it neuropsychiatric difficulties. But enough of that for the moment.

HIV is a small spherical virus; one of the smallest. About 1/70th the size of a red blood cell: 4 millionths of an inch, which allows it to conveniently hide away. This little guy is surrounded by a membrane of fatty material studded with 72 spiky projections. Internally, it has only nine genes, but, oh my, these nine code for proteins controlling its ability to infect a cell, produce new copies and/or cause disease.

These 72 spikes are formed from glycoproteins: a sugar/protein complex. The sugars of this complex are a long string of monosaccharides, called polysaccharides, oligosaccharides, or glycans. Attached to proteins, they become, glycoproteins, and these glycoproteins act as anchors that HIV particles use to latch onto human cell surface receptors. The spikes stick to our cell receptors that then fuse with our cell membranes. The contents of the HIV particles, its nine genes, are then released into the cell, leaving the envelope behind. Once inside the cell, HIV's genes direct our cells to make copies of itself, millions of copies, which then escape the cell heading straight for our T-lymphocytes, destroying them, causing severe immune deficiency. That, dear reader, is the name of this ugly game.

In response to the flood of antibodies released to attack the virus particles, the antigens, the sly particles, shift the location of its glycoproteins to evade detection. It's a game; move and counter move between us humans and one of the planets smallest things. I say things, because a virus is not living in the sense that bacteria and fungi are. Viruses can only reproduce inside human, animal and plant cells. Outside of these cells they can do nothing. But for reasons beyond belief, they have, well, remarkable abilities.

The game goes on. With the shift of its glycoproteins, new glycoproteins arise that can trip them up, by allowing antibodies to attack that are able to target a broader range of viral particles.

Antibodies made by vaccines have had little effect against HIV. Recently, however, researchers have detected broadly neutralizing antibodies-BNab's-in the blood stream of AIDS patients.

As luck would have it, Dr's Penny L. Moore, and Lynn Morris of South Africa's National Health Laboratory, Capetown, found a chink in HIV 's ever-changing armor; a chink that may offer a way for a preventive vaccine. The vulnerable 'spot' open to antibody attack, occurred because of a shift in position of a glycan protein of an HIV particle infecting several of their patients.

As with all microbes, each type, each genera, has a number of strains or species. HIV has so many that no known antibody can kill-off all of them. That's the conundrum defying and requiring solution if a vaccine is to succeed.

This new discovery in South Africa may just point the way to the possibility of developing mixtures, some of them cocktails, of large doses of a diversity of antibodies to use as therapy for AIDS patients, as well as inducing the immune system to produce antibodies capable of destroying the shifty HIV invaders. This production of antibody mixtures would be tantamount to the inoculation of a polyvalent vaccine.

Drs. Moore and Morris, thoughtful physicians and clever researchers, took the next step to see what had changed in their patients HIV-loaded blood streams. To their surprise they found potent broadly neutralizing antibodies circulating there. They also found that a glycan molecule on the surface of the virus infecting their patients had simply moved positions among the lumpy spikes studding the viral surface. That simple shift, that bit of virus cunning, may just trip up the virus, as it allows those BNab's to grab on to the virus, further alerting the immune system to the presence of an invader. Shortly thereafter, phagocytes appeared at the site, ready to engulf and remove the virus.[43]

This elegant piece of clinical research and discovery will surely imbue immunologists to pursue this fascinating lead. What is needed, of course, is a way to develop a vaccine that triggers production of broadly neutralizing antibodies. When that is accomplished, drugs will be a not-so-fond memory, along with their fierce prices. And recall, many vaccines are forever.

Will a vaccine be forthcoming in the near future? Its far too early to speculate as over the past 30 years the field of HIV studies has been strewn with the corpses of failed attempts to develop a cure. However, there is a new and steadfast determination to produce an appropriate vaccine. The Global HIV Vaccine Enterprise is spearheading the search for a preventive vaccine. This non-profit organization, based in New York City, has new leadership and commitment. Bill Snow, its new Director, will be pushing scientists and fundraisers, and leaning on politicians to make a vaccine a reality, eradicating a deadly affliction.

Hold on a moment. In January 2013, a stunning statistic was published. It appears that HIV patients that smoke lose more years of life to tobacco than to the virus. Danish investigators studying three thousand HIV patients, found that a 35-year-old non-smoking HIV patient, was likely to live to age 78, while smokers were likely to die before age 63. When they compared healthy Danes to HIV smokers, HIV made smoking far more lethal.[44]

The researchers urged physicians caring for HIV patients to get them to quit smoking. Sounds like an admirable suggestion, so that they would be around when a new vaccine comes on line.

Dengue Fever

Then there is Dengue Fever, for which there is no vaccine in sight, although not for lack of trying.

Dengue, aka, Breakbone Fever, is well named as the crippling muscle pains and pains in knees, elbows, and hips can be so severe it feels as if some creature out of Star Wars has latched on to your body, tearing it asunder.

This growing and fearsome malady is transmitted with the bite of those flying hypodermics; two different and menacing mosquitoes: Aedes aegypti (the Egyptian), and Aedes albopictus, the white spotted tiger. These beasts prefer to obtain their blood meals from us humans, the blood they need to grow and produce eggs. We also provide them with the water they need for egg laying and for the eggs to mature into larvae, and on to adult mosquitoes. We do this by not emptying rainwater from bottles, pails, pots, and other containers loitering around our homes. We give them what they need to sicken us.

These mosquitoes transmit any one of the four Dengue Fever viruses. Infection with one does not provide protection against any of the others.

Over 100 million people around the world are infected yearly,with tens of thousands of deaths. Here in the America's the mosquitoes and human cases have been moving north from South America, into Mexico and most recently into Florida with confirmed cases there reported in November 2012.

However, India is the mother of all Dengue infections. WHO physicians conservatively estimate that some 40 million cases and a quarter-of-a-million hospitalizations occur there annually. These are only rough estimates as government officials have turned a blind-eye on Dengue cases, preferring to avoid acknowledging the appalling numbers sweeping across Indian cities, with literally hundreds of millions at risk. Worse, these cases become risk for people in other countries as Indians move to nearby countries, and by train, boat and plane to countries around the world. Additionally, vacationers from Europe and the United States returning from sojourns in India bring the virus with them in their blood streams. Often providing the mosquitoes with a free ride to new and unfamiliar habitats they quickly call home.

Thailand is yet another Dengue hot spot where it is believed that no child reaches adulthood without at least being infected twice. In India, estimates also suggest that no one reaches the age of 20 without having a bout of Dengue.

According to Dr. Joseph M. Vinetz of the University of California, San Diego, "a visitor to India has a reasonable expectation of getting Dengue after a few months. If you stay for longer periods, it's a certainty."[45]

This disabling illness has escaped greater worldwide attention because 75-80 percent of cases cause mild, flu-like symptoms. The remaining 20-25 percent are the recipients of the incredibly nasty symptoms-bleeding gums and nose, unbearable joint and muscle pain; searing pain behind the eyes. Depression and fatigue often linger for month after the acute episodes have faded.

For another number of cases, especially after a second infection in which the immune system fails to respond for a time, it responds shockingly with an overwhelming cascade of killer chemicals that often ends in death of the patient. In its attempt to protect, it kills.

In October 2012, two Dengue outbreaks grabbed headlines. Puerto Rico publicly declared the existence of an epidemic that sickened some five thousand people and claimed six lives.

And on the island of Madeira, some 400 hundred miles west of Morocco, more than 1,300 people had Dengue symptoms severe enough to be hospitalized.

A recent trial of a new, advanced vaccine failed badly. At the moment no one believes a new vaccine will be available for a decade, if then, meanwhile, and unfortunately, many new cases can be expected.

Prevention can best be accomplished by judiciously choosing your vacation venues.

Malaria

Every 30 seconds a child dies of Malaria. That's why a vaccine is urgently needed.

Malaria kills over a million people worldwide every year: most are young kids in sub-Saharan Africa. In 2010, there were 216 million new cases, with an uncertainty range of 147-274 million. Either way, the numbers are staggering.

Following hard on the heels of the disappointing Dengue trials, it was learned in mid-November 2012 of the modest, if not yet another disappointing result: The Malaria Vaccine Phase III Pilot Study, that provided only minimal protection for 6,537 enrolled infants. However, because infants die to the grim tune of about 700 thousand annually, while another million become infected with enduring residual developmental lags, and their communities face devastating economic consequences, researchers want to continue using this inefficient vaccine as it can still save thousands of lives. Well, why not!?

This malaria vaccine, known as RTS,S or Mosquirix, produced by London-based GlaxoSmithKline, and funded by the Bill and Melinda Gates Foundation, that has poured over 200 million dollars into the project, is given in three doses. Infants obtain their first shot at 6-12 weeks, followed by two additional injections one month apart. It appears to be well tolerated.

If a million babies are vaccinated with this so-called inefficient vaccine, about 260 thousand new cases will be prevented: a huge number saved no matter how inefficient.[46]

The data from the most recent RTS,S trial was less than heartening, as the vaccine only lowered the risk of clinical episodes 31 percent among 6-12 week old babies who received their first dose. Consequently there is little hope that the vaccine will be widely available by 2015. Nevertheless, GlaxoSmithKline (GSK) that developed it in partnership with the PATH Malaria Vaccine Initiative (MVI) is committed to continued development. The vaccine appears to provide substantial benefit for older babies, but it is for the younger ones that the public health system is set up to administer the vaccine, which also makes it much less costly. At this point, it may be that the younger babies suffer from a still immature immune system. At this juncture, it is uncertain how much more the Gates Foundation will continue to fund this effort.

The RTS,S vaccine, a vaccine specifically formulated against Plasmodium falciparum, the offending microbe carried and injected by Anopheles mosquitoes, contains a protein normally found on its surface. When this protein is injected it stimulates production of antibodies against P.falciparum. When falciparum is injected by that winged hypodermic, Anopheles, the antibodies are there to attack and kill it. Despite that, these slippery falciparum creatures enter the blood stream, making a bee-line for our livers, where they can hide out undetected for weeks, months and years, making it extremely difficult to get at and eradicate. For reasons not yet clear, children under 5 appear to be the mosquitoes primary and favorite target.

Although there are 30-40 different species of these Anopheles, two, An.gambiae, and An.funestus, are the primary vectors; all mosquitoes control efforts are pointed in their direction.

To our everlasting misfortune, there are some 200 types of Plasmodia, but thankfully only four infect us humans: P.vivax; falciparum;ovale, and malariae. It's the vivax that's most widely distributed, and out of Africa as well. A vaccine against it is in an early developmental stage, but is not expected to be generally available until 2018 at the earliest.

Additionally unfortunate, is the depressing fact that infection with P.falciparum neither confers lasting immunity, nor does it protect against any of the other three. Ergo, developing a vaccine against Malaria is both a frustrating and dicey enterprise. Not to say anything about the formidable difficulty of getting the many African countries to agree to allow vaccines to be tested on their children, as is finding the money to keep studies going to increase vaccine efficiency.

With the horrendous number of new Malaria cases annually, the holy grail would be a vaccine with an efficiency of 90-95 percent, and lasting immunity to either falciparum or vivax, but as with all Grails, we can expect that to continue be elusive. Nevertheless, hope does spring. The good news is that another vaccine is being developed that is considered unconventional, as it is based on using the entire P.falciparum microbe grown in laboratory-raised mosquitoes, and killed by radiation. The idea being that the entire Plasmodium may contain a range of antigenic proteins that can stimulate a variety of antibodies. That too, remains a good way down the road.

HPV-Human Papilloma Virus

A recent addition to the vaccine armamentarium was the Human Papilloma Vaccine-HPV- specifically designed to protect young girls and boys from the repugnant consequences of the most common sexually transmitted virus. These HPV's, and there are 150 related types in this group, of which some 30-plus can readily spread via skin to skin contact during vaginal, oral and anal sexual activity.

Although HPV is widely thought of as being primarily a risk for young girls, young boys do not get a free pass. Most of them do not know they harbor the virus: its silent until warts or cancers appear, and during that silent period, they can easily pass the virus to others.

HPV is so common that it's currently estimated that 75 percent of both women and men will become infected in their lifetime. The highest rates are in men 20-24, and in women 16-19. Sexual intercourse isn't necessary to acquire the virus. Any type of genital contact is all that's required. HPV can also infect the mouth, throat, base of the tongue and tonsils producing clusters of warts-Condyloma acuminata–which usually appear as elevated pimples or papules whose surfaces resemble the irregularity of cauliflower.

Growing in the throat, warts can block airways causing difficulty breathing and coarse voice. Fortunately these warts do not become cancerous. Nevertheless, far too many young girls and boys erroneously believe that anal and oral sexual relations offer a disease-free social activity. Not so. A free lunch is decidedly uncommon. According to the Centers for Disease Control, CDC, 20 million people are currently infected, and 6 million become infected yearly. Most don't know they are infected until warts or cancers show up or are diagnosed.

Twelve-thousand-plus women acquire cervical cancer each year: ninety percent of which are HPV-related. Young men will have penile and anal cancers. Clearly a preventive was, and is, needed. Currently two vaccines have been approved by the FDA, and are readily available.

Gardisil, a product of Merck & Company, provides some 90 percent protection against four of the most common types of HPV--6, 11,16, and 18. Although cervical cancer is the most common cancer, the vaccine also protects against vaginal and vulvar carcinoma.

Cervarix, another anti-HPV vaccine, is produced by GlaxoSmithKline. Gardisil appears to be most effective when all three injections are taken by 11 and 12-year-old girls. It also provides protection against genital warts of both boys and girls.

An important study that may help calm parents apprehensive about a relationship between preventing HPV on the one hand, and increasing sexual activity on the other, was conducted at the Emory Vaccine Center, Emory University. Their researchers using an epidemiologic retrospective cohort study evaluated the sexual activity of 1,398, 11-12 year-old girls over a three-year period: 493 had the Gardisil vaccine; 905 did not. Sexually transmitted infections and pregnancy rates were determined for both groups. An association between use of vaccine and increased sexual activity was not found. "It's protection, not an invitation to risky behavior," exclaimed a New York Times Editorial.[47]

These two vaccines, as with others, jolts the immune system to produce protective antibodies. Protection lasts six to seven years at this time, and both, contain inactivated extracts of the HPV.

Gardisil is a quadravalent vaccine providing protection against HPV 6, 11, 16, and 18. Ceravix is bivalent, providing protection against HPV 16 and 18. Both are injected into muscle of the upper arm in three doses: 1st dose-now; 2nd dose-1-2 months later; 3rd dose-6 months after that.

With vaccines documented and certified to be both safe and effective, and with millions of young, sexually active boys and girls at potential risk, use of either of these two vaccines seems to be a no brainer. Rejection reigns. The most preposterous objection raised by religious and social conservatives against having their young girls vaccinated is exactly the reverse of what physician/scientists at Emory University discovered: that the use of vaccine does not encourage promiscuity by vaccine users. The New York Times had it about right.

According to the CDC, as of 2012, only 35 percent of girls 13 to 17 have had the full course of vaccine; three injections over six months. This is a sure sign that women who get cervical cancer could have avoided it. Not a happy thought.

The cost of a full coarse is in the vicinity of five hundred dollars, which could be a gatekeeper, preventing vaccination. However, under our new health care law, the Affordable Care Act, insurance providers are required to cover the vaccine, which removes the barrier.

Currently, HPV vaccination rates vary significantly by state. So, for example, l'il ole Rhode Island has the highest vaccination rate with fifty-seven percent of adolescent girls vaccinated. Vermont and South Dakota follow closely with 50 percent. On the flip side, Arkansas with 15 percent has the lowest rate. Mississippi, Utah and Kansas are a bit higher, with 20 percent completion rates. Considering that HPV is currently the most common sexually transmitted infection in the country, and given the many states with low vaccination rates, cervical cancer appears certain to be a major clinical problem down the road. Yet another concern is throat cancer. "Over the past three decades throat cancer has soared among heterosexual middle-aged men. Some 70 percent of oropharyngeal cancers are now caused by sexually transmitted viruses, up from 16 percent in the 1980's. The epidemic made headlines in June 2013, when the actor Michael Douglas told a British newspaper that his throat cancer had come from performing oral sex."[48]

A recent study done in Costa Rica, supported by our National Cancer Institute, enrolled 5,840 sexually active women aged 18 to 25, provided 93 percent protection against infection with two types of of HPV that cause most of the cancers. Four years after all had been vaccinated with Ceravix only one of the women who had the Ceravix was infected with HPV 16 or HPV 18. Fifteen of the control enrollees, who had gotten a placebo were infected. We now know that this vaccine not only protects against cervical cancer, but it also protects against throat cancer. Isn't that evidence enough to give vaccination rates a major jolt?

Cocaine...of All Things!

Curiously enough, Psychiatrists are looking to vaccines to curb Cocaine and other stimulant drug addictions.

The idea of using the body's immune system to combat addictive drugs compelled Dr. Thomas Kosten of Baylor University's College of Medicine, to combine a harmless component of the bacterium Vibrio cholerae with Cocaine molecules to induce the production of antibodies to the bacterial protein that includes Cocaine.

Injecting his hybrid antigen into a number of his patients, several developed a strong immune response: having a thirty percent greater Cocaine drug-free test, than his patients who either generated a weak response, or had received a placebo. Indeed, the body does treat the hybrid drugs as foreign antigens, producing antibodies that bind to them.

The Cocaine that a patient normally ingested would

have rapidly crossed into his/her brain as a huge dose would now arrive slowly, if at all. Ergo, no more high! No rush! No joy!

The idea behind the vaccine, is more than likely, just what you're thinking: when Cocaine addicts no longer get their high's, they'll stop using Cocaine or other stimulants. That's the general idea, but this has a long way to go, as most of his patients had weak immune responses, and the immunity was brief, requiring a series of booster shots.[49]

A brief digression seems called for at this point. As we've seen, most vaccines provide the immune system with specific microbe-derived molecules to help it later recognize and attack the same intruder. However, some molecules, influenza is a good example, are not capable of provoking strong immune responses. Non-microbial chemicals can be another.

To get around this, adjuvants, chemicals that prompt the immune system to greater activity and protection, have been used. The most common have been aluminum salts, such as aluminum hydroxide and aluminum phosphate. Although these salts rouse certain types of cells, they haven't been able to buck up T-cells.

Currently, researchers are turning to bacteria to prod immune cells to stronger responses, and interestingly enough, the stimulant is not a protein but a lipopolysaccharide obtained from gram-negative bacteria such as our old reliable standby, E. coli, that obtains strong immune responses without toxic side effects.

This may just be the first step to designer adjuvants-curing a specific condition with a lipopolysaccharide adjuvant bound to a vaccine. Researchers at the University of Texas at Austin can be applauded for this work, should it prove itself in further tests. Of course I'm thinking this may be an answer for the Cocaine problem.

Then there is Dr. S.Michael Owens, of the University of Arkansas for Medical Sciences, who prefers not to depend on the uncertainties of responses of a patients immune system. He has synthesized antibodies to Methamphetamine that can be infused into addicted individuals: a classic and provocative example of artificially acquired active immunity. A vaccination by any other name, and why not? Dr. Owens maintains that he can give enough antibody faster, and at the appropriate dose. Here as well, the immune response, as to be expected, fades over time.[50]

Nevertheless, and be that as it may, Dr. Shanker Vallabhajosuela, of Cornell University's Weil Medical School, New York City, believes he can increase the length of the immune response using a virus to deliver genetic material that reprograms liver cells to consistently produce antibodies to stimulant drugs. His belief was demonstrated via brain scans showing that a gene-therapy vaccine blocked Cocaine from entering the brain of monkeys as long as four months after injection. A trial in human addicts is planned.[51]

One thing is certain; there is no lack of creativity around the country, and initial results indicate that a suitable vaccine is not only possible, but will be forthcoming.

As my mother of blessed memory often said, if you can conceive of it, you can create it. She must be smiling up there.

As 2012 was passing into 2013, new research on miss-folded proteins-prions-suggested new ways to treat Alzheimer's, Parkinson's and Lou Gehrig's disease, Amyotrophic Lateral Sclerosis, ALA. Actually, dozens of diseases are now linked to deformed proteins including Cataracts, a type of Emphysema, and Type 2 Diabetes.

Proteins are produced as strings of amino acids that cannot perform their specific functions until those strings become folded. Each of our thousands of proteins has a distinctive three-dimensional fold, or fingerprint, which informs its ultimate function. Curiously enough, a miss-folded, or unfolded protein can cause appropriately folded proteins to unfold or miss-fold leading to brain and other abnormalities.

Deformed proteins can be made right, but new research suggests the real possibility of preventing a miss-folded protein from triggering a domino effect —all falling down. If this domino effect could be prevented, the various miss-folded protein diseases could be prevented: a tremendous possibility and advance.

One possible pathway to prevention is being funded by the Michael J.Fox Foundation for Parkinson's research. This pathway is a vaccine developed by Affiris, AG., an Austrian firm, whose vaccine would induce the immune system to produce antibodies that bind to the toxic Synuclein protein and remove it from circulation. That's a wait and see, and more power to them for a first rate idea.[52]

At the University of Pennsylvania's School of Medicine, an antibody therapy is being tested on animals to see if it would arrest the spread of the toxic alpha-Synuclein. If it succeeds, human trials would be the welcome next phase. Antibody therapy appears to be gaining traction for a number of diseases here-to-fore considered refractory to medical intervention, which leads us directly to young Emma Whitehead.

And so it came to pass that young Emma Whitehead became a prototype and a winner.

In spring, 2011, Emma then 6, was near death from Acute Lymphoblastic Leukemia, and her physicians had run out of options. Desperate to save her, her parents rushed her to Children's Hospital of Philadelphia where she received an experimental therapy never before tried on a child.

Researchers at Children's Hospital used a disabled Human immunodeficiency virus to reprogram Emma's immune system. Essentially, the procedure removes millions of her T-cells for insertion of genes that enable her T-cells to kill cancer cells. The new genes inserted into the T-cells by the disabled virus, direct T-cells to attack B-cells that had become malignant.

The altered T-cells, now referred to as, Chimeric Antigen Receptor Cells, were then placed back in her vein. As all went well, as planned, and expected to do, the new, overhauled T-cells began multiplying and destroying her cancer cells, without harming her healthy cells.

As of the end of January 2013, Emma now 7, is cancer-free! The first child, and one of the first humans whose immune systems can battle and beat cancer, thanks to the treatment devised by Dr. Carl June, leader of the team at Penn.[53]

In addition to Emma, three adults with chronic leukemia received this unprecedented therapy, and they too have remained disease-free. Two of them have been cancer-free for two years. In two other adults, the treatment did not work as well: apparently the numbers of T-cells were insufficient in one of them, while the others B-cell's lacked the needed surface CD-19 surface proteins. Insufficient T-cells can be remedied; the B-cell issue remains uncertain.

With this type of antibody therapy, painful bone marrow transplantations could readily pass into much needed oblivion. Moreover, should this procedure continue to get high marks, it would revolutionize the treatment of Leukemia, and related blood-system cancers.

The highly imaginative approach devised by Dr. June, was to have the new T-cells target the specific CD-19 proteins on the B-cells surface. Unfortunately, such an attack can also trigger an immune storm causing raging fever and chills, which is dangerous, but manageable. Nevertheless, the current procedure avoids the danger of an immune firestorm. Now, the T-cells become living "drugs", antibody "drugs," always present and ready for battle should the need arise. Isn't dazzling the ultimate adjective for our immune system? At this juncture, a new batch of T-cells must be prepared for each new cancer patient. It's highly personalized; using your own immune system's cells to fight your own cancer cells. Now that's huge. One size simply cannot fit all. Those days are on the way out.

Nevertheless, perfection remains elusive. There is a complication. Recall, that B-cells also battle infectious microbes. And, as CD-19 protein is on the B-cell surface, whether they are healthy or malignant B-cells, the chimeric antigen receptor T-cells will continue to attack them. Consequently, until this issue is resolved, and although the cancer has been vanquished, the now cancer-free individual remains susceptible to opportunistic microbes, germs, which in those of us with intact immune systems, can do no harm, but in immunocompromised individuals can be catastrophic. For young Emma, that means regular infusions of immunoglobulins to keep her infection-free.

It is hardly fanciful to believe that not all that far down this road, that problem will also be solved. Not only is it not fanciful, it is quite realistic to assume, to believe that these problems will be surmounted and new therapies born. A vital ingredient is the continued funding of the National Institutes of Healths budgets, supporting creative studies that seek to relieve nature of her secrets.

The Rejectionists...and the Pressing Need for Childhood Vaccinations

The question being bruited about in scientific circles is, could a bird-flu virus mutate sufficiently, enabling it to take up residence and flourish in the mucus linings of our nose and down into our airways? If it could and did, similar to the Spanish Flu of 1918-1919, the mother of all pandemics," would another 50 million or more of us, perish?

Recall, that at the time, no one had had any contact with an H1N1 virus, and thus, not a hint of its "memory" in their immune systems. The population was totally virginal regarding that viral strain. That's one hell of a thought. But it's hardly fanciful, as influenza viruses have an uncanny ability to mutate, given their eight RNA fragments in their viral cores that can rearrange and rearrange. And, along with the many H and N possible combinations, they have the crafty ability to slip under our immune radar. Is there any hope for avoidance? Can the community, the herd, be protected?

An answer may be hiding in plain sight. Underfoot as it were. So, let's ask, who are our primary flu spreaders? Dr. Katherine A. Ryan, of the University of Florida's Department of Pediatrics, maintains that the "schools are virus exchange systems, and children are super spreaders." Ah, I believe she's on to something. She also says that these kids "shed more virus for longer periods than adults."[54] So, are these elementary school kids the means, the weapons, to protect the rest of us? It may just come to that.

Dr. Ryan offers a plan that appears to have worked well in Alachua County, Florida, the home of the University of Florida. There, a free and voluntary, school-based attenuated flu vaccine, FluMist, a nasal spray, was given to students in grades pre K to 12. In both public and private schools that produced a remarkable immunization rate of 65 percent. During the 2010-2011 flu seasons the number of influenza cases in that county was near zero. Who could ask for more?

With the ready availability of FluMist, there remains little reason to avoid flu vaccine, as this nasal spray was approved by the FDA for all healthy children and adults ages two to forty-nine. We owe FluMist to Dr. Hunein Maassab, who was born in Syria and arrived in the US at age 20; studied at the University of Missouri, then on to the School of Public Health, University of Michigan. From there, with a newly minted Ph.D, he began a long career at the National Institute of Allergy and Infectious

Disease, where he worked to develop FluMist. Dr. Maassab died at age 87, on February 1st, 2014. He deserves our gratitude.[55]

Dr. Ryan believes this type of program could easily go nationwide, raising the overall immunization level and protecting all of us. It's doable and it's relatively simple. But if it's free to the kids, who will fund the vaccine, the sprayers and the people to do the spraying? These costs, she maintains, to each state, would not only be minimal, but the savings in hospitalizations, visits to physicians, and lost wages, would be substantial. Seems like a no-brainer. Could that be its demise? Surely there are people in each state who would pick up and run with this ball. It's got to be a public/private effort.

Unfortunately our states have a spotty record getting their children immunized. Washington state, for example, the home of Bill and Melinda Gates, and their Foundation, supporters of vaccines and vaccinations worldwide, was the lowest on the totem pole of all states in the numbers of children vaccinated. Oregon and Nevada are not far behind. California recently had a Pertussis, whooping cough, episode that took the lives of ten children—the worst event in over 50 years. A county in Minnesota had 21 cases of measles in 2011, as many children went unvaccinated because their parents were overly concerned about the safety of the standard measles, mumps, rubella vaccine. Children too young to be vaccinated became infected. No help from the herd, there.

The states, knowing that breaching the wall of immunity was a danger to its citizens, especially its children, and a costly danger to boot, began tightening its opt out regulations. Let us hope that will close the gaps in the wall of immunity.

Far too many people are being misled by false information disseminated by the media and Internet. Far too many parents are unaware of the seriousness of chickenpox, measles and whooping cough.

If Rwanda can do it, why can't we? Most Rwandan children are vaccinated twice against measles, and cases among children in that African country have been near zero for over the past half-dozen years.

Rwanda has been so successful at eliminating measles that it was expected to be the first country to get independent financial support to allow it to go after Rubella in 2013, with the same thoroughness. In Mid-March the Rwandan government planned to hold a three-day vaccination campaign using a combined measles/rubella vaccine that is geared to encompass as many as five million children up to the age of fourteen. With that completed, the combined vaccine will become part of their countrywide health care under their national health service. The Measles & Rubella Initiative will provide the vaccine. If we can't do the same, shame on us.[56]

The virus of Rubella, German measles, causes a rash similar to measles, making it difficult to distinguish one from the other. An infected pregnant woman can lose her infant, or the virus can cause serious birth defects– blindness and deafness are not uncommon. Obviously the Rwandan people, but parents especially, take their vaccinations seriously. We can surely do the same.

Pediatricians and Epidemiologists in Colorado looking to quantify the results of not vaccinating, found hat of the thousands of children in the state, those not vaccinated were 23 times more likely to contract whooping cough, nine times more likely to get chickenpox, and almost seven times more likely to be hospitalized with pneumonia than vaccinated children from the same communities. The numbers fairly jump up and grab you. Is it necessary to point out that vaccines do work?!

Although ten viral and nine bacterial vaccines are currently available, and have combined to drastically reduce both illness and death from their specific diseases, our communications media continue to report on anecdotal claims of harm from vaccines.

Vaccines Currently Available

Bacterial vaccines:	Viral vaccines:
Diphtheria	Measles
Pertussis	Mumps
Pneumococcal Pneumonia	Rubella
Tuberculosis	Influenza
Meningitis	Poliomyelitis
Cholera	Rabies
Tetanus	Yellow Fever
Typhus	Hepatitis B
Typhoid	Shingles (Herpes)
	HPV

The Rejectionists

Babies, the immunosuppressed, those with various types of cancers, along with those with HIV/AIDS, and those on chemotherapy, are not candidates for vaccines. Nevertheless, the more folks in our communities that get their "shots" the greater the protection for all of us because of Herd Immunity. How does it work?

When you're vaccinated before the Flu season begins, you can't pass on a flu virus to anyone around you. You are in affect, a viral dead end. If others in your community are also vaccinated, a "wall" of protection is formed–as a herd of circled Buffalos protects its members against predators. So, in any community, a chain of infection, usually person to person, via respiratory droplets, can be interdicted, when a germ cannot find a susceptible host. This can occur when large numbers of individuals are resistant either naturally, or through vaccination. These individuals limit the spread to others who are susceptible or unvaccinated. However, the degree of protection offered by the herd varies by disease: measles requires a greater number of resistant individuals than influenza. Generally, a population with 80-85 percent of its population resistant can protect the few remaining susceptibles. However, if people refuse or avoid vaccinations, the "wall" is breached and they, and others, can become infected and spread the various germs to the vulnerable among us.

In 2012, the European Health Protection Agency documented 2,016 measles cases in England and Wales, the highest number since 1994. To interdict their most recent outbreak that had sickened more than eight hundred children by the end of April 2013, vaccination teams were sent to every school in an attempt to contain this epidemic. Because measles is so highly contagious, protection of the herd requires ninety-five percent of the public to be vaccinated to protect against an outbreak. That number will not be reached as far too many parents over estimate the risk of vaccination, and under estimate the risks that measles creates.[57]

The benefit of vaccination was again shown, when the CDC announced on March 21st, 2005, that the eradication of Rubella had been achieved: only from the US. Rubella will only be eliminated from the world, if, and only if, Rubella vaccine is faithfully used around the world.

Unfortunately, the numbers of us being vaccinated has been falling since 1998, when Dr. Andrew J. Wakefield, a now discredited British physician, published an article in the prestigious journal, The Lancet, in which he informed the world that childhood vaccines were responsible for Autism. That fraudulent publication was the shot heard around the world. It not only struck the Camel's back, but all four knees. Vaccination rates plummeted. Dr. Wakefield maintained that measles virus from the MMR vaccine (measles, mumps, rubella) spread through the children's intestinal tracks into their skulls causing brain damage. If that wasn't damage enough, parents of Autistic children held that Thimerosal, a mercury-based preservative in vaccines was toxic to the brain, and therefore responsible for Autism.

Neither of these notions has stood up to further evidence and analysis, as mercury in Thimerosal had been removed years before, and Dr. Wakefield lost his license for falsifying data, and The Lancet revoked his publication. Thimerosal, ethyl mercury, an organic mercury compound, was used for some seventy years to prevent bacterial and fungal contamination in multidose vials of vaccine. Advocacy groups forced its removal in the early 2000's believing there was a direct connection with Autism in children. Over the past decade, many research studies have provided overwhelming evidence of its safety.[58]

Nevertheless, the damage was done. The Internet took Dr. Wakefield's fraudulent data worldwide. The U.S., England and Ireland were hit hard by his publication. Ireland had an epidemic in which 300-plus cases of measles were documented along with one hundred hospitalizations and three unnecessary deaths. That was hardly the end of it.

Jenny McCarthy, former Playboy model and MTV star, took up the cudgel, becoming a passionate anti-vaccinationist and rejectionist after her son Ivan, developed what appeared to be Autism. Her best selling book, Louder than Words: A mother's journey in healing Autism, railed against vaccines, as not only unsafe, but causing autism. Her ranting went viral as she exploded on the Ophra Winfrey show purveying her nonsense. She was thoroughly taken in by Dr. Wakfield's publication, before it was recalled by The Lancet as fraudulent. According to the CDC, Jenny McCarthy "was a menace to Public Health."[59]

To make matters even worse, it was later shown that her son Ivan never had Autism; he had Landau-Kleffner Syndrome, a rare neurological disorder. He is currently doing nicely and Jenny has reversed her antagonism to MMR vaccines.

But myths are hard dying. Greater acceptance of vaccines will take time. Far too many will suffer needlessly. Agitators capture the public all to often. Let's try to avoid that.[60]

Rejecting parents are not the only problem allowing measles to spread and inflict its ravages. Doctors Without Borders announced in June 2013, that a measles outbreak "was sweeping Syria's rebel-held north, and that 7-thousand cases of measles had been tallied." They noted too that, "many people have avoided assembling for vaccinations for fear they might attract air strikes or rocket attacks, which would mean many more additional cases," of death and hellish wounds.[61] When civil government becomes a casualty, and public health systems collapse, disease is not far behind.

But hold on: lack of vaccinations has come from yet another, and unsuspected direction: Financial. The cost of vaccines has literally gone through the roof. Pharmaceutical companies keep raising their prices to physicians, and physicians are reimbursed 50 to 70 percent of that cost by insurance companies. Consequently many physicians no longer offer vaccines as part of their practice.

Consider that a number of vaccines require multiple injections. Ergo, the yearly cost to a family can run to thousands of dollars, which many families cannot afford. Current vaccine costs have become an unconscionable burden. If states mandate vaccination for school admission, the state has two options: provide the vaccines free of charge or for a nominal fee, or cap retail vaccine prices at an acceptable level. Transmission of the common childhood viral diseases will be curtailed when all children are vaccinated.

With this early and brief look into the workings of our internal defense forces, and the beneficial microbes that augment it, we turn now to the delinquents, the nasties, worthy of our attention, that have been with us for eons: Some, since we have walked upright. Chapter FOUR guides us along this troubling path.

FOUR

Delinquents Among Us: They Make Us Sick

Infectious disease is not just troubling, it can be downright disagreeable and a contributor to an abbreviated life. At least that's what many of us feel and believe. Nevertheless, of all the known microbial species, only a desperate few are pathogenic. That's an enormously important bit of information.

So, where in the pantheon of our country's leading causes of death do our infectious diseases reside? Just how much of a "player" are they? Let the following tables and their numbers speak to us.

Table 1. Leading Causes of Death, US, 2011

All Causes of death beyond the 10 listed = 2,512,873: 100%

Condition	# of Deaths	% of Total
1. Heart Disease	596,339	23.7
2. Malignant Neoplasms (Cancer)	575,313	22.8
3. Chronic Lower Respiratory Disease	143,382	5.7
4. Cerebrovascular Disease (Stroke)	128,931	5.1
5. Accidents	122,777	4.9

6. Alzheimer's Disease	84,691	3.4
7. Diabetes Mellitus	73,282	2.9
8. Influenza/Pneumonia	53,667	2.1
9. Nephritis/Nephrosis	45,731	1.8
10. Suicide	8,285	1.5
All Other Causes	512,723	20.4%

(Population – July 1, 2011: 308,745,538)

Table 2. Leading Causes of Death, Ages 1-4, 2011

Condition	# of Deaths	% of Total
1. Accidents	1,466	32.9
2. Congenital Malformations	464	10.4
3. Homicide	376	8.4
4. Malignant Neoplasms	350	7.9
5. Heart Disease	154	3.5
6. Influenza/Pneumonia	146	3.3
7. Septicemia	71	1.6
8. Chronic Lower Respiratory Disease	66	1.5
9. Prenatal Issues	58	1.3
10. Neoplasms	53	1.2
All Other Causes	1,246	25%

Table 3. Leading Causes of Death, Ages 5-9, 2011

Condition	# of Deaths	% of Total
1. Accidents	773	30.6
2. Malignant Neoplasms	477	18.9
3. Congenital Malformations	195	7.7
4. Homicide (Assault)	119	4.7
5. Influenza/Pneumonia	106	4.2
6. Heart Disease	97	3.8
7. Chronic Lower Respiratory Disease	64	2.5
8. Neoplasms (Cancer)	40	1.6

9. Septicemia	33	1.3
10. Cerebrovascular Disease	32	1.3
All Other Causes	587	23.3%

Table 4. Leading Causes of Death, Ages 10-14, 2011

Condition	# of Deaths	% of Total
1. Accidents	916	29.3
2. Neoplasms (Cancer)	419	13.4
3. Suicide	259	8.3
4. Homicide	186	5.9
5. Congenital Malformations	169	5.4
6. Influenza/Pneumonia	122	3.9
7. Heart Disease	120	3.8
8. Chronic Lower Respiratory Disease	59	1.9
9. Neoplasms of Uncertain Character	45	1.4
10. Cerebrovascular Disease	42	1.3
All Other Causes	791	25.3%

Table 5. Leading Causes of Death, Ages 15-19, 2011

Condition	# of Deaths	% of Total
1. Accidents	4,807	41.7
2. Homicide (Assault)	1,919	16.7
3. Suicide	1,669	4.5
4. Malignant Neoplasms	644	5.6
5. Heart Disease	335	2.9
6. Congenital Malformations	230	2.0
7. Influenza/Pneumonia	163	1.4
8. Chronic Lower Respiratory Disease	86	0.7
9. Septicemia	61	0.5
10. Cerebrovascular Disease	60	0.5
All Other Causes	1,546	13.4%

Table 6. Leading Causes of Death, Ages 20-24, 2011

Condition	# of Deaths	% of Total
1. Accidents	7,651	40.5
2. Homicide	2,943	.6
3. Suicide	2,702	14.3
	(70.4% from trauma)	
4. Malignant Neoplasms	992	5.2
5. Heart Disease	700	3.7
6. Influenza/Pneumonia	255	1.3
7. Congenital Malformations	227	1.2
8. Pregnancy Childbirth	169	0.9
9. Cerebrovascular Disease	133	0.7
10. HIV (AIDS)	127	0.7
All Other Causes	2.997	15.9%

Table 7. Leading Causes of Death, Ages 25-34, 2011

Condition	# of Deaths	% of Total
1. Accidents	4,062	33.1
2. Suicide	5,320	12.5
3. Homicide	4,222	9.9
	(55.5% from trauma)	
4. Malignant Neoplasms	3,659	8.6
5. Heart Disease	3,174	7.5
6. HIV (AIDS)	881	2.1
7. Influenza/Pneumonia	807	1.9
8. Diabetes Mellitus	604	1.4
9. Cerebrovascular Disease	537	1.3
10. Chronic Liver Disease (Cirrohosis)	459	1.1
All Other Causes	8,777	20.7%

Table 8. Leading Causes of Death, Ages 35-44, 2011

Condition	# of Deaths	% of Total
1. Accidents	15,102	20.2

2. Malignant Neoplasms	12,519	16.8
3. Heart Disease	11,081	14.8
4. Suicide	6,677	8.9
5. Homicide	2,762	3.7
6. Chronic Liver Disease and Cirrhosis	2,481	3.3
7. HIV (AIDS)	2,425	3.2
8. Cerebrovascular Disease	1,916	2.6
9. Diabetes Mellitus	1,872	2.5
10. Influenza/Pneumonia	1,314	1.8
All Other Causes	16,516	22.1%

Table 9. Leading Causes of Death, Ages 45-54, 2011

Condition	# of Deaths	% of Total
1. Malignant Neoplasms	50,616	27.0
2. Heart Disease	36,927	19.7
3. Accidents	19,974	10.6
4. Suicide	8,598	4.6
5. Chronic Liver Disease and Cirrhosis	8,377	4.5
6. Cerebrovascular Disease	6,163	3.3
7. Diabetes Mellitus	5,725	3.1
8. Chronic Lower Respiratory Disease	4,664	2.5
9. HIV (AIDS)	3,388	1.8
10. Influenza/Pneumonia	2,918	1.6
All Other Causes	40,218	21.4%

Table 10. Leading Causes of Death, Ages 55-64, 2011

Condition	# of Deaths	% of Total
1. Malignant Neoplasms	106,829	35.2
2. Heart Disease	67,261	22.2
3. Chronic Lower Respiratory Disease	14,160	4.7
4. Accidents	12,933	4.3
5. Diabetes Mellitus	11,361	3.7

6. Cerebrovascular Disease	10,523	3.5
7. Chronic Liver Disease and Cirrhosis	9,154	3.0
8. Suicide	5,808	1.9
9. Septicemia	4,792	1.6
10. Septicemia	4,628	1.5
All Other Causes	55,858	18.4%

As we run down the list of Table 1, we've got to go as far as position eight to get to a microbial cause of death: a virus, for influenza, and a bacterium for pneumonia. In this instance, influenza and pneumonia (I/P) are joined at the hip, as it were, as they occur together for the most part. Influenza strikes first, preparing the lungs for bacterial attack. This morbid combination usually strikes the very young and the very old. As we see, overall, I/P are responsible for just 2.2 percent of the total deaths from all causes.

As we continue to scan this table, it is obvious that no other source of infectious illness makes it to this table of leading causes, which should give us pause, and a modest degree of comfort.

As we continue on, perusing the leading causes of death by age groups, and scanning ages 1-4, and all the way to 65 and over, we see that I/P are the sixth leading cause for infants, at 3.3 percent of the total, and septicemia, a blood stream infection, in position seven, claiming 1.6 percent of the total deaths in this group. The nastiest problems affecting these infants are accidents and homicide. Does that catch your breath!?

Moving to those 5-9 year olds, the story is similar: I/P in position five, and septicemia in the ninth slot. These youngsters are also afflicted by accidents and homicide. Note well that accidents are their leading cause of death. Disgraceful.

At ages 10-14, I/P occupy the sixth position, causing 3.9 percent of all their deaths, but septicemia is no longer their problem. These young people are surely accident prone. At 29.3 percent of all their deaths, it's their leading cause, and suicide in the third slot tells us they're taking their own lives! Worse yet, in fourth place is homicide: they're also being murdered! Among accidents, suicide and homicide, these traumas are responsible for 43.5 percent of all their deaths. Hard to grasp?

As we glance down the list of deaths for the 15-19 year-olds, the numbers leap up to inform us that I/P in the seventh position claims 1.4 percent of these young people, and septicemia in the ninth slot is responsible for less than one percent. Trauma is also their misfortune: accidents, suicides, and homicide are their top three leading causes of death, at so early an age. Imagine. Almost 73 percent of all their deaths are due to their being killed or killing themselves. Is this madness?

The twenty-year olds, 20-24, die from the same set of traumas: accidents, suicide and homicide. Again up there at 70.4 percent of their total deaths. I/P comes in at position 6 with1.3 percent of their deaths, and HIV/AIDS at the tenth position, now entering the list at less than one percent, along with pregnancy/childbirth another troubling issue responsible for 0.9 percent of their deaths. Shouldn't these types of deaths be seen as a scandalous failure of public health in need of radical change?

And again, as we look at ages 25-34, accidents remain their leading cause of death followed by those deadly twins, suicide and homicide, for a total of 55.5 percent of all their deaths. I/P is in the seventh position responsible for 1.9 percent of the total, and HIV/AIDS adds another 2.1 percent to their death rate.

As we enter the late 30's and early 40's, malignant neoplasms (cancer) and heart disease begin to take their toll, accounting for some 32 percent of the total. But accidents remain number one, along with suicide and homicide, accounting for 32 percent of the total. Here too, HIV/AIDS in the seventh slot, and I/P at the tenth, together, account for four percent.

As age increases, so do the number of cancer deaths. Malignant neoplasms become the leading cause of death for the 45-54 age group, with heart disease a close second and accidents following in third. Together, these three claim 57.3 percent of all deaths, with suicide in fourth place adding another 4.6 percent. HIV/AIDS in ninth place and I/P in tenth are responsible for 3.4 percent.

As we head into the older ages, although 55-64 in this second decade of the 21st century is no longer considered old age, it is the new middle age, and we see ever increasing deaths from cancer and heart disease. Together, the two are responsible for 57.4 percent of the total. I/P have now fallen off the list, and septicemia returns with 1.5 percent, in the tenth slot. It must be evident by now that germs, microbes, infectious disease, are barely a minor problem.

Our last group, those 65 to over 100–those really older folks, many in good health, have pushed heart disease into first place, dropped cancer into second, and together account for 49.4 percent of all deaths. Chronic lower respiratory disease holds down third place with 6.6 percent of deaths. Back on the list in seventh place is I/P, contributing 2.5 percent. Accidents return in ninth place and septicemia holds down the tenth slot with 1.5 percent of all deaths.

Table 11, is a summary table, showing at a glance the positions from 1 to 10 of the leading causes of death by age group. Clearly, accidents are the leading cause of death for all age groups from 1 all the way to 44. I/P bounces around from 5th to10th in various age groups, as does septicemia, which claims lives in five of the ten age groups, but does so most often down at positions nine and ten. HIV/AIDS, another infectious illness, has only been a concern in age groups 20-24, and 45-54, and then well below the fifth position. Does that come as a surprise? Most recently another chronic condition makes its first appearance at the older ages: Alzheimer's assumes the fifth position among those 65 and older.

This summary table offers a quick way to get the overall picture of the major conditions that afflict us.

Table 11. Leading Causes of Death by Age Group, 2011

AGE: CAUSE:	1-4	5-9	10-14	15-19	20-24	25-34	35-44	45-54	55-64	65+
Heart Disease	5	6	7	5	5	5	3	2	2	1
Malignant Neoplasms	4	2	2	4	4	4	2	1	1	2
Accidents	1	1	1	1	1	1	1	3	4	9
Chronic Lower Respiratory Disease	8	7	8	8	-	-	-	8	3	3
Cerebrovascular Disease	-	10	10	10	9	9	8	6	6	4
Suicide	-	-	3	3	3	2	4	4	8	-
Diabetes	-	-	-	-	-	8	9	7	5	6
Septicemia	7	9	-	9	-	-	-	-	10	10
Liver Disease	-	-	-	-	-	-	-	-	-	-
Homicide	3	4	4	2	2	3	5	-	-	-
HIV/AIDS	-	-	-	-	10	6	7	9	-	-
Alzheimer's	-	-	-	-	-	-	-	-	-	5
Influenza/ Pneumonia (I/P)	6	5	6	7	6	7	10	10	-	7
Nephritis	-	-	-	-	-	-	-	-	9	8
Neoplasms (unknown)	10	8	9	-	-	-	-	-	-	-
Congenital Malformations	2	3	5	6	7	-	-	-	-	-

So, what are we to make of these causes of death? What do the numbers reveal? As we move through the second decade of the 21st century, pathogens, those few delinquent microbes, are not the terror we've been led to believe. That has to be a revelation, calling for an adjustment in thinking about microbes that are all around us, and which are the dominant life forms on earth.

The numbers do tell the existing story. Infectious illnesses are few and far between, clinging by their toe nails, to the leading causes of death. Even morbidity, illness, barely makes a dent. Perception simply does not equate with reality. Infections are not the heavy weights we have made them out to be. More than likely it's Influenza, and HIV/AIDS grabbing headlines that has confused us, making infectious diseases larger than life. Time to recalibrate. Pathways of Infectious Disease Transmission

With the numbers behind us, it is relevant to ask: how do infectious diseases spread, move around. How are they transmitted?

Six ways exist for microbes, pathogens, to get to us: six and only six. If they can't get to us b any of these, they can't get to us. So, let's have a look at each, to see how we encourage or deny them entrance. All microbes fit into these categories, and are transmitted by their specific route. Influenza can't be transmitted by food or water, nor can the gonococcus of Gonorrhea, be transmitted by coughing, sneezing, or toilet seats. Toilet seats cannot convey the Treponema of syphilis, nor can it get to us via an animal or insect bite. And West Nile Encephalitis cannot be spread by fomites.

Our bodies have portals of entry as well as exits. Entries include our eyes, ears, nose (secretions) mouth (saliva and sputum) anus, vagina, bruised and or broken skin. We're open to the world, the microbial world.

For a pathogen to spread, the first order of its business is to reproduce, which requires adequate and appropriate conditions for growth. Our pathogens are a fragile lot, requiring warmth (at least 98°F), moisture, nutrients, and of course a place to reproduce. What better than to hole up in us. A suitable animal would do as well. In us, or a diversity of animals, they've got it all. Any reasonable microbe would not want to lose these cozy habitats. Ergo, why kill us? Another good question we'll consider.

But first, the six pathways:

Airborne Transmission

Air is not a fitting growth medium for any pathogen. In air, a pathogen is riding a magic carpet—a dried mucus carpet, a dry fecal flake, or dust particle that can be inhaled into our lungs. This airborne pathogen had to come from somewhere or someone. It could be from soil, an animal, food, or water, or another one of us. Some of these particles are hardier than others. So, for example, Mycobacterium tuberculosis, the pathogen of tuberculosis, can remain desiccated for months after expulsion from an infected individual, and still be capable of infecting another person once inhaled.

Coughing, talking, sneezing, even laughing releases moist droplets into the air. With an unstifled sneeze, the most explosive of all, secretions from our nose and mouth, propelled from behind clenched teeth, lips open, can be ejected with the force of a speeding bullet sailing through the air at the rate of 50-100 meters per second (m/s). This sneeze can eject as many as a million droplets from 10 microns to a millimeter in diameter. The smallest and lightest can reach as far as six feet from our mouths. The larger, heavier droplets fall close to us, and are less of a hazard. The lighter droplets evaporate rapidly, leaving behind droplet nuclei that can remain suspended indefinitely, with the consequent accumulation of large numbers of potentially infective organisms.

Respiratory transmission via droplet nuclei, as you might imagine, is the preferred means of transmission of most human infectious diseases. It is a highly efficient route of passing organisms among crowds, and a highly efficient means for a pathogen to locate new venues, as a means of survival. Charles Darwin had no idea about microbes, but he'd surely see this pathway as fitting nicely with his belief that an organism is free to adopt any strategy that gives it a reproductive advantage. A violent sneeze surely does that.

Those sneezes, coughs, laughs and just talking can send the diphtheria bacillus into the air to be wafted about and inhaled by an unsuspecting child or adult especially in crowded conditions. Then there's Legionnaire's Disease, also known as Legionellosis, or Pontiac Fever, the handiwork of *Legionella pneumophila*. Of course we all are aware of those childhood diseases, all virus borne: chickenpox, rubella, (3-day German measles), mumps and that ever present measles (rubeola) described by Hippocrates in the fifth century bce, and pertussis (whooping cough).

To round off our list, Rheumatic fever, is a Staphylococcal acquisition, and that long-time irritant Streptococcus pneumoniae, delivering Pneumonia to our lungs although we don't see much of it these days, and we're thankful for that. Scarlet fever (Scarlatina) is yet another Streptococcal gift to human discomfort. This organism also conveys Bright's disease known to the medical community as glomerulonephritis, which can play havoc with our kidneys after being inhaled.

Inhaled contaminated air almost killed a Scottish bagpiper. John MacDuffy, not his real name, recently spent a month in a Glasgow hospital in the grip of pneumonia that was resistant to most antibiotics, literally fighting for his life. As was later discovered, his pipe bag was loaded with two fungi, growing luxuriantly inside. Bag- Pipers are supposed to clean their bags regularly with antimicrobials. Mac Duffy didn't, but he's alive to talk about it.

Person-to-Person Spread

We deal here with direct, close, personal contact: mucus membranes, to mucus membranes, as well as skin to skin. This means shaking hands can be an issue if we rub our eyes, or stick our fingers in our mouths, as we often do. Of course sexually transmitted diseases such as Gonorrhea, Syphilis and HIV/AIDS are members of this highly select pathway. Gonorrhea comes to us via sexual intercourse, conveyed by that microbe of antiquity,

Neisseria gonorrhoeae. The Greeks had it right: Gono, means seed, and rhein, means to flow, which it surely does and painfully so, while urinating. Syphilis, recognized in sixteenth century Europe, is also acquired by, and only by, sexual intercourse, delivering Treponema pallidum, a tightly coiled, thin, corkscrew of a germ onto delicate mucus tissues, finding its way to the nervous system where it can induce mental retardation and blindness. It shows no favoritism. It's all-inclusive. Card-carrying members of that non-exclusive club have had as its members, Henry VIII, Adolph Hitler, Al Capone, Francisco Goya, Oscar Wilde, Franz Schubert, Giacomo Puccini, and Kaiser Wilhelm, among many others.

In the mid-sixteenth century, an Italian physician of Verona, Jerome Fracastor, (Girolamo Fracastoro) wrote a poem that made him famous-Syphilis sive morbus gallius-Syphilis, or the French disease. In this poem an unusually handsome young shepherd boy disrespectful of the gods, is cursed by the Sun God, who sends him a facial disfiguring venereal disease. Inhabitants of the surrounding countryside named this condition Syphilis in memory of the first person to suffer from it. Ergo, the name Syphilis, was born.

HIV/AIDS joined this group in 1981, and has been a major contributor ever since. Human papilloma virus, HPV, is yet another member that involves exchanges of saliva, between unsuspecting individuals, as well as the penetration of their tongues into body cavities. This behavior has sent rates of mouth, tongue and cheek cancer skyrocketing.

Genital herpes, carried hither and yon by the Herpes simplex virus type 2, via sexual activity, causes pain and blistering in the genital areas of both men and women. Herpes labalis delivers cold sores and fever blisters, which our friend Hippocrates knew quite well around 400 bce. Of course the Greeks had a word for it too: Herpes, means to creep, which it does around lips, mouth and gums.

This group must also include infectious mononuleosis, another close contact infection, the consequence of kissing and exchanges of saliva. It's important to note that these sexually transmitted microbes are fragile creatures that cannot survive outside the human body, and must be rapidly deposited within a new host if they are to survive and reproduce. Isn't that a welcome circumstance? And not to forget Ebola, exploding to a worldwide dread.

Closely related to direct contact is a pathway that permits transmission via fomites, non-living objects such as bedding, diapers, eating utensils, drinking cups, surgical instruments, catheters, toothbrushes, toys, clothing and other items frequently handled. As we shall see, several of these figure importantly in infections acquired in hospitals and nursing homes.

Common Vehicle Transmission

Water and food are a major means of transmission that can readily snare large numbers of unsuspecting people. Food poisoning at church suppers, picnics, and business retreats can, and have resulted in the illness of hundreds of folks enjoying themselves while consuming, egg, tuna, chicken and shellfish salads, along with meat and dairy products containing pathogenic organisms or their toxins. Explosions of gastrointestinal illness follow anywhere from four, to twelve hours later.

Food-borne Salmonellosis, Shigellosis, and Staphylococcal food poisoning are primary culprits, as is Campylobacter jejeuni, another leading cause of gastroenteritis. Listeriosis, brought to us by Listeria monocytogenes, is often the consequence of improper pasteurization of milk used in the production of Mexican-style cheeses. Food borne illness comes to us when foods are inadequately cooked, or when foods are contaminated by food handlers, shedding their germs directly into the foods as they are being prepared. Too often hands are not washed after a visit to the john. And large batches of luscious, high protein foods kept overnight at room temperatures, or in refrigerators at temperatures well above 40°F, allowing contaminating organisms to flourish and produce their toxins, are ready-made gastrointestinal bombs.

The waterborne route can take down an entire community as Typhoid did to Riverside, California, a number of years ago.

A worker shedding typhoid bacilli and urinating in a trench where water pipes are being connected can also cause a wide and severe epidemic.

Of course Cholera and Schistosomiasis are spread by water. Both are the result of fecal matter containing the specific microbe, being deposited in the water.

Arthropodborne Diseases

Arthopodborne illnesses are delivered by the bites of blood-sucking arthropods-ticks, mites, fleas, and mosquitoes. The diversity of microbes they harbor multiply in the tissues of these creatures without producing illness. We are their preferred blood meal.

Examples follow:

Lyme Disease

First recognized in 1975 in Old Lyme, Connecticut, after a clutch of children were diagnosed as having juvenile rheumatoid arthritis. This is a remarkable disease with a complex life cycle, involving deer, mice, ticks, a bacterium, (spirochete), acorns, and us.

Adult ticks piggybacking on deer drop off to the forest floor, where female ticks deposit their eggs, which hatch the following spring and summer, just in time for the larval ticks to partake of a blood meal from a nearby mouse. It's during this nutritious meal that the ticks imbibe the spirochete. These tick larvae grow into a larger nymph, which over-winters on the forest floor. In spring, a mature tick readily finds a deer on which to hop. Now, at the height of deer-tick activity, hikers, kids, hunters, are fair game for the black-legged tick, which can take a blood meal from either deer or human, but given a preference, its the human who becomes the depository of Borrelia, the spirochete. If susceptible, the victim may show the telltale bull's eye ring known as erythema nigrans, along with one or more flulike symptoms, such as fever, chills, muscle aches, or lethargy. And let's not forget the acorns. An abundance of them every three or four years accounts for the fluctuation of new cases, when the white-tailed deer, the white-footed mice and ticks thrive. How did such complexity come to be!? Something to dwell upon.

It is also worth noting that body lice are not the sole province of young school children. The current civil war in Syria has given lice new breeding grounds. As recently reported in the New York Times, "Often Dr. Yassir Dawish, was jammed into (prison) cells so crowded that prisoners rationed space: in one such cell, he said, each 16 x16 inch tile was allocated to three men and room to sleep assigned in shifts. Everyone had body lice." Indeed, this is the type of environment in which lice, both body and head, thrive.[1]

The living conditions and crowded situations of the homeless, war refugees, and/or victims of natural disasters often provide ideal conditions for the spread of lice, fleas, and mites. The consequences of these relationships appear to be widely underestimated.

Ehrlichiosis

This fever causing, a rather new illness for us, first diagnosed in the US in 1986, is the consequence of a relatively new bacterial species, Ehrlichia chaffeensis. This is transmitted by dogs and deer, which carry the Lone star, or dog tick, that shelters Ehrlichia in its gut. When the tick latches on to our legs, it bites, which we don't often feel, and it injects the bacterium. The newness of the disease, its few number of cases, some 1,500 a year around the country, and the fact that it resembles other febrile conditions, make it difficult to diagnose. Currently it appears endemic, from Maine to Florida, and as far west as Texas and the gulf states.

Chagas Disease

Chagas disease is named after the Brazilian physician Carlos Chagas, and is also referred to as American Trypanosomiasis. It is of course, well known in South America, especially Brazil, Argentina and Columbia, where it infects 8-9 million men, women and children yearly, and kills 10-12 thousand.

The disease is the fruit of being bitten by the Assassin or Kissing bug, Triatoma, a huge fly-like beast, so-called as it takes its blood meal near the mouth while people are sleeping. As it bites, it defecates, leaving the fecal matter containing the Trypanasome parasite near the bite. When the bitten person rubs the wound, the feces are deposited in the wound along with the Trypanasome, allowing it free access to the blood stream. Furthermore, with its painless bite, its salivary proteins can cause immunologic shock–anaphylaxis. Chagas disease can also lead to intestinal infections, heart disease and death.

Although Triatomes are found in the US, primarily in our southern states, they do their damage a bit differently; not defecating along with the bite, but some time after, which does not get the Trypanasome into the circulation as it does in South America. That's why Chagas disease has not made an impression in the US. We can only hope that since global warming has kicked in, it does not bring the blood-sucking South American Assassin up north; a not unreasonable contingency.

African Sleeping Sickness

African Sleeping sickness, also known as African Trypanasomiasis, comes to us on the wings of the blood-sucking Tetse-fly, Glossina, which harbors the

Trypanasome, and spreads it widely. Cattle, wild animals and of course we humans are the preferred blood donors. Thus far, the Tetse fly has remained close to the rain forests of west and central Africa. Here again, it's the bite of the fly, and a painful bite it is, that injects the protozoan Trypanasome, that moves quickly into the lymph stream, then the blood stream, initiating nervous disorders and its characteristic sleepiness, with drooling rom the mouth, and general prostration. Recent research revealing the Tetse flies grim actions indicate that the microbe *Wigglesworthia glossinidia* lives comfortably in the fly's gut where it synthesizes vitamin B-1, Thiamin, which the fly cannot do on its own. Without Wigglesworthia the fly remains infertile and under nourished, unable to perpetrate its hellish business. *Wolbachia*, another gut microbe, has yet to divulge its roll in the fly's gastly enterprise.[2]

This frightful illness places 60 million people in thirty-seven countries at risk, racking up 300-500 thousand new cases annually, and kills 60-70 thousand. It's an unmitigated economic disaster, keeping huge areas of central Africa uncultivated and uninhabited.

In addition to these three diseases, Yellow Fever and Malaria are mosquito borne virus diseases. West Nile Encephalitis virus comes to us on the wings of birds. Both Bubonic and Pneumonic plague arrive on the silent paws of rats and other rodents carrying fleas harboring the Plague bacillus, which will be discussed at length a bit further on.

Eastern Equine Encephalitis

EEE is one of a half-dozen mosquito borne viral encephalitides in the US. Mosquitoes, primarily, Culiseta melanura, which holes up in forested swamps, carry the viruses they pick up while dining on the blood of fowl, rodents, horses and wild birds. As they alight on us for yet another blood meal, they deposit the virus that enters our cells and replicates profusely, crossing the blood-brain barrier, where they induce encephalitis. Although equine encephalitis suggests the disease in horses, we humans are also fair game with fever, headaches, often meningitis and on to coma, often loss of speech and memory, and death.

Eastern Equine Encephalitis, EEE, has occurred along the east coast from Massachusetts all the way to Mexico, Central and South America. The only preventive measures currently available are ridding our area of mosquitoes and their breeding larvae.

Most recently, the over-wintering resevoir for EEE, was discovered. How the virus survived during the winter months was a bewildering mystery. Researchers at the Universities of South Florida (Tampa), and Auburn (Alabama) unearthed the answer: Snakes. Cotton-mouthed rattlers, timber rattlesnakes and other rattlers, harbor the virus during the winter! The virus emerges in summer to be picked up by mosquitoes, transmitting them to horses and humans. But mosquitoes can't pierce a snake's skin. No, they can't. They go through the eye! Surprise! And yes, the snakes contained antibodies to EEE. Its case fatality rate of 35-to 75 percent makes EEE virus the most deadly mosquito-borne pathogen in North America! That must come as yet another surprise.[3] Current concern has it that climate change will drive Culeseta melanura northward into Vermont and New Hampshire. Yet another negative, for climate change and us.

West Nile Encephalitis

First discovered in the West Nile region of Uganda in 1937, it had remained in the Middle East, Africa, and southwest Asia. For reasons not yet known, it crossed the Atlantic in infected birds, swooping into New York City in 1999, with birds dropping out of the sky. Shortly thereafter, human encephalitis cases began occurring. Over the next half-dozen years, some ten thousand people were infected, with about 300 deaths, and not one of our continental forty-eight states was left unscathed.

That Culex mosquito is everywhere, and harbors a great concentration of virus; but late summer and fall are its peak biting seasons. Thankfully, most of those bitten and infected show only mild, flu-like illness. Less than one percent of those infected developed meningitis, an inflammation of the meningeal covering of the brain, or go on to full-blown encephalitis.

Zoonoses: Animal Diseases Transferable to Humans

Most of our diseases, some sixty to seventy percent have been shown to be directly related to a variety of animals. We'll deal with six.

We begin with Leptospirosis. The causative agent, *Leptospira interrogans,* another spirochete, is transmitted by rodents, dogs, horses, raccoons, and cattle. The Leptospire gets to us via contact with urine-contaminated water. Because the bacterium is thin and highly mobile, it can readily penetrate through invisible breaks or scratches in the skin, then spreading from blood to the urinary tract. Fever, muscle and headaches are characteristic. It's rarely fatal, but in those cases that it is, death is due to kidney and liver failure or respiratory distress.

Who gets this organism? Mostly butchers, ranchers, farmers and sewage treatment plant workers who are in regular contact with contaminated water.

Tularemia

Francisella tularensis is acutely infectious. No more than a few cells are required for a full-blown case of Tularemia to occur. Tulare County, California has given its name to this disease, as it was the first place to have been diagnosed in hunters who butchered wild animals.

The organism is tiny, and can easily pass through unbroken skin or mucus membranes. Direct contact with an infected carcass, a tick bite, or biting flies can inject the bacterium that normally lives comfortably in rabbits, ticks and insects.

We can also become infected during animal slaughter, while eating contaminated meat, and drinking contaminated water. Hunters and taxidermists appear to be at greatest risk. As the organism is present in tick saliva and feces, getting the tick quickly can prevent an infection. Those infected usually experience fever, chills, headaches, muscle and joint pain. These common symptoms make diagnoses difficult. In some cases ulcers appear at the point of a tick bite. Tender and swollen lymph nodes can also appear at the bite site.

Curiously enough, in 2004, three researchers working in a high security lab at Boston University became infected with Francisella, which is on the federal "select agents" list because of its potential to be weaponized. We'll meet up with "select agents" further on. How the researchers became infected remains a mystery.

Rabies

Rabies, from the Latin, meaning rage or madness, referring to the people bitten by infected animals, is the result of several viruses that have a morbid affinity for our nervous system.

Rabies has been a terror since antiquity when the cry "mad dog" sent people running in panic. The bite of an animal, foxes, skunks, raccoons, as well as bats and dogs, deposits the saliva-containing virus deep into muscle tissues. Entering tissue cells, the virus begins rapid multiplication, and moves to the nervous system and spinal cord. Characteristic symptoms begin: anxiety, irritability, depression, fever, loss of appetite, then paralysis. In many cases intense and painful throat spasms occur when swallowing liquids...hydrophobia.

Rabies is often referred to as hydrophobia as the mere sight of water can send the infected person into seizures.

For the most part, Veterinarians and lab personnel are at highest risk for rabies. However, in the US, fewer than ten people a year have gotten rabies.

Unfortunately, there is yet another way in for the rabies virus, one that few, if any would suspect: Donor organ transplants. Now that's a horror!

A patient in Maryland, waiting anxiously for a donor kidney to save his life, received one from a donor who died in Florida. His organs went to recipients in Georgia, Illinois, and Maryland.

More than a year passed before the patient in Maryland became ill with rabies and died. Yes, the disease can have a long incubation period. His rabies strain matched that of a raccoon's. As he had no known contact with animals, stored, frozen tissue from the original donor was tested and found positive for the same strain of rabies that killed the recipient in Maryland. The other recipients, still alive, have received rabies vaccine and immunoglobulins. Another point of this problem is that drugs given to prevent tissue rejection also suppress the immune system, leaving the recipient vulnerable to infection.[4] Who knew?

Psittacosis (Ornithosis)

This is a worldwide infectious disease of psittacine birds—parrots, parakeets, macaws, budgerigars, cockatiels, gulls, and others, are readily transmissible to us. Of course those at highest risk are bird lovers who maintain them as pets, and pet store attendants. The infecting organism is a Chlamydia, an intracellular parasite that can only grow when inside our cells; similar to viruses, but not a virus.

Recently, birds other than the psittacines have been found to carry Chlamhydia: chickens, turkeys and ducks are potential transmitters. That is why the disease is also referred to as Ornithosis. Ornis is Latin for bird.

How is this organism passed? Inhaling bird excreta is the well-established pathway. Given that turkeys and ducks are involved, poultry industry workers can be a major risk group. Inflammation of the lungs along with pneumonia and hemorrhaging are diagnostic features. Nevertheless, there are fewer than a hundred cases annually in the US.

Ebola Hemorrhagic Fever

Ebola's name derives from the Ebola river, in the Democratic Republic of the Congo, where it was first identified in 1976. Unquestionably, this is a serious multi system episode in which the vascular system sustains great disruption along with multi-organ failure, resulting in extensive blood loss along with debilitating watery diarrhea.

Infection with this highly virulent virus is deadly. The fatality rate is upwards of seventy percent. Blood loss is so severe that death is rapid. Direct contact with an infected person's skin, blood, saliva, bloody vomit, urine, and/or feces, as well as clothing and bedding is not just sufficient but necessary to transmit the virus, initiating further illness and death.

As of 2012, the bites of the large African hammer-headed fruit bats appear to be the vehicle of virus transmission. However, definitive proof awaits isolation and identification of live virus particles from these bats.

Currently, there is neither a preventive vaccine nor a treatment for this mortal infection, although the drug ZMapp, is in development and vaccines are being pursued, these take time to produce and test in both animals and humans.

ZMapp, a product of Mapp Biopharmaceuticals, San Diego, California, is a form of immunotherapy using antibodies to bind to the virus protein that seeks to stimulate an infected persons immune system to attack the virus. It brings immunoglobulin G, IgG, into play to destroy the virus. ZMapp is undergoing clinical testing to determine if in fact it can subdue Ebola. Unfortunately, even for emergency use, there is precious little ZMapp available, as the antibodies are grown in tobacco plants (Nicotinia tobaccum) which take months to mature during the growing season. Consequently, cases and deaths will continue to increase.

"Dozens Die as Ebola Outbreak Hits Guinea," was a recent headline marking the 86 cases and 60 deaths during the February and March 2014, outbreak. According to health officials on site, these numbers are grossly underestimated, as cases are difficult to locate in the dense jungle, and many go unreported by families to avoid public attention and shunning. Nevertheless, the numbers seemed to suggest a local affair that could be contained. That notion soon took leave.

Guinea, a West African country where cases and deaths are piling up, sits between Sierra Leone and Liberia to its southwest, borders on the Atlantic Ocean. It is the world's ninth poorest country where cholera and measles have been rampant, as their medical system is barely existent: lacking infrastructure, medical personnel-physicians and nurses, resources, and is further encumbered by a communal culture fostering wholesale infections. In an early attempt to quell this outbreak the government banned the eating of Bat soup, as fruit Bats are a known virus reservoirs and bat soup is a popular staple and a favorite dish. Butchering bats for table is an extremely high-risk enterprise, but common and difficult to prevent[5]

By early August 2014, WHO had confirmed 930 deaths, a ten-fold increase, but the rush of new cases is driving the deaths into the thousands. Cross-border transmission between Guinea, Sierrra Leone and Liberia is occurring rapidly as people scramble to leave their infected areas taking their infections with them, and they are difficult to track. Consequently the numbers of cases and deaths continues to increase as those infected rapidly shuttle the virus to new, unsuspecting susceptible populations. Nothing new under that sun.

By the end of October, WHO had documented five thousand deaths, yet another ten-fold increase and nine thousand new cases, in these three countries. These cases and deaths were severely out-running all attempts to cap the epidemic. The people simply would not change their behavior. Their culture required all family members be present at preparations for burial that required washing the body of their dead relatives, placing them at immediate risk of contacting virus-laden body fluids, clothing and bedding. Entire families and even villages perished.

With the ever increasing rate of cases and deaths in these West African countries, WHO believes that by the end of 2014 there could well be 50 thousand or more deaths:not unrealistic numbers, but becoming a catastrophe of unimaginable proportions. If the virus gains entry to a densely populated city such as Lagos, the capital of Nigeria, it could resemble the massive deaths of the medieval plagues: a horror to contemplate.

Ebola should never have left Africa. But it has. To keep it from gaining leverage in Europe and the United States, the epidemic must be controlled in West Africa, and individuals seeking to leave their West African countries by plane must be isolated there for a minimum of fifteen days to assure that they are not incubating the virus. Simply taking their temperatures before boarding flights to Europe and the US is a flawed procedure. Not to be trusted. Individuals from West African nations who have not been isolated and arrive at European and US airports, should be quarantined for fifteen days, otherwise they could become risks to those around them should they develop Ebola. Unfortunately these isolation procedures will not prevail as business trumps health.

Brucellosis (Undulant Fever, Malta Fever)

We humans pick up and become infected with the Brucella bacterium by ingesting contaminated food or water. We can also inhale it, or the bacterium can enter via skin wounds. However, the most common route is by drinking contaminated or unpasteurized milk. Most cases, and there have been fewer than a hundred a year in the US, have occurred among slaughter house workers, meat inspectors, animal handlers and veterinarians.

Most cases have been reported from California, Texas, Florida, and Virginia. Brucellosis is more of a concern in Portugal, Spain, France, Italy, Greece, North Africa and Turkey, where animal control regulations are less strenuous, which suggests that tourists need be cautious about eating cheeses made of unpasteurized milk.

What kind of disease is this? Flu-like symptoms, for the most part, are the first to appear along with muscle and backaches, followed by arthritis, and testicular swelling in men. Depression and meningitis can also occur. Mortality is low. This is not a souvenir you want to bring back from a vacation abroad.

Wound/Parenteral Infections

Wound infections either accidental or purposeful, can occur via nails, thorns, gunshots, stabbings and hyperdermic needles, especially dirty ones, passed from person to person by drug users and abusers, all punctures of one sort or another.

Puncture wounds often introduce Clostridial organisms which live comfortably in soil, and in the intestinal tracts of cattle and in humans where oxygen levels are low. Ergo, deep wounds are to their liking. Tetanus is the model illness for puncture wounds, with its painful contractions of neck and jaw muscles, from whence cometh lockjaw.

Infection may occur whenever a laceration or puncture becomes contaminated with soil. When Kevin Ware, a University of Louisville basketball player fell on the court during the 2013, NCAA March Madness basketball game, his leg twisted so badly that his fibula, the smaller of the two bones of the leg, between the knee and ankle, simply tore through his skin, creating a double open fracture. It was awful. When his leg was surgically set, he wanted to leave the hospital and get back to his team. His surgeons, concerned about the possibility of a Clostridial infection, kept him a day longer to assure that an infection was not incubating. Ware's contact with the floor, with the bone protruding, could easily have been an entry point for the Clostridium. He was safe, and free to go. No problem.[6]

Another toxin producer, *Clostridium perfringens*, also thrives in soil. When blood-carrying oxygen to tissues is interrupted by a puncture wound, ischemia can develop, with tissues becoming oxygen depleted, progressing to necrosis and tissue destruction. Should Clostridium perfringens or tetani be in the neighborhood, gangrene can follow. If not treated quickly, systemic shock, kidney failure and death results.

Healthy tissues do not host these organisms, nor are they invasive. They must be brought into deep tissue by some form of puncture.

An accidental, or unintended parenteral intrusion can occur when a contaminated syringe, needle or fluid used for an intravenous drip is placed in the arm of a hospitalized patient. The parenteral route is not, repeat, not your typical portal of entry. It is a means of circumventing normal portals. By injection, a variety of organisms can be delivered to tissues, especially the blood stream, to be conveyed throughout the body, where they simply do not belong, nor would they be found, and could not get to. Of course, such distribution can become a medical emergency, requiring rapid attention to avoid illness or death.

With such an array of routes into our bodies, all six of them, it is understandable that there is ample opportunity to create havoc. Nevertheless, as is also obvious, we have not only survived, but thrived and flourished. Again, the numbers provided earlier remind us that infectious disorders are disarmingly few, remaining low on the illness and death dealing totem pole. That ought to be a source of comfort in our manifestly confused world.

Moreover, yet another source of comfort comes from a splendid piece of work done by a team of scientists from the University of Colorado, at Boulder. In the first sentence of their publication they indicate that "the microbiological quality of air we encounter daily, and depend upon absolutely, is a little-addressed societal concern." They then inform us that, "the goal of this study was to determine the composition and diversity of microorganisms associated with bioaerosols in a heavily trafficked metropolitan subway environment." Dr. Norman R. Pace and his team studied New York City's, with its billion-plus riders annually. And what did they find down under in those 137 miles of subterranean tunnels and tracks? Analysis of subway air found not a sign nor hint of pathogenic microbes. This has to come as a shocking piece of news to those who believe that microbial nasties lurk everywhere. Of course microbes are everywhere, but nasties are not. The researchers found that subway air was similar to outdoor air, containing a mix of microbes normally found on our skin, in soil and water. Nothing exotic. Furthermore, this in-depth study establishes a baseline, data highly useful for bioterrorism surveillance. Now that the normal everyday microbial quality is known, sudden changes in numbers and types can be appropriately interpreted by Homeland Security. With this good news, frequent subway riders should breath easier. [7]

Then there is the asymptomatic carrier, an individual who usually doesn't know that she or he is shedding pathogenic microbes in their stools, which can place others at risk. Let's we deal with that.

The Carrier

During the first decade of the twentieth century, there were thousands of cases of Typhoid Fever, and hundreds of deaths. Most cases occurred from drinking sewage contaminated drinking water, or eating food prepared by food handlers, cooks, who were shedding the Typhoid bacterium, Salmonella typhi. This is not at all like the Salmonella of food borne Salmonellosis.

Individuals can harbor pathogens and transmit them to others unknowingly, inadvertently, as they are symptomless; that's the problem. Not a sign or symptom of illness. These passers, or spreaders, as they are called, are generally known to public health authorities as carriers, asymptomatic carriers, who can initiate local epidemics: especially if, or when, they become cooks in private homes or food handlers in restaurants.

Mary Mallon, aka, Typhoid Mary, a name living in infamy, can be our archetypal, quintessential embodiment of the asymptomatic carrier, as she was the first person in the US to be identified as such. How did Mary Mallon's work experience foster our public health education?

Mary Mallon arrived in New York City from Ireland in 1874, at age fifteen. For her first quarter-of-a century little is known of her whereabouts or activities. Things were about to change for her. Apparently she was a good cook.

Charles Henry Warren hired Mary in 1906 to be the family cook during their summer vacation at Oyster Bay

Long Island, New York. During that summer one of Mr. Warren's daughters developed Typhoid Fever.

As the Warren's had planned to vacation at Oyster Bay, and in that very house for several summers, they wanted to be sure that the house was not a problem. Consequently they hired George Soper, a civil engineer, to track down the source of their daughter's illness.

Soper quickly zeroed in on Mary. He traced her employment history from 1900 to 1907. Interestingly, she had been a cook in several homes and in each she left before typhoid appeared. She was never suspected. In fact she had worked for several families and had been the cause of twenty-two cases of typhoid fever, with one death.

Soper confronted Mary in the Warren kitchen and pointedly asked her for a sample of her urine, feces and blood. Mary was horrified. Picking up a carving knife and pointing it at him, and moving toward him, he beat a hasty retreat.

Soper then went to see Dr.Herman Biggs, Head of N.Y. City's Health Department. Biggs agreed to have Mary picked up, sending several police and an ambulance to fetch her forcefully to Willard Parker Hospital, to obtain the necessary samples. It was a struggle.

At the hospital, where she was being restrained against her will, and in fact, illegally, samples were obtained and typhoid bacilli were found in her stool samples.

Health Department officials pleaded with her to undergo Cholesystetomy, removal of her gall bladder, where the bacilli were tucked away, and all but impossible to extricate, but she refused, saying, "The Health Department just wants to use that way of murdering me." Of course, this was way before the availability of Penicillin, the first antibiotic to be discovered, and used in the early 1940's. Antibiotics were no guarantee of riddance and surgery would still be required.

Mary was then transferred to an isolated cottage on North Brother Island, in the East River, off 138th street, near the Bronx. Over the next two years, 120 of her 163 stool samples proved positive for typhoid bacilli. Obviously she had been passing the microbe by her hands as she prepared the families meals.

In 1909, after being held at North Brother Island, and without a trial, and having committed no crime, she sued the Health Department. Although the Judge hearing the case held in favor of the Health Department, Mary agreed never to work as a cook again, and was released.

Five years after her release, in 1915, a typhoid outbreak occurred in the Sloan Maternity Hospital in Manhattan. Twenty-five people became ill: two died. Evidence rapidly pointed to the cook, a Mrs. Brown, who was Typhoid Mary, as an article in the Journal of the American Medical Association had dubbed her. Mary had simply changed her name and had continued to work as a cook, despite her pledge.

This time she was again confined to North Brother Island, but under careful supervision, where she remained for twenty-three years. During that time Mary had a stroke, and died at age 79 in 1938.[8]

All told, Mary had been the point source, the cause of 51 typhoid cases and three deaths.

Since her death there have been some 4,500-5,000 new cases of typhoid, with about three percent becoming carriers. The New York City Health Department keeps a watchful eye on known carriers making sure they don't work in restaurants. I suspect most health departments are on similar alert.

Given the paucity of local outbreaks of typhoid, carriers seem few and well controlled.

A Selection of Delinquents

As we have seen there are opportunities to invade, infect, and sicken us. But of the vast thousands of microbes, germs, only about 1,100 types are potential pathogens. So we have:

538 types of bacteria

317 types of fungi

208 types of virus

57 types of protozoa

However, and this a consequential however, only about 100 of these are human pathogens, and of these 100, some 60, possibly 70 percent are zoonotic. We and the many animals around us, are inextricably tied together. I've selected a number that have either been irritating us since biblical times or before, or those that have emerged more recently co-evolving along with the rise of mammals. We begin with Leprosy, a disfiguring malady older than the Hebrew bible.

Leprosy has the distinction of being the first human disease to be related to a microbe. To avoid the frightful images leprosy conjures, the ailment is now referred to as Hansen's disease, named for Gerhard Henrik Amauer Hansen, a Norwegian physician who discovered the rod-shaped organisms in 1873, in skin nodes. That was four years before Robert Koch discovered the Anthrax bacillus in 1877; the first germ found to be the cause of an animal disease. It is the rare individual who knows that Dr. Hansen was the first to make the connection between human illness and microbes.

Norway of the 1860's was a hotbed of Leprosy, with Lepers so disfigured and deformed, they were outcasts, and Bergen, Norway, was the European center for leprosy research. Is that unbelievable? It was into this milieu that young Hansen, a newly minted physician, took up his practice, believing leprosy was caused by a specific germ, when all other physicians were certain it was either the consequence of a miasma (noxious vapor), heredity, or god's visiting an evil upon sinners. Not only was it none of these, but was solely the work of the slow-growing Mycobacterium leprae, a close cousin of Mycobacterium tuberculosis, the second human disease found to be caused by a bacterium.

Leprosy, from the Greek, Lepra, meaning scaley, is a chronic illness, forming thick, scaley nodules on the face is not highly infectious, nor communicable, taking up to twenty years to appear. It is transmitted from person to person, with difficulty, via droplets from nose and mouth during prolonged close contact. Untreated leprosy (yes, it can be successfully treated) can lead to progressive and permanent damage to nerves, causing numbness leading to loss of fingers, toes, nose, and ear lobes, the coolest parts of the body.

The unfortunate problem with the leprosy bacillus, and therefore the disease, is its total inability to be grown in artificial media under laboratory conditions. That inability prevented development of a preventive vaccine and a cure, as it languished in the shadows of medical science.

Today, leprosy is not the leprosy of antiquity. Leprosy is curable and treatment provided in the early stages averts disability. Multidrug therapy has been made available freely to all patients worldwide by the World Health Organization, WHO, since 1995. The triple drug combination kills the pathogen and cures the patient.

According to WHO, reports from 105 countries estimate the registered prevalence of leprosy at the beginning of 2012, was 181,941 cases. The number of incident, or new cases detected during 2011, was 209,075, compared to 228,474 in 2010. Most of the affected are in Brazil, India, Indonesia, and the Philippines. Norway is no longer the problem it was.

As for the US, 150-200 new cases are reported annually. Of these, thirty percent are due to hunters trapping and eating the naturally infected nine-banded Armadillos in Texas and Louisiana, where these burrowing, armored creatures abound. Armadillos are the only animal known to either harbor the bacillus, or in which it can be inoculated and grown under lab conditions.

The best news arrived in January 2013. American researchers at the Infectious Disease Research Institute, IDRIS, of Seattle, Washington, developed a simple, rapid, and perhaps most important, an inexpensive test that can detect the presence of the Mycobacterium well before signs appear. By the way, medically, a sign is objective evidence of disease- a rash, swelling, fever, and in the case of leprosy, numbness. A symptom is subjective indication of disease; pain, headache, anxiety, insomnia, feelings, physicians or nurses cannot see, but surely need to know.

This new test requires only a single drop of blood mixed with a developing reagent in a plastic plate. The development of two dark lines on the side of the plate is a positive test: Leprosy present. A number is also obtained which indicates the person's bacterial burden. Because of the large number of lepers in Brazil, a Brazilian diagnostic company, OrangeLife, is manufacturing the test kit with the proviso that the price of the kit will be one dollar or less![9]

Furthermore, IDRIS is developing a vaccine from the fusion of four key leprosy proteins. They appear to be far enough along to have scheduled a human trial by the end of 2013. With a rapid test available for early detection, and the development of a preventive vaccine, together these could spell the end of leprosy. Is this unbelievable!? Consigned to the dustbin of history after 4,000 years. What a victory for humankind!

Plague

"Oh east is east, and west is west, and never the twain shall meet." Many of course will recognize the opening line of Rudyard Kipling's Ballad of East and West. I've always loved that lyrical poem, but apparently he hadn't heard of the Silk Road.

East and west were meeting, as well as trading and transmitting microbes and their diseases for well over 2,000 years along the vast expanse of trails, paths and camel tracks known as the Silk Road. This 4,000 mile network of interlinking trade routes connected the Far East, especially China and southern and western Asia with the Mediterranean world and Europe; primarily due to the lucrative trade in Chinese silk.

Travel along these trade routes increased and became more organized as the Romans developed a hunger for silk from Han dynasty China, which they received from their eastern neighbors, the Parthians. Trade and contagion, the twins of disease transmission, misery and death.

The first recorded pandemic, the Justinian plague, named for the sixth century Byzantine emperor, Justinian, began in 541 ce, and reached Constantinople (Istanbul) on grain ships from Egypt, where it was first reported near Suez. The question that rises here asks, why did the plague occur at this time having not arisen anytime before. New evidence suggests that the eruption of the Krakatoa volcano on the island of Java was so forceful, having the energy of 13 thousand atom bombs that it sent so much sulfur dioxide into the atmosphere that it was carried northward to the north pole and southward to the south pole. Nothing like that had ever occurred.[10]

The sulfur dioxide in contact with water vapor formed huge clouds of sulfuric acid whose particulates blocked sunlight from reaching the earth, creating a type of nuclear winter, killing great numbers of plants, animals and people. When this winter finally subsided, among the living things that began to grow were rats;rats carrying fleas. These rat populations stowed away on the many ships bringing grain from Alexandria to Constantinople (Istanbul) and the empire of Justinian. Over the next two hundred years bubonic plague helped dismantle the Roman Empire, killing millions as the plague and its rats moved around the Mediterranean, and into the European heartland. For the following six hundred years, the Plague remained localized and dormant.

In June 2013, researchers at German (Mainz & Munich) and Norwegian (Oslo) universities reported on their testing teeth removed from two 6th century skeletal remains from the early medieval Ascheim-Bajuwarenring cemetery, Ascheim, Bavaria, finally laying to rest the ongoing controversy about whether the plague had crossed the Alps, and the specific microbial cause of the Justinian plague. Their results based on genotyping the skeletal DNA teeth and sequencing genomes of Yersinia pestis, clearly showed that the plague had crossed the Alps and severely affected local populations in what is today's Bavaria. They also proved that this first plague was due to Yersinia pestis. End of controversy.[11]

Then the Black Death struck. Starting in central Asia in 1338, plague spread by land on the Silk Road, reaching the Crimea and the shores of the Black Sea by 1346.

Accompanying the flow of silk, spices and grains along the Silk Road were black rats and their fleas. Rats were attracted to the human and animal waste ditched by the caravans, along with the grains, making it easy for fleas to spread from one infected rat population to another. Rats were also able to stash themselves away in the bales of goods the caravans carried.

As the plague marched across Europe, entire towns were wiped out. In many of them, there were not enough survivors to bury the dead. Of course, as people fled, they took their plague with them, along with rats and their fleas. "The Great Dying," as it is often called, continued for three long, miserable years, during which time, one person in three died: some maintain that the total reached fifty million, changing the face of Europe forever. Children appeared unperturbed by the disruption around them, often holding hands, dancing in a circle, and singing:

Ring around the rosies

a pocket full of posies

Ashes, ashes

we all fall down.

The rhyme does suggest the contradictions: life is lovely, but death is sure, swift and nearby.

The third and modern plague also began in China. This time in the 1860's and appeared in Hong Kong in 1894. Over the next 20 years, it spread to port cities around the world by rats on merchant ships, causing another ten million deaths.

It was during this period that Alexandre Emile Jean Yersin, a French physician was sent to Hong Kong to investigate the outbreak there that had the city in turmoil. Yersin arrived on June 15th, 1894, and set up a makeshift lab in a ramshackle, thatched-roof hut. Five days later, on the 20th, he found the causative organism in an infected patient's swollen bubo that he had sliced open, a medical tour de force, if ever there was one. In his honor, the pathogen Yersinia pestis bears his name.

Plague signs and symptoms depend on how a person is exposed to the germ. Exposure can take one of three routes: bubonic, septicemic, or pneumonic. Individuals bitten by an infected flea develop the bubonic form, with sudden fever, headache, chills, weakness and one or more swollen, tender and painful lymph nodes-called buboes, in the arm pit, neck, groin, or thigh. Bubo, comes to us from the Latin bubo, meaning swelling, and the Greek, bubon, meaning groin, where it most often develops. The bacteria multiply in the lymph nodes. If treatment is not instituted quickly, with appropriate antibiotics, the bacteria can spread around the body, with death not far away.

Black death gets its name from the color of blood pooled in the skin that changes from red, to purple, to brown and black, buboes.

Septicemic plague can develop from untreated bubonic plague, or as a primary invasion, with similar early signs and symptoms, but now there is bleeding into the skin and other organs as the bacteria moves throughout the body via the blood stream. The skin turns black and dries, especially on fingers, toes and nose. At this point, death is rapid.

The pneumonic form develops from inhaling infectious droplets, or may develop from untreated bubonic or pneumonic plague after the bacteria spread to the lungs. Shortness of breath is a consequence of pneumonia, with chest pain, cough, and bloody or watery mucus. Respiratory failure and shock may follow. This is the most serious form of the disease and the only form that can spread from person to person, via those infectious droplets.

So, what is the current state of plague in the US today? Plague arrived in the US in 1900 aboard rat-infested steamships from the Orient. The last urban plague epidemic occurred in Los Angeles from 1924 to 1925. It then spread from urban to rural rats and rodents, and became entrenched in our western states. Between 1900 and 2010, 999 confirmed cases occurred. Another few may have occurred that were not reported. Eighty percent of these cases were bubonic, and most occurred in two regions: northern New Mexico, northern Arizona and southern Colorado, and California, southern Oregon and western Nevada.

Over the past twenty years, some 6 to 8 cases have occurred each year, with fifty percent occurring among those 12 to 45 years old.

Around the world, most cases occur in central Africa, and about one to two thousand cases are reported yearly to WHO. These cases occur primarily in small towns and agricultural areas.

The bubonic plague of the 14th century remains an unwholesome memory.

One day on the road in the English countryside, a Clergyman happened to meet Plague. "Where are you going?" asked the Clergyman. "To London," responded Plague, "to kill a thousand." They chatted for a few minutes and went their separate ways. When they chanced to meet again, some weeks later, the Clergyman inquired, "I thought you were going to kill a thousand, how is it that two thousand died?" "Ah yes," replied Plague. "I killed only a thousand. Fear killed the rest."
– Anon

Cholera

A recent account in the New York Times provided the final, and grim account of the remains of 57 young Irish boys in a mass grave, hard by the SEPTA railroad tracks in Malvern, Pennsylvania.

Our story begins, they tell us, in June 1832, when their ship, the John Stamp, brought some 120 young boys into Philadelphia harbor from Derry, in northern Ireland. Not long after, a Mr. Duffy, a local contractor for the Philadelphia and Columbia Railroad, had them at work digging and shoveling, preparing the ground for a rail line. So far, so good. Until. Until the summer of 1832, brought Cholera to a panicked Philadelphia. As the New York Times has it, "Cholera struck the work site by way of a contaminated creek running past the men's crude living quarters." Apparently a quarantine was imposed upon the group of young men, and a number were killed, shot, trying to violate the quarantine. Prejudice against

Irish Catholics contributed to the denial of care to the workers. A bit later, all dead from Cholera, they were interred in a deep, mass grave beside the tracks, and they were forgotten—until 1907 when an enclosure of massive granite blocks was erected surrounding their burial site. Then, not quite a hundred years later, a group of Immaculata College students and their faculty began digging at the site. As they dug, typically Irish artifacts emerged, along with bodily remains.

Today, an historic marker identifying the Duffy's cut mass grave speaks to their deaths. The remains of a body, thought to be young John Ruddy, age 18 at the time, has been returned to Ireland and was properly buried in a church cemetery in Ardara, near Donegal.[12]

We will return to the 1832 Cholera epidemic in America, but first we harken back to the early days of Cholera.

Seven Cholera pandemics have swept around the world since it first exploded out of India's Ganges River delta in 1817. By the 1820's immigration and trade had carried the disease to Southeast Asia, central Asia, the Middle East, eastern Africa, and the Mediterranean coast. British records estimate that hundreds of thousands died, including thousands of their soldiers. By mid1823, it had disappeared.

The second pandemic, 1829-1849, (a pandemic is an epidemic that can last for as long as decades, and moves across continents) was another Indian contribution, reaching Russia by 1830 then continuing into Finland and Poland. A two-year outbreak in England claimed 22 thousand lives.

In the 1830's it reached the US killing some 5,000 in New Orleans. Philadelphia was hit in July 1832. Deaths were high all through August with over a hundred dying every day. The peak days were August 6th and 7th, accounting for 312 cases and 144 deaths. The disease ran its course by September, as thousands fled the city, many taking their Cholera with them. Yet another way of transmitting diseases, which continues to occur.

Irish immigrants fleeing poverty and the potato famine carried Cholera to North America. On their arrival in the summer of 1832, 1,220, died in Montreal and another thousand across Quebec. Another outbreak across England and Wales in 1848 killed 52,000.

In 1849, Cholera spread again from Irish immigrant ships, through the Mississippi region killing another 3,000 in New Orleans, and 4,500 in St. Louis. Also in that year, after four years in office, President James K. Polk our eleventh president, went south on a good will tour, contracted Cholera and died at his home in Nashville. President Zachary Taylor, the twelfth president, died in 1850, after only one year in office, of a raging gastroenteritis, that may have been Cholera, but remains undetermined.[13]

The third pandemic, considered the most deadly, was yet again another Indian benefaction devastating large swaths of Asia, Europe, North America and Africa. But 1854 was a banner year, although 23 thousand died in England. It was that year, that Dr. John Snow, a thinking man's physician who had been studying and analyzing death rates from two British Cholera episodes, inferred the existence of a "Cholera poison," transmitted by contaminated water. He noted too, that the cause of the disease must be able to multiply in water, and that consecutive cases suggested a means of transmission, more so than could be accounted for by coincidence. He also tells us "that diseases which are communicated from person to person are caused by some material which passes from the sick to the healthy."[14] Of course he was right, but he couldn't know why. Not in 1854. But he was close. Furthermore, "the morbid material is ingested through the mouth, multiplies in the gut, and is excreted with feces." Brilliant! An incandescent insight. Nevertheless, few, if any physicians believed that Cholera was a water borne disease. Nonetheless, 1854 had to be seen as a good year, although Cholera struck

Chicago, taking 3,500 lives, 5.5 percent of its total population.

Where did the fourth wave, 1863-1879, arise? From the Bengal region of India and from which Indian Muslim pilgrims visiting the holy cities of Mecca and Medina, spread Cholera to the Middle East. From there it was carried to Europe and North America. We are informed that 30 thousand of the 90 thousand pilgrims died of the disease.

The fifth pandemic, 1881-1896, also originated in the Bengal region, and this time in addition to taking in Asia, Africa and South America, hit hard in France, Germany and Russia, taking upwards of 200 hundred-thousand lives there, than rolling into Japan, where another 100-thousand died. Clearly no country was exempt, including 50-thousand deaths in the US.

With the arrival of the 20th century, the sixth wave took the lives of more than 800-hundred thousand in India. In the US, the last outbreak occurred from 1910 to 1911, when the steamship Moltke brought infected Italian immigrants with eleven deaths, from Naples to New York City. By 1923, Cholera had receded from most of the world, but many cases were still present in India.

Unlike the six pandemics, the seventh, 1961-2010, came roaring out of Indonesia, ravaging populations across Asia and the Middle East. By 1973, it had arrived in Italy. In 1994, it killed thousands in the Democratic Republic of the Congo, and in 2008, attacked Zimbabwe, and by the end of 2008, there were 12-thousand cases across Africa.

Finally, this last pandemic appears to have receded after dealing a mighty blow to the Haitians, sickening some 100-thousand, and killing 22 thousand, possibly more. And that was after a volcanic eruption devastated the island, killing more than 200-thousand. Perhaps the most disturbing thing about Cholera's deadliness in Haiti was the fact that there had not been an epidemic in Haiti for a hundred years, and there was no reason for it to occur in 2010. How did this happen? The volcanic eruption with its tremendous wreckage and loss of life, brought in Nepalese army troops to help the Haitians, and with them came the introduction of a south Asian variant of the microbe, Vibrio cholerae, that the Nepalese introduced via their feces into the drinking water, and the epidemic was off and running, that exemplifies the on-going threat of this two-hundred year-old scourge[15]

So, what is this Cholera infection? Obviously Cholera is an acute intestinal infection causing profuse watery diarrhea, vomiting (the body, in its wisdom, is trying to rid itself of the bacterial toxin, from both ends) circulatory collapse and shock. It is an extremely virulent infection that can kill in hours. There is no such thing as living with cholera. You either die quickly, or somehow recover.

Brackish and seawater generally are natural environments for the Vibrio, but they rarely exist by themselves in a body of water. It has been discovered that V.cholera cells colonize the surfaces of tiny invertebrates, crustaceans, called Copepods. These Copepods depend on the Vibrios to eat through their chitinous egg cases, releasing their young: a mutually beneficial relationship. But that's only part of the story. These bacteria from human feces can also attach themselves to the hard-chitinous shells of crabs, shrimp, clams and oysters, which can imbibe them, with the gallons of water they take in daily, that can be a source of infection when these seafoods are eaten raw or undercooked.

Cholera is most often found and spread in areas with inadequate water treatment systems, poor sanitation, and inadequate hygiene.

It can now be successfully treated by replacement of lost fluids with glucose/saline solutions either orally or by IV rehydration. If done promptly, less than one percent of patients die.

For the US, water-related spread has been eliminated by modern water and sewage treatment. However, travelers to parts of Africa, Asia, India and Latin America are at risk. Caution is called for.

For 2011, the number of Cholera cases reported to WHO was 589,854 from 58 countries, with 7,816 deaths, but these are considered way under-reported. Estimates suggest the true figures are closer to 3-5 million cases and 100-200 thousand deaths annually. If the seventh wave is believed to be over, are these huge numbers the beginning of an eighth wave? In today's world, it is suggested that smugglers pass Cholera around. In fact, there is no way for smugglers to cause that many cases. What ever it is, won't be unknown for long.

Toxoplasmosis

Can cat poop be sequestered? It certainly needs to be, if Toxoplasmosis is to be curbed. We'll pursue that. Most people who become infected with Toxoplasma gondii, the single-cell parasite that induces Toxoplasmosis, are not aware of it. Some who have the condition may feel as though they have the "flu", with swollen lymph glands, muscle aches and pains that last a month or more. So just what is this curious illness?

It is estimated that more than 60 million people in the US, women, children and men carry the organism but few have either signs or symptoms as our immune system tamps down the parasites ability to cause overt illness. Nevertheless, pregnant women and those with compromised immune systems are at increased risk as a Toxoplasma infection can cause serious health problems. Severe Toxoplasmosis can cause brain damage, and eye problems with blurred vision, reduced vision, tearing and redness, from an acute infection, or one that occurred earlier in life and is now reactivated. Severe cases are more likely to occur in individuals whose immune systems have been weakened by other diseases.

Curiously enough, in the US, Toxoplasmosis is the leading cause of death attributable to food-borne illness. Primary suspects are eating undercooked, contaminated meat, especially pork, lamb, and venison, or eating food that was contaminated by knives, utensils, and using cutting boards that had contact with raw, contaminated meat. Drinking water contaminated with T.gondii is yet another avenue of infection, as is the accidental swallowing of the organisms via contact with cat feces that often contain Toxoplama parasites. How could that happen? All to often it is the consequence of cleaning a cat's litter box when the cat has shed Toxoplasma cells in its feces, or accidentally ingesting contaminated soil, by not washing hands after gardening, or eating unwashed fruit and veggies from a garden where cats have roamed.

Pregnant women can keep their cats, but must be cautious, ensuring their cat's litter boxes are changed daily as the parasite does not become infectious until one to five days after it is shed. It may be best to avoid changing the litter box. Better yet, if someone else can do it for you while wearing disposable gloves and washing hands with soap and water. If possible, keep your cat indoors, and feed it only canned or dried commercial food, or well-cooked table food, not raw or undercooked meats.

Toxoplasmosis is not passed from person to person, except in instances of mother-to-fetus (congenital) transmission, blood transmission or organ transplant. A woman who is newly infected during pregnancy can pass the infection to her fetus. She may not show signs or symptoms but there can be serious consequences for the unborn child: stillbirths, spontaneous abortions, blindness, jaundice and anemia. Most infants who are infected while still in the womb have no symptoms at birth, but may develop them later in life. A small percentage of infected newborns have serious eye or brain damage at birth.

It can't be overstated: cats play a major role in the spread of Toxoplasmosis. They become infected by eating infected rodents, birds, or other small animals. The parasite is then passed in the cat's feces, which can only be seen under a microscope. Kittens are also major contributors to fecal spread, shedding millions of T.gondii cells in their feces for as long as three weeks after infection. Pregnant women want to avoid playing with kittens, and surely not to adopt one, or take in a stray. Simply stated, the only known definitive host for T.gondii, are domestic cats and their relatives.

Recently, a new dimension has been added to T.gondii's bag of tricks. Researchers at Imperial College, London, and Leeds University, Leeds, England, have shown that these parasites may manipulate behavior. Infected rodents become fatally attracted to the odor of cat urine, losing their fear of cats, resulting in their early demise. Apparently T.gondii targets regions in the brain associated with fear, which helps to explain why they lose their fear of cats. These researchers also suggest that we humans may also be compromised causing some cases of schizophrenia.[16]

Researchers at Charles University, Prague, in the Czech Republic, report that personality changes have been documented in cases of Toxoplasmosis, and that these changes become more pronounced over time. This new science of neuroparasitology, as it matures, may offer ideas to pharmaceutical companies looking for new drugs for mental disorders. Meanwhile, let's be mindful of those kitties and cats.[17]

Yet another new concern. A new term, Pollutagen, is being used to describe a disturbing trend: marine life exposed to human microbial pathogens are becoming ill, and dying. Our terrestrial microbes are entering the seas in such profusion that we are seeing new forms of pollution: polluting pathogens, hence pollutogens.

Strangely enough, one of these pollutogens is, yes, T. gondii, which has been killing Dolphins, and sea Otters off the central California coast and Hawaiian Monk seals and Guadaloupe fur seals, in Mexican waters, and the culprits are, you guessed it, those feline house pets–cats.[18]

It is well known that cats can shed as many as 100 million T.Gondii larvae-like parasites in their feces. When cat poop is flushed down a toilet, 70 percent of it enters the sea, and seventy percent of dead sea Otters have been found to have T. gondii which can only come from cat feces. More recently, T.gondii has been isolated from Beluga whales in Arctic waters. It's become a worldwide menace, and needs to be abated. Can that be accomplished? We ask again, can cat poop be curtailed? It surely needs to be. Creativity is called for.

Tuberculosis

Tuberculosis, TB, is the world's leading cause of death, and thirty percent of the world's population is infected. That's nothing new. In 400 bce, Hippocrates wrote that phthisis (Greek, for consumption, and an old term for TB) was the most wide spread disease of the time. Still earlier, ancient Egypt was afflicted. Mummies, from 3,000 to 2400 bce show clear evidence of spinal tuberculosis.

TB is both old and new: new in the sense that its become resistant to our armamentarium of anti-TB drugs, including antibiotics. So, lets back up and have a look at this continuously troubling malady.

As noted earlier, Tuberculosis, TB (short for tubercle bacillus), is the contribution of Mycobacterium tuberculosis, which prefers lung tissue, but can assault kidneys, spine, and brain as well. Person to person spread via airborne droplets from nose and mouth by way of coughs, sneezes and even singing, is its choice means of transmission. Shaking hands won't do it. Neither will kissing, sharing toothbrushes, food or drink, or fomites such as bed linens or toilet seats.

Most importantly, not everyone infected with the Mycobacterium becomes ill. Consequently, there are two TB-related conditions: latent TB, and the frank disease.

Most of us who inhale the bacilli do not become ill; our immune system sees to that. We have no signs or symptoms. We are not, repeat, not infectious, and cannot spread the germ to others. But, yes, there is a but; should our immune system weaken, our latent infection becomes active and the organism multiplies, causing us to become tubercular. And, another but: this is a rare event.

TB's symptoms and signs are classical: chest pains, chronic coughing, and weight loss. This is consumption kicking in. The body is being consumed. Additionally, there is loss of appetite, weakness, coughing up blood, fever and night sweats. Once the microbe is active, chances of developing a frank disease increase if a person has diabetes, an HIV infection, abuses alcohol, or uses illegal drugs.

Two types of tests are available to check for the presence of the bacterium: a skin test and a blood test. A positive reaction to either leads to other tests to determine if there is latency or actual disease. A negative test indicates the body did not react and that there is neither a latent nor an active infection.

Although TB is declining in the US, it has become a serious complication for individuals with HIV/AIDS. The twinning of diseases is being called syndemic, and is currently the leading cause of death among those living with AIDS.

South Africa appears to be in the throes of a syndemic explosion as many individuals with AIDS are also battling multiple-drug resistant TB–MDRTB–as well as, XDRTB, extensively drug resistant TB, which means resistance to four normally powerful anti-tubercular drugs. Its become that difficult; meaning, few options remaining.

Our prisons are hotbeds of TB transmission and frank disease. Five percent of all TB in the US occurs among prison inmates. If they fail to take the drugs that can halt their infections, which many of them fail to do, they become spreaders when released.

Just under eleven thousand frank TB cases, were reported in the US in 2011. Both the case rate and deaths declined from 2010. And since 1990, TB has declined well over fifty percent. Nevertheless, over sixty percent of all TB cases and eighty percent of the MDRTB cases are in recent immigrants who bring their germs with them, and they to, can become spreaders. US rates of MDRTB are inching up as volunteers return from hot-spot countries.

Around the world however, the numbers are grim: a third of the world's population are infected, with a million-and-a half deaths yearly. Eastern European countries are the very hot spots: Belarus, Kazakhstan, and Kyrgyzstan hold the top spots, followed by Estonia, Uzbekistan, Azerbaijan, and Russia. All are the victims of alcoholics, drug users, and HIV patients who infect the wider populations. Western Europe is beginning to see drug resistant TB strains, as populations move from east to west. India is in the midst of a TB epidemic, and with many Indians leaving the country they too, will be spreaders as they enter other countries.

Our 2,000-mile border with Mexico is another hot spot for drug resistant TB. Both California and Texas report increased rates of resistance as Mexicans with TB move across and around the border until they become too weak to work, but in the process become transmitters.

The one bright spot was the recent announcement in January 2013, that the FDA approved the first new TB drug in forty years. Bedaquiline, also known as Sirturo, was developed by Janssen Pharmaceuticals of Titusville, New Jersey, a unit of Johnson & Johnson, for use by MDRTB patients, but requires two years of treatment. Because the Mycobacterium can develop resistance to single drugs used against it, Bediquiline will require combining with other drugs. Although this is a major step forward, TB will not be eradicated easily. In fact, the latest numbers developed by researchers at Harvard Medical School and Brigham & Women's Hospital,

Boston, tell us that about one million children worldwide contract TB annually and that these are under age fifteen. Furthermore, young children are affected differently; some thirty percent develop TB in parts of their body other than their lungs. They also develop the illness faster than adults and become much sicker. It is also evident that they are being infected by their family members. Obviously there is a worldwide pediatric TB epidemic that has been missed.

Staphylococci

"Staph," short for Staphylococcus, from the Greek, grape-cluster or berry, was first identified in 1880, in Aberdeen, Scotland, in pus from a surgical abcess in a knee joint. However, and nevertheless, it is a common bacterium, with over thirty types, and frequently found in the human respiratory tract, and on the skin.

Estimates indicate that twenty percent of us humans are long-term carriers of Staph.aureus. Staph aureus also causes most Staph infections including: Pneumonia, food poisoning, Toxic Shock syndrome-TSS, Bacteremia-blood poisoning, and skin infections.

Staph.aureus is an unusually successful and adaptive human pathogen that can initiate epidemics of invasive disease despite its status as normal skin flora.

Over the past hundred or more years, it has been responsible for outbreaks in hospitals (each year some 500-hundred thousand patients in our hospitals contract a Staph infection) and in the community schools and gyms, and has developed resistance to every antibiotic sent against it. So, it's worth having a look at this collegial/harmful microbe/germ.

Skin infections, pimples and boils are its most common bequests. They may be red, swollen and painful, and at times have pus or drainage. Boils and carbuncles are painful pus-filled bumps that form under the skin

198

when these bacteria infect and inflame one or more hair follicles. These boils–also known as furuncles, can rupture and drain. Carbuncles are clusters of boils that form a connected area of infection under the skin.

Boils can occur anywhere on skin, but appear mainly on our face, neck armpits, buttocks and thighs: hair-bearing areas where we're most likely to sweat or experience friction. And boils usually form when one or more hair follicles become infected with Staph, which enter through a cut, scratch, or other break in the skin. As that occurs, neutrophils, white blood cells, arrive at the site to battle and engulf the Staph, which leads to inflammation and the formation of pus, a mixture of old white blood cells, bacteria and dead skin cells.

To the question, who gets Staph infections, the response is fairly clear: infections are most common among children, teenagers, and young adults. Impetigo, in which the skin becomes red and crusty, accounts for one in ten of all reported skin infections in children.

Staph aureus can cause illness by toxin production as well as by infecting both local tissue and the systemic circulation. Accordingly, transmission can occur in several additional settings as follows:

Gastrointestinal: Staph strains, as we've seen, can cause acute episodes of food poisoning via preformed enterotoxins, as discussed in Chap.6. Food items likely to be infected by these organisms include meat and meat products, poultry and egg products; salads, such as tuna, chicken, egg, potato and macaroni; cream-filled pastries, cream pies, and chocolate eclairs; sandwich fillings, and milk and dairy products. Just about anything we adore. For us it's just a race to see who gets these goodies first. Hey, they love protein as much as we do.

Systemic infections: Staph commonly cause infective endocarditis-inflammation of the lining of the heart in IV drug users, Osteomyelitis, inflammation of bone marrow, as well as sinus infections, and epiglottis- inflammation of the flap covering the entrance to the larynx- in young children.

Nosocomial Infections: Methicillin resistant Staph aureus, MRSA, is a strain of bacteria, now all too frequently implicated in hospital-acquired infections. Risk factors for MRSA colonization or infection in hospital settings include antibiotic use, admission to an intensive care unit, surgical incisions and exposure to infected patients.

Resistance to methicillin is also resistance to penicillin, amoxicillin, oxacillin, Nafcillin, Cloxacillin, and other antibiotics of the same class of organic ring compounds. Resistance to these antibiotics has anointed these Staph with the sobriquet, Superbugs. MRSA has also moved outside of hospitals to the community, where additional risk factors include, again, antibiotic use, more than likely, overuse, sharing of contaminated items, towels, razors, athletic benches, mats, having skin diseases or injuries, poor hygiene, and living in crowded conditions.

MRSA infections are often mild, superficial infections that can be treated successfully with proper skin care and antibiotics. They can also be difficult to treat, progressing to life-threatening blood or bone infections as there are now fewer effective antibiotics to deal with an overwhelming infection.

All penicillin-like antibiotics are organic ring compounds, whose most crucial feature is the beta-lactam ring, essential for their antimicrobial activity. The Cephalosporins, another family of antibiotics, also have the lactam side ring and consequently, this group of antibiotics is also ineffective against the superbugs. With all these no longer useful, Vancomycin, a glycopeptide, a totally different type of chemical, was considered the antibiotic of last resort, and was successful for a time. Unfortunately it, too, is losing ground to the ever-evolving S.aureus.

The race is now on to develop new antimicrobials, chemicals, that either defy resistance, which is almost too much to hope for, or prolong the time to resistance. Failure is not an option.

With that as the high water mark, scientists at Rockefeller University, New York, have turned to viruses that naturally infect bacteria, and have created a drug that mimics a cell-wall bursting viral enzyme called lysins. Epimerox, this new combatant, is to begin its clinical trials within two years, 2015. Should the trials prove safe and effective, the drug could be available for human use by 2020. In the meantime, we can hope that yet another bold advance will enter the fray.[20]

Antibiotics and Antibiotic Resistance

1928 was the year. September, the month, and the Prince of Serendip was in the neighborhood, along with Dr. Alexander Fleming, who had just returned to his lab at St. Mary's Hospital, in London's Paddington area, after a brief vacation.

During his absence agar-containing Petri dishes that he had inoculated a week before with Staphylococcus aureus had grown nicely, covering the entire agar surface: almost. A blue-green mold had floated up from a lab just below his and settled on one of his plates. A clear zone around the mold was obvious. Something produced by the fungus, the mold, had inhibited growth of the Staph around the mold. Other than that clear zone, the Staph were growing luxuriantly on the agar.

In the process of cleaning up his desk space, Fleming almost lost this plate as he placed them in a lysol solution to disinfect them for reuse. That clear area caught his eye.

Using this fungus, he found it effective in killing disease-producing bacteria and noted that it appeared non-toxic to white blood cells and living tissue. But with little chemical background, he could do nothing with the crude substance he called Penicillin, and simply left it, and went on with his other bacterial studies. By the way, under the microscope, to the early Penicillium researchers, the mold resembled a paintbrush, so they named the mold Penicillium from the Latin, Penicillius, meaning paintbrush.

Twelve years after Fleming's accidental discovery, as World WarII was heating up in Europe, two established biochemists/pathologists, Howard Walter Florey, and Ernst Chain, searching for antibacterial substances, rediscovered Fleming's work on Penicillium and carried it forward.[21]

"At 11:00 a.m. on Saturday, May 25th 1940, eight white mice received approximately eight times the minimal lethal number of Streptococci. Four of these mice were set aside as controls, but four others received injections of Penicillin (that they had been able to isolate and purify, either a single injection of ten milligrams, or repeated injections of five milligrams.

All four of the controls, the un-injected mice, had died by 3:30 a.m. On Sunday morning, May 26th, three of the penicillin-injected mice were frolicking nicely. The fourth was not doing so well, but survived for two more days. Animal experiments on a much larger scale soon made it evident that Penicillin had great potential life-saving importance.

In September 1940, an Oxford police constable, Albert Alexander, provided the first test case. Alexander got a scratch on his face working in his rose garden. That scratch, infected with staphylococci, spread to his eyes and scalp. Feverish with a virulent infection he was treated for five days with the only small supply of Penicillin available. He showed steady signs of improvement until the Penicillin ran out–even recovering it from his urine and re-using it. It just wasn't enough. He died. But it showed that Penicillin could be used effectively even for advanced stages of infection.[22]

Fast forward to the US, 1942, and the National Academy of Sciences, Northern Regional Research Laboratory, NRRL. Penicillin had proved itself, and if it was to be used to treat infections and war wounds among the allied troops, it had to be available in large quantities. Two things were necessary: find a strain of Penicillium that would yield far larger quantities of Penicillin than Fleming's original strain, then scale it up for mass production.

At the NRRL, the search was on for a high yielding strain. Women were asked to search the markets in and around Peoria for a blue-green mold growing on fruits or vegetables. One was found growing blissfully on a cantaloupe. It proved to be a great producer of Penicillin. The pharmaceutical companies, Merck & Company, and Charles Pfizer, were capable of large-scale fermentations.

Penicillin was brought to Europe proving to be "just what the doctor ordered," reducing wound infection deaths by over ninety percent.

After the War, Penicillin became commercially available. It's worth remembering that all industrial/ commercial strains of Penicillin used today are descendants of the original strain found growing on that cantaloupe in Peoria.

Trouble was brewing. "Because of its potency and non-toxicity penicillin is the paradigm of antibacterial substances, but it's not without snags."[23] All microbes have developed defenses against harmful environments: chemicals. To protect themselves against penicillin which prevents microbes from synthesizing intact cell walls, without which they simply burst and die, many microbes produce penicillinase, a penicillin-destroying enzyme. Initially the use of penicillin caught the delinquents unaware and killed them–at least most of them. The use of antibiotics exploded. We were using antibiotics excessively and the pathogenic bacteria they were used against, began to change, found ways to neutralize the antibiotics. They were becoming resistant. Antibiotics are supposed to protect us. Why aren't they working? That's the issue. Why aren't they working? Lets back up a moment.

We have taken antibiotics for granted. As Professor Robert L. Dorit of Smith College put it, "We are marinating the world in antibiotics." In the process we've forgotten Charles Darwin and evolution. Recall that in his Origin of Species, he reminded us that, "It isn't the strongest of the species that survives, nor the most intelligent that survives. It is the one that is the most adaptable to change." Our magic bullets are being blunted. As we shall see, pathogenic microbes are becoming bulletproof; they are adapting.[24]

So it is fitting to ask, what are antibiotics, and how do they work? Simply put they are chemicals, drugs, produced by microbes that are being used against them to prevent them from harming us. Yes, indeed, we're using their natural metabolites, their chemicals to fight them. It's warfare. Us against them.

Antibiotics are small molecules that inhibit important functions in microbial cells; functions that impair their survival. All microbes are not equally susceptible to an antibiotic. An infectious organism can require one or more different types to knock it out. These chemicals can disrupt cells in several different ways. Some destroy the cell's walls. Others interfere with enzymes that affect DNA activity. Still others prevent protein synthesis. Several antibiotics block folic acid synthesis needed by many microbes. And some antibiotics block the functioning of metabolic pathways.

Recently it was found that many pathogens have a natural defense against antibiotics, producing an enzyme, a protein, with the curious name NDM-1. This enzyme binds to, and breaks, a chemical bond that antibiotics need to function. Talk about tricks! Currently, the search is on to find a way to block this enzyme's binding capacity. That could become an appropriate new antibiotic. It shouldn't be all that difficult now that the connection is known. Maybe.

Each class of antibiotic seeks out a single major target in a microbial cell—a target that it disrupts. No one antibiotic is, or has been effective against any or all pathogens. Antibiotics have had to be selective–effective against specific germs. Each type or class of antibiotic uses one of these targets, which are usually enzymes that are the movers and shakers of all cells to which the specific antibiotic latches onto–preventing that enzyme from accomplishing its function. It's the old monkey wrench in the works–the Sabot in the machinery. Sabotage.

Our many antibiotics worked just fine for the 60 or so years we've sent them against our microbial enemies, and we were winning: fewer disabling infections and deaths. But they were not totally destroyed. Not all. Each time an antibiotic was used it killed off most of the susceptible cells, but there were a few naturally resistant cells in the mix, and these resistant ones began to grow into larger populations. Therein hangs the tale. The pathogens were gaining on us.

For Professor Roberto Kolter of Harvard Medical School, antibiotic resistance makes perfect sense. It's evolution at work. Evolution in action.[25] It's different with microbes whose generation time varies from twenty minutes to half-an-hour. In that short frame, one cell becomes two, and two four; four become eight, and within twelve hours, with 24 geometric doublings, you've got 8,388,708 bacterial cells; and after 24 hours, 48 divisions, there are multiple billions, with only a single cell! We humans are not like that. For mammals, including us, evolution takes eons of time. Ergo, those invisible microbes, those germs, can perfect evasive tactics in hours, and they have.

Trillions of microbial cells in our bodies are multiplying endlessly, and evolving constantly. The idea, the thought, has to be mind-blowing. Evolve fast enough to meet changing conditions, or become extinct. To avoid extinction, microbes became resistant to our antibiotics. Resistance is simply the failure of antibiotics to destroy all pathogens. It usually begins with a large population of microbes that is confronted by a specific antibiotic. Within that population are a small number of cells, mutants, which are naturally resistant having thrived over millions of years in harsh environments. It's reasonable to assume that they have worked out, developed, mechanisms to defeat a world of chemicals thrown against them. It's worth recalling that we are dealing with living things of only a single cell! How to explain that!

The naturally resistant cells are being selected for over and over, by excessive use of antibiotics, resulting in huge resistant populations. It had to happen. The once susceptible populations have been replaced by resistant populations. Bacterial evolution has inevitably followed Darwin's principles with unforeseen, but inevitable consequences for us.

Darwin suggested that living things contained "variants." He didn't know about genes (not having read Gregor Mendel's account of genes) that can increase, or decrease in frequency subject to selection. So, if Darwin was right, and we were listening, we would have known that antibiotics could do at least two things: totally eliminate some bacteria, if these bacteria had no resistant variants within them, or if some bacteria did in fact contain resistant variants, constant use of an antibiotic would select out for resistance as susceptibles were wiped out, resulting in large and resistant populations. And so it came to pass. Darwin had it right. The goals of life are the same for fleas, fish, foxes, and female humans–males also: avoid death, and reproduce your DNA.

Are we helpless? At the moment we are in trouble. Too many of our antibiotics are unavailing. Moreover, it has now been shown that "the major cause of resistance to Vancomycin is horizontal gene transport-HGT-of a set of genes from other microbes, that remove the antibiotics normal cell wall target, replacing it with an alternative cell wall building block, that carries out the same function, but is not sensitive to Vancomycin. HGT is a major factor for the spread of resistance. Who knew?

Who knew about the inordinate ability of these single-cell creatures to out-maneuver us multicellular creatures! This must give us pause.

Their creativity doesn't end there. Some organisms have developed a pumping system that enables them to pump out an antibiotic as it flows into their cells. Another cunning example of resistance, and the evolutionary desire to live and reproduce.

Too many physicians fearful of losing a patient, or more interested in running a lucrative business than practicing responsible medicine, gave antibiotics to anyone who asked for, or demanded them. This has contributed significantly to resistance.

Furthermore, there is evidence that the excessive use of antibiotics in cattle-cows, sheep, pigs, goats and poultry, to promote growth, to bring them to market faster, to turn a quick profit, and to clean up infections, has transferred antibiotic resistant bacteria and/or genes from these animals to us. Antibiotic residues in animal tissue, appears to be another culprit. Worse yet, livestock use as much as 25 million pounds–13,000 tons–of antibiotics yearly in animal feedstuffs, which are discharged by the animals onto soils and into waterways, eventually finding their way into community water supplies.

Antibiotic resistance, natural selection, and microbial evolution: Darwin would be stroking his long, white beard. He never knew about these wee creatures, and HGT would have come as a complete surprise. So, at this juncture, where are we? Perhaps it is safe to say we are at a crossroads.

If Dr. David Hughes, an Irish geneticist, a Dubliner, working at a genetics institute in Sweden, is correct, when he says, "we are now in a long-term war against the entire bacterial world, which is unfortunate, because not only is the bacterial world overwhelmingly stronger in terms of total numbers of species, and total biomass," but, he goes on to say, "it also contains what is probably the greatest diversity of chemical and enzymatic activity on the planet."[26] That has to be humbling, and we had better be careful and prepared the next time.

No, we are not helpless. At the moment we are in a bit of trouble, but as noted earlier, creative minds in academia are pushing the envelope into new frontiers to remedy this ticklish situation. Pharmaceutical companies have lost interest in developing new antibiotics, as they do not see them as a profit source. Collaboration among our universities, the federal government and the pharmaceutical industry could readily swing the battle our way. Will that happen? It remains an open question. Sadly.

Nosocomial Infections

Hospital acquired infections are just that, infections occurring as a consequence of being a patient in a hospital; a nosocomium, from the Greek, meaning a place where the sick are cared for. And nosocomial is an illness occurring in such a place. Ergo, hospital infections are not a modern phenomenon.

With a hospital infection, it's not unreasonable to expect to remain in the hospital days or weeks longer, incurring additional harm, even death, and of course, additional costs.

According to the CDC, in 2002, their last survey year, under two million infections occurred in our nations 5,724 registered hospitals, with about 100 thousand deaths: a mortality rate of approximately five percent.

High by any set of criteria. But these numbers are estimates, reasonable estimates, nevertheless estimates. More than likely the numbers are higher, given the state of the reporting system. Furthermore, those illnesses and deaths added $28-33 billion to our national health are costs. Such numbers and costs demand attention, and changes are called for.

Having said that, it must also be noted that in 2009, the CDC reported there were 25 thousand fewer blood stream infections (from indwelling catheters), and they also inform us that over the period, 2001-2009, 27 thousand lives were saved and about $1.8 billion in excess costs saved. Now that's a tidy sum, and needs to be extended.

Interestingly, there does not appear to be a predilection for one sex over another. For both male and female hospital infections are an equal opportunity circumstance. No biases there. Nor do hospital infections favor one age group over another. Equality reigns there as well. It's the type of infection that does favor one group over another.

Blood stream infections, followed by pneumonia and urinary tract infections are most common in children. Urinary tract infections are the most commonly acquired infection in adults; usually the result of catheters that can deliver bacteria into areas where they do not belong or, would normally invade.

Hospitals are not hotels, although some people treat them as though they are. Far too many visitors bring their collection of microbes into the hospital on their clothing, shoes, hands, and gifts. Far too many arrive with colds and runny noses. Unfortunately there are no STOP signs for them.

Physicians, nurses, technicians, and porters carry and distribute their organisms especially those who fail to wash their hands with soap, as they move from patient to patient. How many physicians medical students and other assisting personnel are in and out of the hospital, walking the streets near their hospital, wearing their green or blue scrubs, then returning without changing booties, headwear, or uniforms. Again, no STOP signs.

Of course hospitals are loaded with equipment. Some of it is easily cleaned and sterilized; some just cleaned-sanitized, some neither. Then there is the hospital environment itself. Air conditioning can carry microbial particles from floor to floor if filtering systems are not in place or are overloaded. Waste is another potential source of organisms moving about the hospital, if allowed to sit around, or dragged around uncovered. It's worth remembering that we are dealing with workers and their behavior, which runs a wide gamut.

Latex gloves can be a secure barrier against infectious agents, but if not changed frequently, they can become detrimental spreaders. Let's not forget the patients themselves, who can readily contribute germs from their noses, mouths, gastrointestinal tracts and genitourinary systems. Unquestionably, there are good and substantial reasons why hospitals are often loaded with assorted microbes. The fact that there is only a five percent infection rate, that is, five people in a hundred, is remarkable. Nevertheless, this seemingly low number does embrace millions of people. Hospitals can do better—a lot better. As we shall see, the most formidable problems are people problems; problems that can be solved, but inertia holds them back.

Ninety-five percent of pneumonia cases picked up in hospitals are the result of contaminated respiratory ventilators. These devices are devilishly difficult to sterilize, and if not sterilized between patients, infections can circulate from patient to patient. If the numbers are trustworthy, some 75 percent of urinary infections come from urinary tract catheters that have been inadequately cleaned and sterilized, or mishandled after sterilization, during insertion.

Central lines, central venous catheters, are tubes placed in a large neck vein, in the chest, groin, or arm to supply fluids, blood, or medication. These central lines can remain in place for days or weeks, even months, and with that, the risk of infection increases. IV lines, used to deliver medication are used for shorter periods, and thus are less likely to be a problem. That doesn't mean they aren't.

Surgical site infections can occur a month after an operation when the patient is home. If an implant was placed, an infection could take up to a year before becoming evident. Surgical site infections can be superficial, involving only the skin around the site. They can also be a good deal more serious, involving deep tissues, organs, and the implant as well.

In 2002, the CDC published a revised, "Guideline for Hand Hygiene in Health-Care Settings." They concluded that commercially available alcohol-based hand disinfectants were more effective for standard hand washing or hand antisepsis than soap or antimicrobial soaps. They noted too, that alcohol-based liquids or gels were far more bactericidal against antibiotic-resistant pathogens than soaps or antibacterial-containing detergents.

That was a decade ago, but is still pertinent. All too often, however, these Guidelines are overlooked, or ignored. Not used. Hospitals and other health care facilities where microbes are always in abundance should have multiple alcohol-based dispensers on every floor, especially in ICU's and surgical suites. We need not return to Dr.'s Semmelweis, or Lister, with their potent chlorine solutions, that did the job nicely, but frequent use of alcohol-based products, will do as well, offering the additional benefit of softening the skin, keeping it from cracking.

Moreover, alcohol-based disinfectants destroy viruses. Now that's a plus. I use the word destroy, because you can't kill something that is not alive. Recall that a virus can only reproduce itself and cause trouble when inside a living cell where it highjacks the cell's machinery, initiating the process of infection. That dear reader, is also why antibiotics have no effect on viruses: there's nothing on either the outside or inside of a virus for an antibiotic to disrupt. Antibiotics are only effective and useful against living things. Thus, using alcohol-based disinfectants destroys viruses before they reach our cells. Hospitals and other health-related facilities where large numbers of virus are often present, would do well to use alcohol-based disinfectants as a primary line of defense;or attack. After all, 80 percent of all infections are transmitted by hands.

Unfortunately, nosocomial infections are a far greater problem than our communications media suggest. That may be because hospitals are loath to allow rates of infection and deaths to creep out. That information may not make hospitals look good to a public wondering what hospital would be best, when needed. Consider this: if nosocomial infections were considered a disease, which it isn't, with 100 thousand deaths annually, it would be the sixth leading cause of death, following accidents. Unfortunately it's not widely known.

So what does the future hold? Can hospitals substantially reduce their infection and death rates? The short answer is yes, if behavior can be modified, and new and novel developments introduced. So, for example, hospital physicians can now use microbial DNA sequencing, as detailed in Chapter TWO, to trace disease outbreaks in a matter of hours. This can be an absolute game changer, once they get used to the idea and procedure.

Another of these novel developments is the Flexicath, a product of Misgav, an Israeli company[27] that has developed a sterile catheter insertion system that appears to solve the difficult and expensive problem of in-dwelling catheters. The Flexicath is designed to eliminate both airborne and touch contamination during placement, reducing the risk of catheter-related septicemias. Let's remember that catheters are the leading cause of hospital-acquired infections, accounting for some forty percent of all infections. For patients requiring a catheter for longer than a week, 25 percent develop a urinary tract infection, requiring a longer hospital stay, increased risk of a spreading infection, and of course increased cost.

Sharklet Technologies of Aurora, Colorado, produces the Sharklet-patterned urinary catheter, a catheter manufactured with a micro-pattern resembling a shark's skin, which prevents the survival and migration of bacteria into the urinary tract. This micro pattern appears to reduce bacterial attachment to surfaces inhibiting survival, and hindering touch transference. Sharklet is also developing textured films for "high-touch" countertops that can inhibit bacterial growth. The compelling feature is that there is no need for disinfectants. This is a supplement to, not a substitute for standard infection control.[28]

Richmond, Virginia, is the headquarters of EOS surfaces, which has joined with Sentara Health Care and Cupron to evaluate the clinical and economic effectiveness of using antimicrobial copper-based hard surfaces and textiles in hospital settings, which include bed rails, IV poles, and hospital tables. The trial began in April 2013, at Sentara Norfolk General Hospital, and Sentara Leigh Hospital. Sentara, a not-for-profit health system, operates more than one hundred sites serving residents across Virginia and North Carolina. By the end of 2013, a portion of these hospitals will be control facilities without the copper surfacing, while another portion will be enhanced with copper surfaces, and copper-containing textiles to determine the effectiveness of copper in reducing the microbial load of hospital rooms, countertops, lavatories, and furniture. EOS conducted a clinical trial of Cupron-enhanced textiles in Israel that resulted in positive outcomes for chronically ill patients.[29]

The Cupron company investigates novel methods of delivering the antimicrobial properties of copper compounds in textiles, solids and other polymeric materials that may provide protection against a broad range of microbes.[30]

Combating hospital infections is a multi-tiered process. The entire clinical environment needs to come under the microscope. Each of the above developments has a role to play. Clearly, the environment is taking on a new prominence, as it surely should. Nevertheless, it cannot replace hand washing. Hand washing, above all else, is essential. There's no getting around that.

"A few years ago, Long Island's North Shore University Hospital, New York, had a dismal compliance rate with hand washing; under ten percent. After installing cameras at hand washing stations compliance rose over ninety percent, and is still there."[31] If it takes cameras to achieve results, let a thousand cameras bloom. But be sure they too, are disinfected regularly.

As the past Director of Hospital Infection Surveillance, at a major hospital-medical school in Philadelphia, I'm all for the above developments, but when the chips are down, the greatest reduction in infection rates will only come from changes in the behavior of all healthcare personnel.

So, for example, too many hospital-based personnel are eschewing flu vaccine: maintaining it to be an infringement on their liberty. Many are being discharged, fired, as hospitals maintain, and rightly so, that their patients come first, and if they are going to care for their patients, they must be vaccinated. That's not asking too much, and hardly infringes on their liberty.

That's part of the behavior problem. Dr.Peter Pronovost, a critical care specialist at Johns Hopkins, has been trying tirelessly to change physician behavior to reduce infection rates. He has been able to make changes that are being taken up at hospitals across the country, but far too slowly. Therefore, we give him the last word.

According to Dr. Pronovost, many troubling hospital issues can be eliminated, yes, eliminated, by use of checklists. Imagine, something as simple as that. Unfortunately, people, physicians, nurses, med techs, janitors either forget, are in too much of a hurry, or believe they know it all. With his lists in place, in several hospitals, rates of pneumonia, medical errors and IV catheter infections plummeted. Moreover, good teamwork, collaboration, means safer care and fewer infections. At Johns Hopkins hospital, a course in hospital safety has been inaugurated for medical students, which emphasizes the importance of teamwork and collaboration. These physicians of the future are being trained in a way the "old guard" wasn't. For the older traditionalists, independence and confidence were the watchwords. Also unfortunate is the fact, yet another entrenched tradition, that no nurse would tell a physician that he/she was not following the new protocol.

Far too many hospitals have central line blood stream infection rates ten to fifteen times the national average. As we see from our list of leading causes of death, septicemia takes more than 25 thousand lives annually. That need not continue. A checklist can reduce that mightily.

Dr. Pronovost is also quick to note that check lists must be based on evidence, and updated regularly. Unless and until there is public reporting of infection rates, public pressure can't be mounted against hospitals. That too needs to change, and it can be done by state and federal governments withholding payments to hospitals, as well as facing financial penalties for septicemias. Dr. Pronovost is right on target when he says that most infections are preventable. If rates don't come down there should be penalties. "We have the knowledge to prevent infections, but it's just not being used or getting the attention it deserves, and that's astounding."[32]

No more need be said.

Weaponized Microbes: Bioterrorism

It's ugly! It's malignant human mischief, purposely disseminating known, deadly microbial pathogens on unsuspecting populations. That's bioterrorism defined; in a nutshell. A 21st century creation, it is not.

Our kind has known disease since we walked upon the earth and gathered together. We may have thought about sickness as punishment for any number of sins, but we also came early to the idea that we could visit it upon our enemies, for our benefit.

Bioterror weapons disseminate disease-causing bacteria, fungi, and/or their toxins, to harm or kill us and our food, animals and crops. These repulsive agents, as we have seen, are typically found naturally, but we've learned to modify them, alter them, to increase their virulence and make them unresponsive to antimicrobial drugs.

How and when did this begin? Historians tell us that those ancient Romans threw feces into their enemies faces. Although that hardly fits today's scenarios, the fecal/oral route appears to have been compelling early on. During the 14th century, Bubonic plague was used to defeat enemy cities. Hurling of diseased animal carcasses and human cadavers, clothing and bedding, over city walls, or into wells to contaminate water supplies were common. Obviously transmission of disease was well known. Writing in the Bulletin of the History of Medicine, Prof. Joseph Duffy informed us that, "The Colonists were well aware of the potency of smallpox as a weapon against the Indians, and on several occasions deliberate efforts were made to infect the Redmen. One of the instances occurred during the Pontiac Conspiracy in 1763. The British Commander, Sir Jeffrey Amherst, added the following postscript to a letter to Col. Henry Bouquet, "Could it not be contrived to send the smallpox among those disaffected tribes of Indians? We must on this occasion use every stratige in our power to reduce them." Bouquet replied on July 13, 1763, I will try to inoculate the...with some blankets that may fall in their hands, and take care not to get the disease myself."[33] Just how successful Bouquet's attempt was is not known.

Fast forward to 1915 and World War 1. Shortly after the start of the war, Germany launched a biological sabotage campaign in the US, biowarfare against the Russians on the eastern front, and the French on the western.

A German national, Anton Dilger, was sent to the US carrying cultures of the Glanders bacillus, *Burkholderia mallei*, a virulent disease of horses and mules. Dilger set up a lab in his home in Chevy Chase, Maryland, and used stevedores working the docks of Baltimore to infect horses with the Glanders bacillus as they were waiting to be shipped to England. Glanders is just what it sounds like: problems with glands, swollen glands. Horses and mules sicken and die from inflammation of the mucus membranes lining their noses and throats, as breathing becomes impossible.

Although the government was on to Dilger, he managed to slip away to Spain, where he died during the influenza pandemic of 1918. Was it poetic justice that a virus did him in?[34]

Germany and its allies infected French cavalry horses and Russian mules, thereby hindering artillery and troop movements along with supply convoys.

Under President Franklin D. Roosevelt, a biological weapons development program began in 1942, lasting until 1969, when President Richard M. Nixon shut down all programs dealing with offensive use of biological weapons.

In his Executive Order, he declared that, "Biological weapons have massive, unpredictable, and potentially uncontrollable consequences. They may produce global epidemics and impair the health of future generations." Nixon went on to say that, "in recognition of these dangers the United States has decided to destroy

217

its entire stockpile of biological agents and confine its future biological research program to defensive measures, such as vaccines and field detectors."

This declaration was one of the motivating forces for the founding of the Biological and Toxic Weapons Convention (BTWC) in 1972, which described bioweapons "as repugnant to the conscience of mankind." Its statement of purpose, contained in its Article One, was unequivocal. It effectively prohibits the development, production, acquisition, transfer, retention, stockpiling and use of biological and toxic weapons and is a key element in the International Communities efforts to address the proliferation of weapons of mass destruction. It was the first multilayered disarmament treaty banning an entire category of weapons, touching every base. A golden opportunity appeared to be at hand to rid the world of bioweapons. Could it accomplish its grand mission?

Currently 168 countries have signed on. The BTWC is now subsumed under UNODA, the United Nations office of Disarmament Affairs. Does that have meaning for its effectiveness? Between 1975 and 2011, the BTWC has had five international conferences during which the discussions seek to raise awareness of bioweapons and biowarfare, among its hundreds of participants, who would then motivate their governments to forsake biological weapons.

No question the BTWC set the world a great challenge. It also had a great failing. In its forty years of existence, four decades of pushing and exhorting for prohibitions against bioweapons, its most obvious and utterly surprising weakness is its stated inability to monitor claims that bioweapons have been destroyed, and that member states are not researching new ones. Verification is not in its founding documents. In fact, some member states are adamantly opposed to verification. Does it require a high degree of cynicism to believe that the BTWC conferences are no more than shams, and that their treaties are only so much paper, and another grand opportunity was, is, going nowhere. Where does this leave us? Clearly, we must be prepared, as verification is nowhere in sight. What are we to prepare for? What are we up against?

A full historical account of biological agen ts in warfare has been ably captured by Stefan Reidel and should be required reading by anyone concerned or interested in their use.[35]

Types of Bioweapons

Almost any disease-causing microbe can become a potential weapon. That's the fact of it. With our scientific and technical creativity however, these microbes can be weaponized, enhanced to make them suitable for mass production, storage and dissemination. Consider too, that these weapons are invisible, highly virulent, readily accessible, and most disturbing, relatively easy to deliver. Biological agents can be carried easily in vials and tubes or in an envelope in a jacket or vest pocket, undetectable, as a harmless looking person passes through any number of detectors or pat downs. They become the virtual stealth bombers, with their ability to sow fear, panic, illness and death.

Being invisible, odorless, and tasteless, few, if any would know that an attack was underway. As aerosolization is a known means of dissemination, such low tech methods as spray tanks fitted to planes, cars, trucks and boats, as well as backpack sprayers, even purse-size atomizers can spread fine powders or droplets effectively over and among large numbers of people. Then, of course, water and food-borne dissemination can incapacitate huge numbers of us. Therefore, the burning question is, what microbial agents are we, should we, be concerned about. Beyond that, the deeper question that follows is, are we prepared?

Under current US law, bioagents that have been declared by the Department of Health and Human Services to have the, "potential to pose a threat to public heath and safety," are officially defined as "select agents." The CDC categorizes these "select agents" as A, B, & C, and administers the Select Agent Program, which regulates laboratories that may possess, use, or transfer agents within the US.

Category A's six agents included here are the highest priority agents that pose the greatest risk to our security. They can be easily transmitted and disseminated and culminate in high illness and death rates. They have the potential to spawn a major public health impact, public panic, and require special action to be prepared for and combat.

Tularemia. Rabbit fever, as noted earlier, has a low fatality rate if treated rapidly, but can grievously incapacitate. If the bacterium Francisella tularensis were made airborne for inhalation, severe respiratory illness would occur, including a fulminating pneumonia, and systemic infections. However, making a suitable aerosol requires considerable sophistication. This is not a garage activity.

Anthrax. This delinquent could arrive as either inhalational or cutaneous Anthrax. Inhalational is the most serious, beginning with flu-like symptoms, followed by acute respiratory complications. Exposure to airborne spores could initiate symptoms as soon as two to three days, or as late as six to eight weeks. Once symptoms appear, antibiotics may be of little to no avail. Cutaneous Anthrax begins with a swelling resembling an insect bite, but progresses to an ulcer forming a coal-black scab. If not treated, the infection can spread and become fatal.

Smallpox. Since the 1980's it has been holy writ that the only Smallpox virus was safely frozen and locked away at the CDC in Atlanta, and at Koltsovo, in Russia. Apparently the CDC holds 451 vials of the virus, while Russia maintains 120. Although it was recommended in 2011 that both countries reduce their stocks to ten vials each, that remains a recommendation. However, rumor has it that with the expiration of the Soviet Union, and mother Russia again resurgent, Smallpox cultures may have fallen into other hands. If so, this puts Smallpox high on all lists of bioweapons as none of us, repeat, none of us have any existing antibody immunity, except military and certain medical personnel. Recall that Smallpox virus is transmitted from person to person via airborne particles, and as a virus, is not amenable to antibiotic treatment. On the other hand, many Smallpox experts believe that today Smallpox would not be the menace it was decades ago.

Pneumonic Plague. This ancient scourge, along with its twin, Bubonic plague, that swept away half the population of Europe in the 14th century, has long been on the back burner, so to speak, of those pondering bioweapons. The pneumonic form surely calls forth pneumonia with its high fever, chills and cough is almost one hundred percent fatal if not treated within twenty-four hours of onset. This too, is a person-to-person transmission via coughs and sneezes. The fact that there is no substantive treatment currently available, places it in this top category.

Botulism toxin. Will we be dealing with a highly potent Botox? We may not think of it as such, but botulism toxin is all over the place, and so easily obtained. This protein is one of the most poisonous known. To be an effective bioweapon, the toxin would be delivered as an aerosol, or in food. Depending upon the severity of the exposure, symptoms progress rapidly to generalized muscle weakness and respiratory paralysis, as the toxin blocks the neurotransmitter, acetylcholine. The Clostridia organisms produce seven toxins, labelled A to G, which can be dealt with by injection of antitoxin, specific to each. Without antitoxin, it's fatal within 24 to 72 hours. As luck would have it a new strain dubbed "H", has recently been discovered by scientists at the California State Department of Public Health. Because of its exquisite toxicity the Department decided not to release genetic sequencing details about this organism's toxin for fear that terrorists would latch on to it and use it for whatever nasty purpose they have in mind. However, once an antitoxin becomes available, the genetic details will be published.[36] Nevertheless it's hard to imagine how any of these eight toxins could disrupt a city. Of course, creative minds, thinking outside that metaphoric box may conjure up something. Vigilance remains a top priority.

Viral Hemorrhagic Fevers. These are the purveyors of a diverse group of deadly viruses: Ebola, Marburg, Yellow, and Lassa fevers. Here again, illness begins with flu-like symptoms; fever, fatigue, head and muscle aches and dizziness, which make for difficult diagnosis early on given the fact that few physicians have had experience with those exotic fevers. Nonetheless, severe infections lead to dire complications from massive blood loss and systemic shock due to damage to blood vessels. And again, no antibiotics are effective against these esoteric viruses.

So, those are the big six. The ones to be expected should some state or non-governmental terrorist group, or lone nut-jobs lose their grip on reality.

Category B, the second tier holds another thirteen possible agents including Cholera, that could possibly initiate a waterborne epidemic. However, our nation wide system of water and sewage treatment suggests why this potential agent is not in Category A.

Category C, with its five viral agents including HIV and Influenza also need to be inhaled if they are to be effective agents. Any flu strain would have to be a highly mutated, virulent strain to bring a city to its knees. HIV is a "dark horse" as there has never been an inhalational form of this virus. Yet, knowing how disruptive to our immune system it can be, places it among potential bioweapons.

Categories A, B, and C, deal for the most part with non-genetically re-engineered microbes, but scientific and technological advances could make these organisms far worse. Not wanting to be victims of hardening of the categories, we need to be prepared for changes that could come via genetic manipulation.

The Human Genome Project, as noted in Chapter TWO, has decoded the alphabet of life and published a human molecular blueprint. Moreover, the complete genome sequences are publicly available for hundreds of viruses, dozens of bacteria and fungi. For those concerned with bioweapons, those published genomes would certainly allow the development of far more virulent and resistant organisms. Indeed, virtual parts lists of useful genes for a genetic Leggo are readily available for anyone to build, construct, a totally new organism. Now that's scary. It may be only a matter of time until creative and malevolent individuals develop synthetic genes, synthetic viruses, and even devise new organisms never before known on our planet: Chimera viruses and bacteria! Biowarfare would enter a new dimension; a new and pernicious phase.

Megalomaniacal terrorists are looking for original ways to surprise and devastate an enemy. Consequently, we need to be highly attentive to these new and malignant developments. However, many scientists believe it's in the best interests of society to produce these synthetic organisms as a means of learning more about them. With that reasoning, molecular biologists at The State University of New York, Stony Brook, recently synthesized a Polio virus from materials readily available from biological supply companies. After piecing together sequences of RNA to form a full-length polio virus genome, they replicated and translated this polio genome, and the resulting nucleic acids and proteins assembled themselves into a fully functioning infectious virus.[37] It can be done. Good and bad news.

Furthermore, we must realize that there is a delay between exposure and onset of illness–days to weeks.

Hence, a bioweapon would likely be chosen for the longest incubation period, allowing exposed individuals to spread the disease far and wide, as they go about their business. As illness developed, these people would get to medical facilities where unsuspecting physicians and nurses would themselves become exposed and infected. Hospitals would be swamped and unable to cope with the sick and dying.

The communications media would contribute to public fear, and panic would grow with ensuing civil disorder; a scenario terrorists would die for. Not a pretty picture.

Unquestionably, agents in these three groups are meant to cause fear and panic among populations, shutting down the economy, causing wide spread chaos. That's the madness of bioweapons, and the BTWC can do nothing about it!

Thus far we've said nothing about our agricultural resources whose critical features make it vulnerable to terrorist attack. Our livestock industry is highly concentrated, as is the centralized nature of our food processing industry, which suggests that pathogens and toxins could be intentionally inserted at a number of points along the farm-to-table continuum. Even the threat of an attack could adversely affect the public's confidence in the safety of its food, and destabilize our export market.[38]

An excellent example is the aggressive virus of Foot and Mouth Disease (FMD) capable of causing countrywide economic turmoil, as occurred in the 2001 and 2007 episodes in the UK.

In the spring and summer of 2001, more than 2,000 cases of disease occurred on farms around the northern countryside. About seven million sheep and cattle were killed in the successful attempt to halt the devastation. By the time the disease was under control, it was estimated to have cost Britain thirteen billion dollars, costs shared by agricultural as well as supporting and

224

related industries.

What made this outbreak so severe was the amount of time between the infection's recognition and the time when counter measures were instituted, such as bans on trucks and then detergent washing of all vehicles and personnel entering livestock areas. The epidemic was more than likely caused by pigs that had been fed infected garbage that had not been properly heat-sterilized. The garbage appeared to contain remains of infected meat that had been illegally imported. It was later found that there had been extreme overkill as many disease-free animals were culled.[39]

FMD struck again in August and September 2007. This time the virus was identified as one having escaped from a nearby laboratory in the Surrey area, that was developing FMD vaccine. It escaped from the drainage system connecting the vaccine lab by way of fomites and deposited itself on the road leading to the farm where trucks and cars and people easily carried it into the farm. There's always a pathway. And to isolate the virus, again all cattle were culled and a protective zone with a radius of some two miles out from the farm was imposed. No cattle or pigs could be moved in all the surrounding area. Again, financial losses were tremendous: sixty-one million dollars to the government, and 169 million dollar loss to the local farmers. By the way, to cull, is a verb most often meaning to select, pick or glean; here we mean, slaughter.

When FMD strikes a farm, vesicles appear in the mouth and on the upper lip of cattle as well as on the coronary band of the foot, and on the mammary glands and areas of fine skin. It's visual misery, and can't be missed. These vesicles burst, leaving painful red erosions. Secondary bacterial infections of the open vesicles can also occur in the mouth and lips. Large quantities of virus are eliminated in saliva, which is esponsible for both environmental and airborne spread. Viruses can also be spread widely in drinking water, inhalation of aerosols, and eating contaminated food. All are links in a chain of spread that terrorists can exploit.

Farmers know that they and the many other people living and working on the farm can become transmitting sources (vectors) carrying the virus on boots, wheel barrows, and truck tires. Their dogs and cats can also spread the virus via their contaminated paws. If infected animals are not spotted quickly, and culled from the herds, spread and financial ruin are inevitable.

The 2001 episode caused suicides among farmers who saw their livelihoods go up in smoke. Add to that the fear of air and water pollution from disposal of animal carcasses. As the outbreak occurred in August, it totally wiped out tourism as the tens of thousands of tourists who had planned to arrive, cancelled their reservations. Yet another blow to an already fragile economy.

After the 2001 British epidemic, our Department of Agriculture calculated that an FMD outbreak could spread to 25 states in as little as five days. A simulation by the National Defense University in June 2002, predicted that an FMD episode could spread to more than one-third of the nation's cattle herds.[40] Let's understand that we are an open society with wide open ranges, allowing someone, or several, disaffected malcontents ready access. Nor have we said anything about the very real possibility of the destruction of our corn, wheat and rice crops.

These types of disastrous events suggest that it may not be necessary to disseminate a virulent microbial agent in one of our crowded cities. Loss of major food supplies can cause the panic and disruption terrorists seek to inflict. It's a vile business that no country wants to have visited upon it. Yet there is no worldwide prohibition, or force to prevent it. Each country is on its own to protect itself, which raises the original and deeper question, are we prepared?

We are, if our Department of Homeland security (DHS) can accomplish its stated mission: to protect the nation's health security by providing early detection and early warning of bioterror attacks.

This now 12-year-old Department, set-up in 2002, combined twenty-two different federal departments and agencies into a unified, integrated Cabinet agency, which surely had to be an auspicious beginning. DHS set four essential pillars of our (their) national biodefense program. These are: *Threat awareness; Prevention and protection; Surveillance and detection; Response and recovery.*

These do appear to cover the gambit of issues. They also appear to have learned hard lessons from the 9/11 muck-up in which our gaggle of intelligence agencies failed miserably in sharing vital information. Homeland Security shares public health and intelligence information dealing with their four core concerns, with state and local partners through seventy-seven local fusion centers.

Their intelligence analysts and biodefense experts at the National Biological Threat Characterization Center conduct studies and lab experiments, filling in gaps to be ready to counteract current and future biothreats.

Guarding the physical safety and security of "Select Agent" facilities is another of their concerns and responsibilities. Visiting these facilities regularly allows them to ascertain vulnerabilities and how to remedy them. By way of sharing, they provide funding to state and local law enforcement, who will be first responders should an incident occur at these facilities. That makes sense. The major question whenever a public disaster occurs is who's in charge? If that question has to be asked, if or when a bioterror event occurs, we're in trouble.

Moreover, of highest concern is early detection and early warning of a bioterror attack. The Department's

National Biosurveillance Integration Center is set up to do just that, enhancing the government's capability to rapidly identify and monitor biological episodes of national concern.

To deal with their core concern of Response and Recovery, their National Bioforensic Analysis Center is set up to quickly analyze forensic evidence to assure identification of the attackers and to prevent a recurrence.

Closely related to this, and of utmost importance, they have developed means of rapid federal responses supporting state and federal jurisdictions that places medical counter measures nearer to those medical personnel who will need to respond to critical situations. That, too, makes sense. To ensure that officials at all levels of government are able to carry out their functions, NBAC developed and conducted a series of biodefenseexercises involving over a thousand state and local officials. So, we know who knows what needs to be done. And we appear to know who's in charge.

Let's hope that none of this needs to be done, and that Homeland Security's activities remain just exercises. By the way, they continue to look for sharp minds to play a vital role in securing our country, keeping it safe.[41]

The bombing at the Boston Marathon on April 16th, 2013, could be a model of reactions that could occur in any city. Boston's was a barbaric attack, unsuspected if ever there was one. Surprise, shock, fear, panic followed shortly by calm and intense desire to help those in trouble. The people, young and old, were resilient, and plan to have the Marathon again in 2014. And they did! 35,671 to be exact; runners, walkers and wheelers not to be denied!

Boston also showed understanding of the need for cooperation among enforcement agencies. Consequently turf wars never occurred, and the culprits were killed or captured amazingly fast. The swift resolution was unprecedented. It's my considered opinion, that as 2015 approaches, our people will deal with bioweapons in much the same way. We are prepared, and Boston was another great learning experience for HLS.

As a postscript, while HLS is doing what it does, creative souls in academia are also searching for ways to protect us. Would you believe that retroreflectors on bicycles are getting a new role and responsibility: detecting biothreats and diagnosing disease organisms should they be in the neighborhood.

Prof. Richard Willson of the University of Houston, in cooperation with the University of Texas, and Sandia National Labs, is developing an ultra-sensitive, all-in-one device utilizing retroreflectors to rapidly tell first responders exactly which disease-causing microbe is in the area. First responders will love it. This group of researchers is also developing procedures for use in a physicians office where reflectors could provide a rapid on-site diagnosis of infectious diseases, getting the results in under an hour.

These reflectors can be designed such that two hundred spots would fit in the dot over the letter i. Additionally, they have biochemically treated surfaces capable of detecting pathogens making them a lab-on-a-chip with minute channels that can process small amounts of blood and other fluids. So, for example, as a sample of blood flows through a channel, parts of the reflector would grow dark, indicating the presence of a specific agent. In a negative test, the reflector would remain bright. Can we hope that this is too good to be true?[42]

I'm encouraged that ample biodefenses are in place, and our country is as secure as it can be. Perhaps you'll agree.

Having squared-off with the nasties, the delinquents, we now take on those food spoilers and poisoners that crave our food as much as we do.

FIVE

Racing for the Chow: Our Food is Their Food

Call him "The Little Corporal, "The Corsican," or "Emperor," either way Napoleon Bonaparte, General of Le Grand Armeé, knew that "an army marched on its stomach." If his quest to conquer Europe and march on Russia was to succeed, his troops needed food that would remain edible for extended periods.

Spoilage was the bane of troops in the field and sailors at sea. But no one knew why spoilage occurred. And, no one would know for 6-7 decades until the discoveries of Louis Pasteur that microbes were the culprits, and that sufficient heat could stop them cold. Nevertheless, in 1798, Napoleon offered a prize of 12,000 Francs, ($48,000 in current dollars) to anyone who devised a practical way of preserving meat and veggies for the army during its forays into hostile territory.

Nicolas Appert, son of an innkeeper, and apprentice Chef at the Palais Royal Hotel in Chalons, east of Paris, knew next to nothing about food preservation, or the existence of microbes, nonetheless he took up the challenge. The airtight bottling process he invented was directly responsible for the huge array of food now available the world over.

Appert's successful experiments heated foods at temperatures well above that of boiling water, 212° F (100° C). To climb above 212° F, he used a gussied-up pressure cooker that, for the 1790's, was simply astonishing: what stroke of creativity would suggest higher temperatures? I'm stuck on that one. That's what he did, and it worked. His use of steam under pressure actually sterilized food: removing all living things. The process was time consuming, taking up to five hours to achieve preservation.

He placed his thick, loosely corked, wide-mouthed bottles containing meats and vegetables in pans of water in his autoclave, locked it, turned up the pressure and set them cooking. After five hours, the bottles were allowed to cool and were tightly corked, sealed with fish glue, and wired shut a la' Champagne. It would be revealing to read his notes, if they exist, to learn why he wired them. It's not too much of a stretch to suspect that in many unsuccessful trials corks flew off from internal pressures generated by microbes dinning on the tasty vittles. Nevertheless, his autoclaving worked. Preservation was achieved.

1804 was a very good year. Appert opened the world's first canning factory in Massy, south of Paris. By 1809, he was ready to present his findings to the Directory, the executive branch of Napoleon's government, and claim the prize. It wasn't that easy. To receive it, he was required to publish his work, which led to the world's first cookbook on modern food preservation: Le Livre de tous menages, ou l'art de Conserver pendant Plesieurs annees toutes les substances Animales et Vegetables, "The Art of Preserving All Kinds of Animal and Vegetable Substances for Several Years," was published in 1810, in time for Napoleon's army's march on Moscow in 1812.

However, this does raise questions. With a five hundred-thousand man army, and let's assume only six bottles per man, which is barely enough to get a hungary soldier five miles down the road, that's three million bottles, for a march of 1,500 miles from Vienna to Moscow. That couldn't possibly be adequate over those long weeks of marching. Were the roads and fields littered with empty bottles? Of even greater concern, could Appert have made or gotten three million bottles? That's a bit of a stretch. So, after winning that huge prize, did the project go any further, and did any preserved food go along to Moscow? Or was this just another grand idea that went nowhere? The archives are silent on this. It does however, as Hercule Poirot, would say, "It gives one to think."

It was Peter Durand, however, another Frenchman, and a brilliant technician, living in England, who switched bottles for metal cans because of breakage. But it had to await the invention of the can opener, in 1855, for the canning industry to take off. Nevertheless, Appert is considered the Father of Canning, and for the longest time his process was called Appertization. A bronze statue of Appert was erected in Chalons in1991, In his honor the French government had declared 2010, the 200th anniversary of Appert's award, a national celebratory year.

So what do we know? We know that some foods can be made microbe free and remain edible almost forever. We also know that lots of foods spoil. Some 30-plus percent of all food is lost to spoilage. Of that percentage, 80-90 percent can be chalked up to microbes banqueting on our food! Spoilage knows no boundaries. People everywhere must contend with spoilage; its part of the cycle of life because microbes require the same nutrients we do, and as our foods are nutrient-rich, its been a constant race between them and us to make sure we get those victuals first, in an edible condition. Because we lose the race so often, we've had to be creative to thwart the spoilers.

So, what's going on here? Two questions jump out and beg for answers: why do foods spoil, and perhaps most important, are spoiled foods harmful? Most people think they are, and believe they'll become deathly ill if smelly foods are eaten. Wrong. False. Not true. Answering the second first, our spoilers are nuisances and irritants, nothing more. They are neither pathogenic nor illness producing. But let's get to the first than back to the second, as the devil is in the details.

Obviously some foods spoil faster than others. Why: Because of their intrinsic chemical content. Yes, you read that right. Chemicals are the defining characteristic. All foods, animal and plant (crops) are organic, which means they are, were, living things, and as such, they, as we, consist of a plethora of organic chemicals, meaning they all contain the ubiquitous carbon atom. If carbon was removed from our world it would resemble the barren surface of the moon. If carbon were removed from animals, plants and us, what would remain would be a bucket of water, albeit a small one, and a handful of minerals. And yes, our carbon-containing chemicals are natural. They are no different than their man-made counterparts. Sucrose, glucose, fructose and maltose for example, all sugars that make up carbohydrates, cannot not be differentiated from the same sugars made in a laboratory or food company. As the lady said, a chemical, is a chemical, is a chemical.

Living things consist of thousands of chemicals. Over a thousand have been identified in a cup of coffee. Among the vast flock of chemicals in all living things are enzymes, proteins that speed up cellular metabolism, assist plants and animals to grow and mature, and produce fruits and vegetables in plants. Understand too, that proteins are the master chemicals of all living things. But, and this is a substantial but, when microbes munch on them to obtain their daily rations, breaking them down to their constituent amino acids, and then on to amines, (am-eens) hold your nose.

As milk has been one of our earliest foods, and

earliest to spoil, it deserves pride of place. Microbes love milk. It has all the water they crave, the proteins, fats, carbo's and minerals they need, but none of the acidity they detest. On the debit side, cows, horses, sheep, goats, camels and buffalo, the major milk producers, are host to a diverse population of microbes, just as we are. Ergo, heat treatment of milk is necessary to remove, kill off, the nasty Mycobacterium tuberculosis, responsible for TB, and others such as Brucella and Brucellosis, as well as the bacterium that delivers Typhoid Fever. Drinking raw milk is asking for trouble. Allowing raw milk to clot, ferment, while often delivering an elegant beverage, is inadequate to the task of removing the Mycobacteria as the lactic acid of fermented milk is too weak an organic acid. Consequently heat must be applied–but carefully.

Pasteurization at 63° C (140° F) for 30 minutes, the traditional Holding Treatment, far from its boiling point, maintains its sweetness, and ensures removal of the Mycobacteria along with many other microbes, but not all. That's critical. Pasteurization is meant to markedly reduce the number and types of microbes, including the spoilers, but is not meant to sterilize: the total absence of all living things. After pasteurization, milk requires refrigeration to keep the remaining organisms from multiplying too quickly. Why the need? Let's do the math; or is it arithmetic? Most microbes we'll meet have a generation time of approximately half-an-hour, which means they double their numbers in 30 minutes. And they prefer a geometric progression. One-1- becomes 2 in 30 minutes, and 4 at the end of an hour; 16 after 2 hours, and on to 32, 64, 128, and in 12 hours there are 5,158,704 from the original one, which may not sound all that bad in a full quart of milk. Or does it? However, by law in all fifty states, freshly pasteurized Grade A milk can have up to 20,000 bacteria per milliliter (ml). Just what does that translate to when we purchase a quart of milk and fetch it home? Well, with 946 ml in a quart, and possibly 20,000 in each of those 946, and if our multiplication is faultless, we are looking at 18,920,000 bacteria in that container of freshly pasteurized milk. Therefore, in each 8 ounce, 239 ml, of a glass of delicious cold, sweet milk, there will be as many as 4,780,000 microbes. Given the number of glasses of milk we've consumed over the years, it doesn't seem much of a stretch to conclude that those potential spoilers are, well, benign. There's an important message in that bottle. Let's bear that in mind, and let's also remember that with each passing day, the number of bacteria in that original container continue to multiply geometrically. Yet it remains sweet and drinkable...until it isn't. Doesn't that help reduce some of the fear of microbes? It's much the same with all foods. They're there, but of no real concern, no bother. And what do those expiration, sell by dates, really mean? They refer to peak freshness, not a gauge of safety. After the date passes, the milk or other food item, should still be safe if your refrigeration temperatures are correct.

Pasteurized milk is expected to have a refrigerated shelf life of two weeks or more, but psychotrophic, cold-loving bacteria, such as the pesky and ubiquitous Pseudomonads can reduce that time markedly as they grow well at 35-40° F. Nevertheless, maintaining your fridge at 40° F or below, is your optimum protection.

These Pseudamonads live in soil and water, and find a natural habitat on the warm teats and udders of cows, even after washing and sanitizing. Water used to clean and rinse milking equipment provides ready entry into bulk milk. Both good reasons for ratcheting up the temperatures as these organisms are uniquely fragile.

More recently food scientists seeking to reduce the numbers of bacteria in milk and extend its shelf life shifted pasteurization to a High Temperature Short Time (HTST) flash process in which milk is heated to 72° C (160° F) for 15 seconds. Even higher temperatures are used in the UHT, ultra high process that heats milk to 82.2°C (180° F) for all of two seconds. This reduces microbial numbers a bit more without coagulating proteins a la´ fried or poached eggs, and doesn't require refrigeration until the container is opened, which can be as much as a year. These unrefrigerated milk cartons are now common items in our markets, going by the name Pamalot, and the taste appears quite acceptable.

Spoilage is not limited to the pseudamonads. A clique of others with such intriguing names as Micrococcus, Aerococcus, and Alcaligenes, have an awful habit of making milk bitter, rancid, sour, malty, ropey and coagulated. None of which are harmful, but the off-odors and tastes are sure signs that the contents require flushing. Need I note that offensive odors, to paraphrase badly, are in the nose of the inhaler. What are we to make of Limburger cheese, a semi-soft gift of the Belgians, which for me, is a vile nose-bending odor, but for many others, a highly prized delicacy, for which they are more than willing to pay top dollar. Let it be widely known, and I do hesitate to mention this, *Brevibacterium linens*, the microbe that supplies Limburger its fascinating aroma, is the identical, repeat, identical bacterium thriving odiously between our toes, and which rocks our socks. Go figure! Getting to know the names of a number of these rascally microbes can make them less mysterious, less threatening. We might even begin to think of them as allies, which would be a sea change of robust proportions.

With its high fat and low moisture content, its difficult but not impossible for butter to become rancid, sour and soapy tasting from the growth, albeit slow, of those few organisms that can dine on fat, producing free fatty acids with their typical off-taste: nothing you'd want to coat your toast with. But again, if you did, it's not harmful. And taste buds do vary markedly among us.

Cheese is one of our oldest foods. Indications are that cheeses were made five to six thousand years ago. Possibly longer. Currently, a bewildering, parade of cheeses, are prepared around the world. Over 2,000 types have been documented, and all the work of microbes.

Hey, you've got to give the wee beasties the credit due them. They are remarkably versatile creatures. But they also spoil those lovely foods for us. All too often Lactobacilli initiate gas production in Mozzarella, while other lactos soften it, as a consequence of the loss of protein. This softened cheese can't easily be sliced or grated and doesn't melt properly. Hold the pizza! Propionibacteria, now that's a moniker to remember, are well known contributors of pink spots and off-odors on Swiss cheese. Most importantly, its their delivery of carbon dioxide that begets Swiss its holes; most often just the right amount. Too often just one huge hole, as too many of these bacteria, gobbling overtime produce far too much gas. That sliced Swiss in our refrigerators can be colonized by a variety of colorful molds. However, before consigning any to the trash, carve off the troublesome area. If what remains tastes as Swiss should rather than soil, munch away. If you like the taste of soil, well…

Cheddar cheese can develop fruity flavors from the growth of Lactococci. This fruitiness heralds the presence of ethanol along with ethyl butyrate and ethyl hexanoate. Unfortunately it's the odd individual that appreciates fruity cheddar. Chemicals are everywhere, even where they shouldn't be.

Cottage and Pot cheese, two widely consumed soft white cheeses, with high casein content, the primary milk protein, will effuse a fecal-like stench when left for two weeks or more in the fridge. It's those putrid amines again that even dogs eschew. Farmer cheese, another soft, white cheese, and one of my favorites, is a candidate for the slimy, pink growth of Serratia and Bacilius subtilis, with an accompanying fetid bouquet. But again, not harmful—except to your dignity.

The three H's, hair, hide and hoofs, along with a cow's gastrointestinal tract provide microbes ready access to our steaks and hamburger. The grinding and mixing of hamburger and sausage meat, including my favorite hot-dogs, as well as the many comminuted luncheon meats noted in Chapter SIX, increases surface area for the wee beasties to grow on, and distribute themselves throughout the meats ensuring rapid putrefaction. If improperly handled by individuals shedding potentially harmful organisms, the evil ones may also enter the picture. We'll have more to say about that further on.

Ham, bacon, and corned beef pickled with salt to withdraw moisture from both meat and microbes, often allows the salt-tolerant Lactobacilli to grow and produce its acid that sours the meats along with slime formation. Hydrogen peroxide formation over time can also change the meats hemoglobin red color to greenish brown, suggesting poor quality. Right, yet not at all harmful.

Spoiling, and spoiled meat, poultry, and fish, offer excellent examples of the odorous chemistry of putrefaction. Putrefaction, the complete bacterial decomposition of protein, releases the fetid and fecal smelling cadaverines, putrescines, skatols and indoles, whose very names induce cringing. For the longest time these odious chemicals were called Ptomaines, from the Greek, Ptoma, meaning corpse or cadaver. These creepy chemicals do not, repeat, do not cause poisoning or illness. Ptomaine poisoning is a hangover from times past, and needs to be laid to rest. Unfortunately, as long as proteinaceous foods are with us, and we surely don't want to lose them, these foul smelling chemicals will also be with us, courtesy of our invisible collegues.

Removed from the sea, fish die quickly and bacterial decomposition waits for no one. That awesome ammoniacal fishy odor emanating from the fish you've had in the fridge far too many days is, TMA, trimethylamine, yet another amine brought to us by bacteria chomping away on fish tissue. Given that the seas the world over are loaded with microbes, TMA can be expected to reach our nostrils if fish and seafood are not quickly iced and/or frozen and rapidly brought to market, cooked and eaten.

Surprisingly enough, chicken innards are mostly free of microbes, but chickens ready for market gather their cadre of bacteria from skin, feathers and feet, and both raw and cooked, will decompose, putrefy, much the same as cattle meat, ushering in and signaling the presence of the vile amines. Speaking of chicken, reminds me that the bacterium Proteus, can digest the sulfur-containing amino acid cysteine, releasing hydrogen sulfide which blackens eggs, and delivers its wicked sulfurous odor we're all too familiar with.

Veggies and fruits with little to no protein are a different kettle of fish. Is that mixing a metaphor? With the exception of rhubarb, most vegetables are acid neutral and brimming with moisture, which invites a range of bacteria, most often Aeromonas and Erwinia. These two, are to veggies what E.coli is to meat. Both enjoy cut, moist surfaces and quickly take up residence, producing their slimies–biofilms. Bell peppers, green, red, or yellow, scallions, onions, lettuce and cucumbers also offering that perfect acid-neutral environment, quickly becoming slimy, soft and mushy in 3 to 4 days. But not to worry. Cut away the slimy areas and their ready to eat. Here again, wrapping in paper toweling will markedly increase shelf life. To keep cut celery slime-free, wrap separate stalks, or the entire stalk in paper toweling and cover with aluminum foil. That will hold down moisture limiting bacterial growth for weeks. The trick with all these is to keep them as dry as possible. Drying buys time, and cuts down losses.

Tomatoes, with their high acid content need little to no help. I'm a tomato lover and can eat tomatoes from dawn to dusk, so I'm pleased that no self-respecting bacterium would consider a tomato whose skin is all but impervious. However, a bruise, more like a cut, exposing interior tissues would be all Alternaria and Fusarium, two acid-tolerant fungi would need to creep inside and turn that tomato to mush.

Lycopene, the chemical pigment bestowing the rich, fire-engine redness to tomatoes is not known for any antimicrobial activity, but was hailed as an antioxidant that would prevent benign prostatic hypertrophy, an enlarged prostate in men. All the hype never panned out. With no special claims for it, except the gratifying fact that recently Cis-3 Hexanal with its intense grassy aroma, is the major volitile organic compound in ripe tomatoes and gives tomatoes its characteristic scent and taste. Ah, those chemicals.

The high sugar content of fruits, along with their high acid and moisture levels extend invitations to yeasts, which are both acid and sugar tolerant. Yeasts need a little time to get the bubbles of carbon dioxide going. Those bubbles indicate that sugar is being metabolized to alcohol. I can't wait to get to the half-filled jar of apple-sauce residing at the rear of our refrigerator. Its been there for some 3-4 weeks and is bubbling with the compelling and fragrant aroma of apple "wine," telling me I'm going to have a ball for a week or so as the alcohol level builds to a peak as the sugar in the apple sauce is converted by my invisible cronies. No sir, no throwing out that good stuff. I recommend the same approach should slices or chunks of pineapple, cherries, and other berries, be left over. Wow! Don't be so fast to trash peaches that have signs of microbial growth. Yeasts and some bacteria give peaches memorable peachy alcoholic flavor. De-lish! Taste before trashing should be your new mantra.

Its extremely high sugar content, lack of moisture and oxygen put jams off-limits to all but a few hardy fungi. Even for them it takes considerable time to form a fuzzy or hairy mat over a jam's surface. Lift off that wooly growth and taste the jam. If it tastes or smells of soil you know the fungus had extended its tentacles, its mycelia, deep into the interior. Trash time.

More often than not, that greenish-bluish fuzz growing on and softening oranges, lemons, grapefruit and low-acid cantaloups, is Penicillium, from which the antibiotic penicillin was originally obtained. How bad can that be? Not bad at all. Slice off the soft part, and, yes, taste. Filling up the trash bucket need not be your goal.

It's worth remembering that although we refer to a great diversity of plants and animals as food, all food, is nothing more than chemicals, strung together in myriad ways to form potatoes, spinach, steak, shrimp, berries, corn, chicken,you name it. We now know that many of the chemicals in plant and animal tissue are there to inhibit potential invaders–insects, worms, mites and microbes, predators seeking a tasty meal. Plants and animals,not unlike us, prefer not to be irritated,or consumed. Preservation is the name of the game. So, for example, eggs are rich in the protein lysozyme that has antimicrobial properties. Lysozyme also occurs in human tears. Although they didn't, couldn't, realize it the folks in ancient India, and continuing today, used the spices cinnamon, mustard, and oregano with their antimicrobial chemicals, to protect their food from spoiling. That's why spices were so highly prized in Europe, well before the advent of refrigeration and other means of preservation. Besides, these spice contributed tempting aromas.

Before taking on the poisoners, let's remember that refrigerators should be kept at 35-40°F (1.6-4.5°C). At these temperatures milk will remain sweet for 10-12 days, if we don't allow cartons of milk to remain on tables while we chat and read. Put the milk back in the fridge and go on reading.

The freezer compartment needs attention. Freezing does not kill microbes. It just slows them down lengthening their generation time, which translates into longer edible shelf life for all the good stuff in there. Keep the freezer at 0-5°F (-17.8 to-15°C). From time to time place a thermometer in the freezer and on refrigerator shelves. Check several areas to assure that cold air is flowing evenly. It will pay dividends.

So, what are we looking at? We're looking at a clutch of signals: wicked tastes, slippery textures, and wretched aromas that tell us singly or in combination, that this food item is not what we want to eat. But if we did, for some obscure reason, neither illness, aches, or pains will befall us. Spoiled or rotten food fails the esthetic test, but there's no harm in that. It's the silent ones that arrive on cat's paws without so much a whiff that do us in. We now take on the silent sickeners.

Food Poisoning: The Sickeners Among Us

Two salient questions come front and center: why do foods become a source of illness and death, and how does it happen? This all too often, deadly duo, strike directly at the core of the problem. The answers, and there are several, can be gleaned from the cases that follow. And it will be evident that our senses are no help, and we will state emphatically that most food poisonings need not occur. Nevertheless, the number of poisonings are appalling:

48 million food poisoning events annually.

28 thousand hospitalizations annually.

3 thousand deaths annually.

Moreover, the Department of Agriculture's Economic Research Service informs us that the bill, the direct costs for this morbidity and mortality has reached $6.7 billion. An intolerable and needless waste!

An appropriate solution is waiting, has been waiting, to take its place along with canning, freezing, and drying to protect our food from both the poisoners and the spoilers. But first, let the cases speak to us.

With a splitting headache, numb mouth, deafness in her left ear, and burning sensations shooting through her body, Teresa Holbrooke, not her real name, lay curled quietly in the darkened confines of a bunk below deck in her 41-foot aluminum centerboard sloop Elan. Teresa was in terrible pain and needed expert medical help. But she and her husband Will, were anchored off Vaka'eitu, an island in the VaVa'u Group, Tonga, in the far Pacific east of Australia and New Zealand. Teresa was airlifted to Bishop Auckland General Hospital in Auckland, New Zealand, where a battery of tests were done. CAT scans, MRI's and lumbar punctures were negative for bacterial and viral meningitis. Additional tests finally indicated that Teresa had parasitic meningitis—rat lungworm meningitis. She had ingested the rat lungworms while eating coleslaw made from raw vegetables. Eating insufficiently cooked escargot, ingesting raw crabmeat, freshwater shrimp, fish or frogs legs have all been culprits. Teresa got hers from insufficiently washed and disinfected cabbage she used for coleslaw.[1]

She was not alone. On the island of Jamaica, 12 of 23 Chicago medical students on spring break became infected in varying degrees from a single shared meal that included raw vegetables. In 1993, the first case of parasitic meningitis was diagnosed in North America, when on a dare, an 11-year-old boy from New Orleans ate a raw snail, became severely ill, but luckily recovered fully in a week. How did these illnesses occur?

Adult lungworms reside in rats' pulmonary arteries. The worms lay eggs that circulate to lung capillaries, hatch, and migrate to the trachea, then down the esophagus, into the gastrointestinal tract, and eliminated in their feces. The feces-encrusted larvae are eaten by land and aquatic snails, crabs and slugs which crawl over fruits and veggies. Teresa, the medical students and the young boy ate raw vegetables and a raw snail picking up Angiostrongylus cantonensis, a worm that readily penetrates the gastrointestinal wall, making its way to central nervous system tissue—usually getting into the fluid-filled spinal cord. Now for the real trouble. Worms begin to die, and the body musters its immune defenses against a foreign protein, and cerebral spinal fluid pressure increases on tissues and nerves, causing great pain.

Because of immune responses, tissue injury can

cause fever, nausea, photophobia, vertigo, stiff neck, and partial paralysis: a roaring cascade, which, in the most serious cases can last for months and years. At this point you understand that all this can be avoided by cooking vegetables. But most of all, there are no signals, no indication that the food contains anything nasty; something about to cause huge trouble. That's a major message.

Botulism, perhaps the deadliest form of food poisoning, is the consequence of ingesting a neurotoxin produced by the bacterium *Clostridium botulinum.* This sublimely potent chemical is the most toxic natural poison known. Most often the foods involved are eaten at home, which accounts for the extensive family involvement. The toxin is rapidly absorbed in the upper intestinal tract, and symptoms usually appear 12-36 hours later.

Typically, the toxin has an affinity for the cranial nerves that control the head and neck. Double vision, difficulty swallowing, and slurred speech are a characteristic triad. Paralyzed neck muscles induce respiratory failure and death. Over 70 percent of cases result in death because treatment with antitoxin is started too late, as emergency room physicians are not thinking, food poisoning, until a family member offers the suggestion.

Around noon on December 12th, a 59-year-old woman in New York City ate a meal that that included eggplant, mushrooms, and peppers that she had jarred at home. That evening she had vomiting, distention and abdominal pain.

December 13th: She called her family doctor, who gave her suppositories, which produced diarrhea.

December 14th and 15th: Complaints of swallowing difficulties.

December 16th: Difficulty breathing.

December 17th: Hospitalized. Admitting diagnosis, bronchitis and respiratory failure.

Between December 17th and 22nd, developed a myocardial infarction and died on the 22nd.

While in the hospital she complained of burning eyes and was unable to close her eyes.

After the funeral the family, 22 in all, returned to her home and ate the same food. On December 24th the daughter-in-law complained of swallowing difficulties and on the 25th had difficulty talking and swallowing. Her father-in-law called the family doctor, whose impression was that her symptoms were hysterical and a placebo was prescribed. The father-in-law then called Emergency Services. Paramedics got her into the hospital on the afternoon of 26th where she had a myocardial infarction and respiratory failure.

Inquiring among family members, health department investigators found that mushrooms, eggplant and peppers were usually cooked in vinegar, to boiling, cooled, and placed in olive oil for storage at room temperature. What happened? *Boiling was inadequate.* Clostridial spores from both the mushrooms and peppers, which easily obtain bacteria from soil, were still viable when they were place under the olive oil. The depth of the olive oil prevented oxygen from penetrating, which was just fine for the Clostridia that can only grow in the absence of oxygen. Microbiologists call them anaerobes. The temperature of the room was just right for continued Clostridium multiplication and toxin formation. Of course the mushrooms and peppers had the traditional taste so they were gobbled up…by some.

Curiously enough, Alaska has had a steady increase in Botulism cases since 1985. Despite its elfin population, it has more cases than any of the other continental 48. However, the cases fall disproportionately on the Eskimos because of their traditional practice of allowing whole fish, fish heads,

Walrus, Sea Lion, Whale flippers, Beaver tails, and birds to ferment for months in sealed plastic containers which provide the Clostridia a luxurious, oxygen-free environment in which to grow and produce toxin. In the old days, a grass-lined hole contained their delicacies, which had sufficient air to prevent bacterial growth. So much for progress. And again, no warning of possible problems.

Pomatomas saltatrix—Bluefish—is seldom suspect. Nevertheless, for the five physicians who sat down to lunch at a New Hampshire Inn, that was cold comfort. Although such non-scombroid fish as Amberjack, and Mahimahi have been implicated in poisonings typical of the Scombridae family, Tuna, Mackerel, and Bonito, Bluefish have not. Nevertheless, within four hours of eating they developed headache, flushing, redness of their upper bodies, diarrhea, abdominal pain, and pounding hearts. Need I say, they required medical attention.[2] What happened here? Bacterial growth on the surface of the unrefrigerated Bluefish decomposed histadine in the fish muscle tissue forming histamine, which caused tightness in their throats, vomiting, along with a metallic and peppery sensation in their mouths as well as the other symptoms. They got the full treatment. Of course the fish looked just fine and tasted great.

After Martha Jefferson–not her real name–a 34-year-old devotee of Sushi, a trendy Japanese dish often containing raw fish, experienced continued pain, she relented and went for X-rays. Embedded in the mucosal lining of her stomach was an inch-long third-stage larva of Anisakis simplex. Raw Salmon is considered its most likely source. This and other parasitic worms, are frequent inhabitants of raw salmon, tuna, mackerel and other fish. The operational term here is raw, but tasted great. Getting medical care, alleviated her pains.[3]

It was a malicious, malignant and premeditated attempt to control the outcome of a municipal election by sickening and killing enough voters that the

Bhagwanshree Rajneesh commune (cult) would win the upcoming election and thereby control community zoning and other community issues.

In Oregon, the Rajneesh religious community had its headquarters in The Dalles, county seat of Wasco county, a community of some 11,000 people, located near the Columbia River, on Interstate 54. Between September 9th and October 10th, 1984, 751, adults became ill with a Salmonella-induced gastroenteritis. All had eaten at salad bars in some 10 restaurants. It took more than a year to accumulate evidence linking the commune with the epidemic. FBI agents found a vial of Salmonella typhimurium (a bacterial culture obtained for a small fee from the American Type Culture Collection, Baltimore, MD) in the commune's clandestine laboratory. On March 19th, 1986, two commune members were indicted for poisoning food in violation of a federal anti tampering act, and were sentenced to substantial prison terms. They admitted that they had intended to make enough citizens sick to prevent them from voting. They also admitted sloshing cultures of Salmonella over foods in salad bars, and in coffee creamers. Salad bars are of course open to all.[4] Who would know? Who could tell that any food was compromised? It was so easy, so uncomplicated. That's the beauty, or is it stealthiness, of bioterrorism. In addition to the illnesses related directly to a specific microbe, there will be psychiatric casualties. Bioterrorism, as discussed in chapter FOUR, is an ugly business.

Vanilla ice cream. Imagine. America's favorite food was the source of the largest outbreak of Salmonellosis and the largest food poisoning episode in American history, September of 1996. The centralized condition of our country's food distribution network lends itself to endangering huge numbers of us.

Commercial Ice cream producers use only pasteurized milk; as well they should, and be expected to.

No problem there. And, as we know, pasteurization readily kills Salmonella. It's the homemade ice cream, often made with raw milk that allows Salmonella to grow and deposit its pernicious exotoxin in ice cream. How, then, could ice cream become the vehicle for inciting the gastroenteritis that laid low so many thousands of ice cream lovers? Let's be up front and open about it. Salmonella bacteria are fecal inhabiting organisms contributed by animals and we humans: that's the sad part.

Tanker trailers hauling thousands of gallons of ice cream made from base premix had hauled unpasteurized liquid eggs to processing plants before taking on the ice cream. That would have been okay had the tanker drivers not broken established work rules requiring tankers hauling unpasteurized liquid eggs to be thoroughly washed and sanitized before loading the ice cream premix. In this instance, tanker after tanker was found to have bypassed the protocols, allowing the Salmonella-contaminated liquid eggs to contaminate the premix, which was not repasteurized after transportation. 224,000 vanilla ice cream lovers became unwilling half-steppers.[5] Can this happen again? Will it happen again? Yes, to both. Why? Human behavior. Don't be surprised when headlines scream, Salmonellosis in thousands!

In 2011, the Center for Disease Control and Prevention, reported that Salmonella infection causes more hospitalizations and death than any other bacteria, and noted that from 2004 to 2008, the major sources of illness caused by Salmonella were poultry, eggs, pork, beef, vine vegetables, fruits and nuts: an exceeding collection of our food supply. Salmonella can cause severe diarrhea, fever, and abdominal cramping. These organisms do not produce toxin in the foods they contaminate. No. They wait until we've eaten, then, in the warm confines of our small intestines they begin their dirty work. Using what resembles miniature syringes, they inject more than 60 proteins into our intestinal cells, allowing them to spread from cell to cell spitting out toxin, prolonging the agony. Who wants that!?

Staphylococcus aureus, the golden one, growing as it does with its glistening golden-yellow pigment, is an exotoxin producer if there ever was one, ruined an excursion for 627 vacationers, many of whom became violently ill as their train rolled into the station at Spartanburg, South Carolina.

We Digress for Toxin: Exo and Endo

Staphylococcal toxins, chemicals toxic to us, not to the Staph, are water-soluble proteins that mix readily with our blood, and consequently are rapidly transported from head to toe. Not only is this toxin among the most lethal chemicals known, but Staphylococci growing in highly nutritious, agreeable environments such as chicken, turkey, tuna, ham, egg, and shrimp salads, release six different toxins as part of their digestion— a waste product no less! Custard-filled cakes and meat pies offer similar luxurious environments.

How did these invisible poisoners get into these otherwise enjoyable foods? Easily. From toxic staphylococci on boils, carbuncles, abscesses, and blisters on hands and fingers of those preparing the salads and meat pies, as well as droplets falling onto foods from those with dripping noses where exotoxigenic Staph frequently hangout, or in. With the passage of a few hours these contaminated foods become virtual bombs.

It's the toxin, not the bacteria, that induces the violent vomiting and diarrhea that the body, in its wisdom, is trying to expel–rid itself, at both ends, simultaneously. For Staph toxin, the violence usually occurs 4-6 hours after ingestion.

Then there are the endotoxin producing nasties, such as Salmonella whose toxin is part of its cell wall. Ah, but these are not proteins. Their toxin is a lipopolysaccharide; lipids, fat, attached to a string of sugars. Who would have thought?

When a food containing Salmonella is eaten, the Salmonella die in the stomach's high acid environment. As they die they release their toxin to do its dirty work. The degree of dirty work depends on the dose, the number of bacterial cells ingested. And how do the Salmonella get in to our foods? It's not nice; via Salmonella-infected food handlers who may be asymtomatic, but still shedding organisms, or actually symptomatic, but telling no one. In either case hands are not washed, or improperly washed after a session in the John. Trouble is about to brew. But no beer in sight.

How toxic can bacterial toxins be? The Clostridia are at the top of the toxin-producing totem. One milligram, a thousandth of a gram, (there are 28 grams in an ounce) of Botulinum, the toxin of Clostridium botulinus, can kill one million Guinea pigs, and quite a few humans, as our lady with the mushrooms and peppers found out, or her family found out.

Let's Rejoin the Folks on the Train

Its been erroneously assumed that high salt concentrations act as preservatives and prevent bacterial growth. Maybe. But not with Staphylococci. Enterotoxigenic strains of Staph can grow in salt concentrations as high as twenty percent. Consequently, ham cured with the usual 3.5 percent offers little challenge to the type A, one of the six, toxin producing species.

On June 11th, of that fateful year, 40 hams were delivered to a small restaurant in Erwin, Tennessee, and stored in a walk-in refrigerator at $14^{\circ}C$ ($57^{\circ}F$)

On the 12th, they were cooked, deboned, separated, and returned to the refrigerator for another day. Out again for slicing, then back in.

On June 14th, the slices were preheated at $350^{\circ}F$

(175°C) for one-and-half to two hours hours—
a treatment that cannot inactivate toxin—then boxed with
other items and delivered to the Erwin railroad station.

On June 15th, 627 hungry passengers on an
excursion between Kentucky and South Carolina
descended on the station at 12:30 pm, for a box lunch.
By 5:30pm, when the train reached Marion, South
Carolina, on its way to Spartanburg, 93 were vomiting
and diarrhetic: 36 required hospitalization. By midnight,
over 200 had become ill. Type A Staph were isolated
from four ham samples, as well as the sickies stool
samples; direct evidence of a cause-effect relationship.
Toxin formation and inadequate refrigeration had struck
again.[6]

Let's keep on this track.

In Tokyo, 343 unsuspecting passengers boarded a
Japan Air Lines 747 Jumbo Jet for a flight to Paris. On
the weekend of February 1st, that year, a cook in Alaska
with Staphylococci-infected finger blisters had prepared
205 portions of ham, for ham and egg omelet trays.

The portions were kept at room temperature for at
least six hours prior to completing the trays.
On completion, the trays were stored overnight at 50°F
(10°C) awaiting the arrival of the 747. Staphylococci
were growing and toxin was accumulating in the ham.
The plane arrived and trays were loaded aboard, and the
plane took off for Copenhagen, its next refueling stop
before Paris.

Six to seven hours later, the trays were heated in
300°F ovens for 15 minutes. Wholly inadequate, to
destroy the toxin. Breakfast was served. As the plane
touched down in Copenhagen, nausea, vomiting,
cramping and diarrhea prostrated 143 passengers who
had to be carried from the plane. Another 50 would be
carried off in Paris.

In this episode, the crew remained unaffected.
That would be of great interest to Epidemiologists

investigating this out break. The new crew that came aboard in Anchorage had already eaten breakfast and had no reason or desire to eat the prepared omelets. In a similar situation pilot and copilot could easily become victims with an outcome unpleasant to contemplate.

Following investigation of this incident, Kenji Kawabata, Executive Director of Inflight Catering International, committed suicide. Are lessons being learned?

Can we say farewell to the toxin producers without a nod to that ever-present bacterium inhabiting our intestines as well as the intestines of many of the animals around us? Certainly not.

Escherchia coli, aka, E.coli, does concern us. That E, is in honor of Dr. Theodor Escherich, a Pediatrician who discovered the 'bug' in feces from a case of travelers diarrhea, in 1885, while an attending physician at Children's Hospital in Munich, Germany. So much for history. Suffice it to say, most types of E.coli, there are many, are harmless. A few incorrigible strains such as E.coli O157:H7 can cause severe bloody diarrhea, abdominal cramping, and kidney failure. Raw vegetables and undercooked ground beef are the leading culprits. Adults usually recover from their twin toxins that suppress our immune defenses, but it's the kids and their grandparents that get walloped with life threatening forms of kidney failure.

The bacterial strains that release these toxins are referred to as Shiga toxin-producing E.coli, or STEC. You may even hear or see them called Verocytotoxic E.coli, VTEC, or enterohemorrhagic E.coli, EHEC, that cause the hemolytic uremic syndrome,HUS. Who would want to skip all this good stuff with those tongue-twisting cognomens?

This dreadful complication usually occurs 3-4 days after eating a contaminated food. It could also be as short as one day, or as long as10. How do we lay hold of it? STEC reside in the guts of cattle, goats, sheep, deer and elk, but for most of us the major contributors are cattle, which do not make them sick. Pigs and birds can also pick up STEC and help spread it around in their droppings. For us to become infected we've got to ingest feces, a microbiological requirement. Not the greatest thought in the world, but we do. It occurs more often than we prefer to believe. Raw milk is a hefty contributor, as is unpasteurized apple cider, and soft cheeses made from, you guessed it, raw milk; undercooked rare hamburger, and even lettuce can convey the microbe and its toxin straight to us. Eating food prepared by those who fail to wash their hands properly after visiting the toilet, become an added risk. What goes on, or doesn't go on in the restroom, can undo many of us.

How about this? As of 5:00 PM, Monday, January 4th, 2010, 21 people infected with O157:H7 had been reported from16 states. Most became ill between mid-October and late November, and range in age from 14 to 87.

Nine have been hospitalized, one with hemolytic uremic syndrome. Thus far none have died. On December 24th, 2009, the Department of Agriculture's Food Safety and Inspection Service, (FSIS) issued a notice of recall for 248,000 pounds of beef distributed by the National Steak and Poultry Company, that was contaminated with O157:H7. It's an on-going problem that needn't be. We'll deal with that shortly.[7]

Cyclospora Cayetanensis
(Sy-clo-spore-uh Kye-uh-tuh-nen sis)

Are there better ways to transplant a foreign parasite than bringing it home with you, or flying it in as air freight? Americans with diarrhea returning home from Nepal, Haiti, and Mexico, brought Cyclospora and its illness Cyclosporiasis unannounced through immigration. Additionally, food importers are flying contaminated fruits and vegetables in at an increasing pace to keep up with demand for those foods.

Before 1996, Cyclosporiasis was seen only sporadically and limited to foreign travelers, but in the spring of 1996, some 1,500 cases erupted around the US and Canada, and another 1,000 in 1997, all attributed to eating feces-contaminated raspberries from Guatemala where this esoteric diarrhea is endemic.

Although blackberries, raspberries, and vegetables were implicated in these massive episodes, cases have also been related to undercooked meat and poultry. An airline pilot became ill when he brought food on board that had been cooked in a Haitian kitchen.

It's well known that waste water in sewage lagoons has been used to irrigate pastureland, as well as vegetable and berry fields. Unless and until it is amply demonstrated that imported fruits and vegetables have been grown by standards deemed appropriate in the US, we consumers might well stay with domestic produce, a reasonable preventive strategy. Rinsing fruits and vegetables does not reliably remove Cyclospora's reproductive cells. No one is immune. All ages and both genders are equally at risk. Travelers heading south of the border to tropical and subtropical areas are at increased risk as Cyclosporiasis is endemic in a number of developing countries. Watery diarrhea and explosive bowel movements, loss of appetite, bloating, and on and on, is what Cyclospora is about. Ergo, vigilance is the price of a calm digestive tract. For the six hundred new cases of Cyclosporiasis in twenty-two states, in June 2013, due to eating salad mix packed by Taylor Farms, in Mexico, a calm digestive tract would be a bit longer in coming. And these new cases had the CDC and FDA racing to prevent additional infections. You just never know.

From the Centers of Disease Control, CDC, we learn that Listeriosis is now a challenging public health problem, especially for pregnant women who are not only at increased risk, but are also 20 times as likely to become infected than women generally. Some 30 percent of all Listeria infections occur during pregnancy. And, it's the newborn infant that suffers the affects, many dying within a few hours of birth. Those who survive may have long-term neurological damage and/or delayed development.

They are not the only ones at increased risk. Immune suppressed individuals, especially those with AIDS are 300 times as likely to become ill. Fever, muscle aches, headaches, stiff neck, confusioin and loss of balance, the prominent symptoms, indicate central nervous system involvement.

Listeria monocytogenes, the organism that causes this wretched illness is common in both wild and domesticated animals whose fecal droppings are deposited in soil and water. Vegetables and meats become contaminated with soil and manure often used as fertilizer. Raw milk, and cheese made from raw milk, are notorious sources of these Listeria.

In adults the illness may take any number of forms, occurring as meningitis, pneumonia, and endocarditis, or in its milder forms, abscesses, skin lesions, and conjunctivitis, severely complicating diagnosis. Fortunately Listeria are readily killed by the heat of pasteurization and cooking. Isn't it our poor choices that get us in trouble? Nevertheless, the FDA, and the Department of Agriculture's Food Safety and Inspection Services offer the following advice for pregnant women:

Do not eat hot dogs, luncheon meats, or deli meats unless they are reheated until steaming hot.

Avoid getting fluid from hot dog packages on other foods, utensils, and preparation surfaces, and wash hands after handling hot dogs, luncheon meats, and deli meats.

Do not eat soft cheeses such as Feta, Brie, and Camenbert, blue-veined cheeses, or Mexican-style cheeses such as Queso Blanco, Queso Fresco, and Panela, unless they have labels that clearly state they have been made from pasteurized milk.

Do not eat refrigerate pate´ or meat spreads.

Do not eat refrigerated smoked seafood unless it is in an ingredient in a cooked dish such as a casserole.

Do not drink unpasteurized milk, or eat foods made of unpasteurized milk.

All this may be a great deal to ask a pregnant woman to forego, but it is worth a healthy baby. Can there be more then that one response?

Isn't it our poor choices that get us in trouble? As the kid said, "we've met the enemy, and he is us" is about right. Would it help if feces were green?

Many of us know that raw oysters are a high demand delicacy. We gobble them up by the bucketful. Wasn't it Sam Weller, Charles Dickens appealing character of Pickwick Papers fame, who ate so many oysters that his stomach rose and fell with the tide? Unfortunately, however yummy they may be, raw and undercooked oysters carry risks. The CDC estimates that annual infections are as high as 45,000, with a substantial death rate.

Among healthy people who ingest the troublesome pathogen *Vibrio vulnificus*, they can expect vomiting, diarrhea, and abdominal pain. But those folks with existing medical conditions such as diabetes, HIV/AIDS, kidney disease, cancer, immune disorders, and chronic liver disease, are eighty times more likely to develop blood stream infections that can lead to death.

This *Vibrio vulnificus*, a close relative of Vibrio cholerae, that has brought us cholera for centuries, is also related to Vibrio parahemolyticus, responsible for a violent diarrhea. A dreadful family to be shunned. Vulnificus, from the latin, meaning, inflicting wounds, and well named, grows exceedingly well in the warm Gulf of Mexico, and along the southern states that border it. Not only does it grow well, there has been a 115 percent increase in oyster-eating *Vibrio vulnificus* infections since 1998. Although the FDA would like those gulf coast states that harvest and ship oysters to employ a post-harvest mild heat treatment, a low-temperature pasteurization, compliance in those states has been spotty at best, as those states do not have the capacity to process all the oysters for raw consumption that are harvested during the seven months from April through October.

It has yet to be determined how long it will take to put in place the equipment required for the low-temperature pasteurization. Consequently, raw and undercooked oysters remain a significant risk. Oyster gobblers be warned. Caution is your watchword.

In its wisdom, the CDC not only collects info on microbes involved in food borne illness, it makes good use of them. So, for example, they have given us the top five pathogens contributing to food borne illness in order of their importance. They are:

Norovirus (Norwalk Agent)

Salmonella (non-typhoidal)

Clostridium perfringens

Campylobacter

Staphylococcus aureus

Norovirus just happens to be the most common cause of acute gastroenteritis in the country, infecting painfully, some 21million of us, sending 70 thousand to hospitals, and another eight hundred to their graves. Norovirus has become a cruise ship company's worst nightmares; trapped between a rock and a hard place, because for the most part it's the passengers that bring the virus on board. But it's the ship and the cruise line that take the brunt of the awful publicity.

We also have the list of the top five pathogens that give no warning of their presence, but contribute to the 70,000 hospitalizations annually. And the winners are!

Salmonella (non-typhoidal)

Norovirus

Campylobacter

Toxplasma gondii

E.coli (STEC)

Also now available are the top five contributing to illness resulting in death. These are:

Salmonella (non-typhoidal)

Toxoplasma gondii

Listeria monocytogenes

Norovirus

Campylobacter

The CDC also reminds us that the Salmonella are responsible for approximately 1.2 million illnesses annually, with $365 million in direct medical and related costs every year. The many different types of Salmonella, 28-hundred strains have been identified, have different animal resevoirs and food sources that make control particularly challenging...read, difficult. Clearly, the need for improved methods of food protection and safety require a higher priority, which leads directly to the new Food Safety and Modernization Act, which will be followed by a discussion of food preservation by irradiation, that can readily prevent or greatly reduce the infections and spoilage wrought by microbes. It's a winnable battle. That's another take away message.

The Food Safety Modernization Act, signed into law by President Obama, on January 4th, 2011, is the most sweeping reform of our food safety laws since 1943. FSMA, seeks to ensure that our food supply is safe by shifting the focus from responding to contamination, to preventing it. This means that contamination controls will be set up and implemented in food production facilities as well as controls for foreign food supplies, which also means that all imported foods meet US standards.

These preventive measures will take time to kick-in, as we get food from over 150 countries, the best and the worst. Furthermore, for the first time, FDA will have the authority to order a recall of food products. Except for infant formula, FDA has had to rely on food manufacturers and distributors to recall food voluntarily, which was a dicey business.

For all of us, the FSMA is a long deferred, and auspicious beginning for a new era in food protection at the source.

Food Irradiation: Elevating Food Safety

Consider these numbers:

47,800,000

127,839

(62,529-215,562)

3,037

(1,492-4,983)

These potent numbers provide a painful and discouraging narrative. 48 million is an estimate of the number of women, children, and men that become ill with a food borne disease every year. That's close to sixteen percent, of our total population! One in every six of us!

128 thousand is an estimate number of women, men and children that, food borne illnesses, send to hospitals around the country every year. The CDC's data suggests that a more realistic number could be as low as 62,529, and as high as 215,562.

Three thousand are the number of men, women and children estimated to die of food borne diseases every year. Here, the CDC indicates that the range estimate is

1,492 to 4,983. All these numbers, these people, are for a single year.

Before digging into food irradiation, a comment about the numbers seems appropriate.

The margin of error bands, 62,529 to 215,562, and, 1,492 to 4,983, are so high, 300 percent or more, that the specific numbers down to the last digits are truly questionable. Wouldn't it be more appropriate to say, 63,000 to 216,000, and 1,500 to 5,000, until much firmer numbers are obtained? After all, numbers do have consequences.

Furthermore, in five and 10 years those numbers, the toll, is grim, but worse, it need not occur. Not when a proven safe and effective means of food preservation is at hand.

Food irradiation is a relatively new food safety process that can eliminate most spoilage organisms and just about all the sickeners such as E.coli, Salmonella, Listeria, Staphylococci, Clostridia, and a host of others. The process provides the extra benefits of inhibiting sprouting in vegetables, delaying ripening of fruits, obviating the need for chemical preservatives, and increasing safe and edible shelf life from days to weeks.

The effects of irradiation on the food and on animals and people eating irradiated food have been studied extensively for more than 40 years, and clearly show that when irradiation is used as approved on foods:

Disease causing microorganisms are reduced or eliminated

The nutritional value is essentially unchanged

The food does not become radioactive

These benefits have galvanized 40 countries worldwide to permit food irradiation of some 40 different foods. Consequently more than 500,000 tons of food are irradiated annually. Because irradiation destroys disease causing bacteria, the process is used in hospitals to sterilize food for immunocompromised patients.

Irradiation is also used for sterilizing medical products such as surgical gloves, destroying bacteria in cosmetics, nonstick cookware coatings, purifying wool, performing security checks on hand luggage at airports, and making tires more durable. Is it necessary to note that none of the above become radioactive?

To become comfortable and familiar with this newest method of food preservation, we begin with the fact that the sun delivers a tremendous amount of energy daily, most of which travels to earth as radiation. Radiation simply means radiant energy. It has nothing, repeat, nothing, to do with radioactivity. It refers only to the transmission and absorption of radiant energy that moves through space as invisible electromagnetic waves with differing energy levels: a completely natural phenomenon. Consequently different types of radiant energy, visible light, microwaves, radio and TV waves, infrared, ultra violet, X-rays and gamma rays can be distinguished from one another by their wavelengths. At one end of the electromagnetic spectrum, we have cosmic, gamma, and X-rays, with the greatest penetrating power, and at the opposite end, FM, radio, TV, and microwaves, with the lowest energy levels and least penetrating power. Visible light, the only energetic wave we can see, exists as a narrow band between ultraviolet and infrared. It's at this end of the energy spectrum that we use the low energy levels to toast bread and cook food.

The radiant energy used in food preservation is called ionizing radiation or irradiation, and is among the shorter more penetrating wavelengths, and are capable of damaging the DNA of the microbes that spoil our foods and initiate disease. As with the heat of pasteurization of milk, irradiation reduces but does not eliminate all spoilage organisms. But it does destroy the more fragile pathogens.

Irradiation exposes food to short bursts of high electromagnetic energy. When microbes are irradiated, the energy from the wave is transferred to the water and

DNA in the bacteria, fungi and insects, creating short-lived, reactive chemicals that prevents their multiplication. They die. As the dose of radiation is so small, there is no chance of the food ever becoming radioactive. Furthermore, the food never touches a radioactive substance. As irradiation is essentially a cold process, producing virtually no heat within the food, taste, aroma, and texture remain unchanged.

At moderate doses of irradiation, nutritional losses are less than, or about the same as cooking or freezing. At lower doses, loss of nutrients are either unmeasurable or insignificant: amino acids, fatty acids, and vitamin content, if altered at all, are so minimal as to be insignificant.

The question that follows appears to be, how are foods irradiated? Two things are required: a source of radiant energy, and a place to confine the energy. Really quite simple. Nothing out-of-the-ordinary. The two irradiation processes currently available, Radioactive Isotopes and Electron Beams, produce energy differently.

Radioactive isotopes, are natural, and the oldest form of irradiation, using radiation emitted by the naturally radioactive chemical Cobalt-60, or Cesium-137, which emit gamma rays that can readily penetrate deeply into food of any density. These gamma rays do not produce neutrons, which means that nothing in their path can become radioactive. You never want to forget this. It's that important! It may help to recall that those of us who receive radiation treatments for medical problems do not become radioactive. Moreover, NASA's astronauts regularly eat foods that have been sterilized at radiation levels 45 times that of commercial levels. They've been doing so for some 40 years and have never experienced adverse reactions. They eat irradiated food to avoid any possibility of a food borne illness while on a space mission.

As both Cobalt-60 and Cesium-137 continually emit their naturally occurring gamma rays, high-energy photons, they are stored in a pool of water that harmlessly absorbs the radiation. When needed, they are raised out of the pool and moved to a room with massive concrete walls that harmlessly absorbs the radiation. Foods to be irradiated are wheeled into the room and exposed to the radiation for a defined period. After use, the isotopes are returned to the pool and the food is sent on its way. The process is clean and fast.

Beams of electrons or "e-beams" are streams of high energy electrons propelled out of an electron gun, the same—but larger—version of the device at the rear of our household TV tubes, before the arrival of flat screens, that propel electrons into the TV screen at the front of the tube, making it light up. With the the e-beam generator radioactive isotopes are not involved, nor is massive concrete shielding needed, as gamma rays are not at all involved.

Electrons, with their far less penetrating energy can go only inches into food so that irradiation via electron beams require either thin sections of food, or the process must use two beams, one above and one below to irradiate thicker portions. An added benefit is the fact that all foods are irradiated in their final packaging which means there's no chance of recontamination. Now that's a compelling feature.

The electrically charged particles emerge from a linear accelerator at speeds approaching the speed of light. As they flash through the foods, they create particles, ions, and free radicals that disrupt microbial and insect DNA, destroying most, but not all of them. The irradiated hamburger we've been purchasing from our local Wegman's supermarket is processed by electron beams. We've been eating and enjoying it for years, knowing that our burgers are free of E.coli and other nasties. With food irradiation, rare hamburger can return to our buns. Electron beam processing is becoming the process of choice, replacing radioactive isotopes.

While meat, poultry, pork, potatoes, fish, seafoods, (not oysters), grains, onions, fruits and veggies are readily amenable to irradiation, some foods are not.

Irradiation causes egg whites to become milky, and more liquid, which makes the egg look like an old egg, and does not do well in recipes. Lettuce and spinach wilt which, at this time seems to be a matter of dose. As irradiation is a form of pasteurization, not all spoilage organisms are removed. Consequently, consumers need to take the same precautions used with all foods–proper refrigeration, appropriate handling and cooking.

By law, all irradiated foods must carry the Radura, the international symbol for irradiation, with its simple green petals (representing the food) in a broken circle (representing the rays from the energy source). This symbol must be accompanied by the words, "Treated by Irradiation," or "Treated with Radiation."

Yes, it does: food irradiation sounds like a wonderful use of nuclear chemistry principles. Although it's routinely used in Europe, Canada, and Mexico, we in the US of A have been hesitant to adopt it widely. It makes no sense. With so many people around the world using it regularly, how is it possible that so many of us think it harmful. Are we in denial? I'm convinced that if the public had gotten information supporting food irradiation in understandable manner, fears would have melted away.

So, for example, in their review of food irradiation, the US General Accountability Office, (GAO) had this to say:

"Despite the benefits of irradiation, the widespread use of irradiated food hinges largely on consumer confidence in the safety and wholesomeness of these products. The cumulative evidence from over four decades of research, carried out in laboratories in the United States, Europe and other countries worldwide, indicates that irradiated food is safe to eat. The food is not radioactive; there is no evidence of toxic substances resulting from irradiation; and there is no evidence or reason to expect that irradiation produces more virulent pathogens

among those that survive irradiation treatment.

In addition, nutritional losses from irradiation are similar to other forms of processing and would not adversely affect a food's nutritional value. "[8]

GAO is not alone in extending high regard for irradiation. The American Medical Association's Council on Scientific Affairs published its Report No.4, Irradiation of Food, as far back as 1993. After a full discussion of the process of food irradiation, it informed its membership and Journal readers that irradiated food was not only safe and efficacious, but also a desirable addition to the pantheon of food preservation processes. It concluded by stating: "The Council on Scientific Affairs recommends that the AMA affirm food irradiation as a safe and effective process that increases the safety of food when applied according to governing regulations."[9]

In similar fashion, the American Dietetic Association, a national and international professional association of thousands of dietitians and nutritionists, published its position on irradiated food, stating that, "The ADA encourages the government, food manufacturers, food commodity groups, and qualified food and nutrition professionals to work together to educate consumers about this additional food safety tool and to make their choice available in the marketplace."[10]

If those were not kudos enough, the Food and Agricultural Organization (FAO) and the World Health Organization (WHO), both UN affiliates, have endorsed food irradiation unreservedly, as had the American Gastroenterological Association, whose thousands of physicians are highly knowledgeable about our gastrointestinal tracts.

The list of endorsers is long and impressive:

US Government Agencies:

The Food and Drug Administration

The Public Health Service

Centers for Disease Control, CDC

US Scientific Organizations:

American Veterinary Medical Association

Council for Agricultural Science and Technology

Institute of Food Technologists

National Association of State Departments of Agriculture

International Organizations:

International Atomic Energy Agency

Codex Alimentarious Commission

Scientific Committee of the European Union

The United Nations

Wow! and Wow! again. Manifestly, and palpably, food irradiation has gained many friends: important friends who know that irradiated food is safe and beneficial. How then, has the American public alone come to fear, and reject it? It's perverse. Is it possible that food irradiation is deemed so unacceptable that 48 million illnesses a year are acceptable? That's too much of a stretch—or is it?

Confidence building needs to begin soon. But it will not happen if newspapers such as The New York Times, my favorite newspaper no less, doesn't get behind food irradiation an provide the public with the essential facts and supporting organizations and agencies. Why the New York Times?

Early in October 2009, The Times ran a long and vivid story headlined, "The Burger That Shattered Her LIfe." Its two-plus pages recounted in harrowing detail the hellish experience of this young, otherwise healthy, vibrant women who ate a hamburger containing E.coli O157:H7 and became paralyzed. Nowhere among its thousands of words did the writer even hint at the possibility of food irradiation preventing such occurrences. On October 10th, a Times editorial declared "Eating a Hamburger Should Not Be a Death-Defying Experience." Indeed, it should not. But again, not a word suggesting there was a food safety process that could prevent this misery, and that it was time to unveil it.

Not a letter to the editor suggesting the use of food irradiation was published. I know, because I sent two: one to the letters column, and when that wasn't acknowledged, I sent another to the Public Editor, which also garnered no response. Given the many national and international organizations are on record supporting food irradiation, it would have been reasonable, at the very least, for The Times to let the public know why it is silent on food irradiation.

I'm disappointed that The Times and other newspapers, and the mass media generally, have given food irradiation short shrift, in the face of the many positive statements by our top medical and scientific organizations. Its as if they don't exist. The silence is deafening while death and illness prevail–unnecessarily.

Too often programs and processes that have the greatest impact on health get the least attention. It's time to make things happen, to lesson the morbidity and mortality rates. Here's hoping we don't miss the wave.

I remain hopeful, knowing that food irradiation can markedly reduce the toll of illness and death. Its' time cannot be far off.

Time now, for a 180 degree twirl. We now join those germs, those microbes that deliver joy, fill our stomachs, and provide relaxation.

SIX

Germs Of Endearment

Germs have captured our attention. We are wary of them. But as we have seen, the delinquents are not only a minority population, they are low, very low on the totem pole of leading causes of death. Therefore, it's time to turn our attention to the many and diverse benefactors that provide for us in myriad ways barely, if ever, noticed.

If not for them, yea, without them, life would be dull, boring, and for the most part unlivable; more than likely, impossible. They are that crucial. So, let the repertoire unfold.

What's Going on Here??

Wisconsin just became the first state to adopt a microbe: yes, adopted a microbe right up there with the state motto, flower and flag. *Lactococcus lactis* is now the official state microbe. And about time. It's the bacterium behind all that cheese, without which Wisconsin would be reduced to the Green Bay Packers sans Aaron Rogers. And Iowa is about to adopt and honor the soil bacterium, *Bradyrhizobium japonicum*, that allows soybeans, "to grow tall and green and produce plenty of beans." If Florida honors *Dunaliella salina*, responsible for the stunning pinks of their tasty shrimp and eye-catching Flamingoes, the race is on—to honor others.

Our gulf coast states are surely indebted to those microbes that gobbled up the oil flowing from a broken well, saving their coastal beaches, tourism, and seafood industry.

Oil-hungry *Alcanivorax burkunensis*, how's that for an arresting moniker, is emerging as the star "cleaner-upper" of the greatest oil spill in American history: a microbe that loves to chow down on hydrocarbons. With its voracious appetite for alkanes, a primary ingredient of crude oil, most of the oil in the Gulf will not have the devastating impact many predicted. We surely do need their untiring craving. Praise be to them.

However, pride of place may just belong to *Bifidobaterium longons*, a resident of human breast milk, which coats the intestinal lining of newborn infants protecting them from potentially harmful delinquent germs. These shining paragons are but the pinnacle of our beneficial microbial universe.

Moreover, our microbes, our germs, do gussy-up our habitats. Who knew that the lush crimson Pointsettia, so colorful at Christmas, owe their luxuriance to the microbes residing within them? Joel Roberts Poinsett, of Charleston, South Carolina, appointed by President John Quincy Adams, as our first Ambassador to Mexico, originally brought them back from Mexico, but he certainly didn't know about this symbiotic relationship as it has only recently been revealed. And when the phytoplasmas, as these bacteria have been dubbed, take up residence in Peonies, the typical bright-red and/or yellow flowers become delicate greens.

Those exotic Orchids we all admire and cherish,

have dust-like seeds that will only grow if nourished by groups of root fungi that grow into the roots of our delicate Orchids which then digest the fungi to obtain needed nutrients.

Nor can we overlook those highly coveted and artistically varigated tulips with their intricate stripes, bars, streaks, featherings and flame-like colorful effects: their breath-taking mottlings–gold and burgundy; purple and whites, reds and whites: green and white streakings, all produced by viruses. While previously the consequence of virus transmission via Aphids, these spectacular tulips and lilies, are currently produced by breeding. These impressive flowers do beautify our world and are a desirable addition.

The list of microbes and their benefits is long and often accompanied by remarkably rewarding consequences.

The Weizmann Organism

It is not too much of a stretch to say that *Clostridium acetobutylicum*, a commercially valuable soil bacterium, often called, "The Weizmann Organism," was directly responsible for the historic Balfour Declaration of November 1917, which led to the creation of the State of Israel. How could that be?

It was 1914: the world was at war; Britain versus Germany. The vital war at sea required huge numbers of shells for the Royal Navy's big guns, as well as its thousands of artillery pieces. These guns needed cordite, which produced smokeless powder that didn't reveal the gun's firing position.

Cordite, made of cellulose nitrate and nitroglycerine-gun cotton had to be combined into a paste with acetone and white petrolatum, petroleum jelly. The essential ingredient was acetone. But the normal supply of charcoal used to make acetone by way of distillation, was simply unavailable. A new way had to be found to make acetone, or Britain could not resist the German onslaught.

Prof. Chaim Weizmann, an organic chemist at Britain's Manchester University, had been working on a microbial fermentation of sugar to make isoprene for rubber. His work was well known at the Scottish branch of the Nobel explosives firm that supplied the Navy with, cordite. When acetone supplies became acute, the Scotts rushed Weizmann to London to meet with the First Lord of the Admiralty: none other than Winston Churchill. They got on famously, and Churchill made sure Weizmann got what he requested to make the huge gallonages of acetone and butyl alcohol he was sure his microbes could produce. Also needed were great quantities of maize, corn, for the starch the Clostridia would chow down on converting the starch to acetone and butyl alcohol, as well as a large distillery with its tanks where large-scale fermentation would occur. He got what he needed, and for the next two years, worked on this Herculean task, a one-man creation of a completely new industry: industrial fermentation.

The process depended upon the bacterium he was the first to isolate, and which, after countless culturings, improved its yield of both acetone and butyl alcohol.

When German U-boat warfare interrupted overseas supplies of corn, Weizmann switched to horse chestnuts that were equally appetizing to the Clostridia. School children were asked to collect the chestnuts, "conkers" they called them, which they eagerly did. For every hundred pounds, they received about seventy-five cents. Some 4-5 thousand tons were colleceted for the war effort.

Between 1914-1918, the Navy fired 200 million shells, and acetone was being produced at about a hundred thousand gallons a year. Remarkable! Given appropriate nutrients microbes can be coaxed to produce almost any biochemical substance by fermentation; changing one organic chemical into another.

Undeniably, Weizmann kept the Royal Navy's gun's firing by taking his Clostridia to Canada where there were unlimited supplies of corn, and continued to churn out all the acetone needed. When the US entered the war in 1917, the process was adopted here in the huge distilleries in Terre Haute, Indiana.[1]

Without a doubt, Clostridium acetobutylicum was an essential ally in winning the war. Microbes to the rescue!

Who was this Chaim Weizmann who saved the day for Britain?

Chaim Azriel Weizmann, world-famed chemist, statesman, leader of a forceful political movement, Zionism, and a great humanitarian, was the first President of the State of Israel.[2]

Weizmann, a Russian-born chemist, taught organic chemistry at the University of Geneva, Switzerland, then moved to Manchester University where he became a student favorite, and widely popular with the faculty. But he will be forever remembered as the chemist who inaugurated the industrial fermentation industry, and the man who was joined at the hip with a bacterium.

Bioremediation

The greatest oil spill in American history occurred in May 2010. Crude oil and gases erupted into the Gulf of Mexico during the explosion of British Petroleum's Deep Water Horizon's offshore drilling rig. The flow of oil and gas from the fractured Macondo well was enormous and unprecedented, and continued for eighty-seven days.

Given the immensity of the spill, over 300 million gallons, a number of scientists predicted that the oil would likely persist for years. They were wrong! By October 2010, propane, ethane, and methane gases along with the crude oil were gone, gobbled up by voracious microbes.

According to Profs. John Kessler of Texas A&M, and David Valentine of the University of California, San Diego, the mix of microbes not only cleaned up the Gulf (in short order I might add) but prevented a major greenhouse gas (methane) from getting into the atmosphere. Which "proves that the bacteria play a vital role in preventing heat trapping greenhouse gases on the ocean floor from entering the earths atmosphere"[3, 4] That's bioremediation in the service of humankind unparalleled.

As noted earlier, one of the most ravenous microbes was Alcanivorax, which dotes on alkanes-straight chain hydrocarbons. Abetting Alcanivorax was Cyclolasticus, which prefers aramatic hydrocarbons-those with at least one six-membered benzene ring.

After the Macondo well was capped, the methane dieters took over. Methylococcus, along with other methylotrophic populations such as methylophaga, the primary consumers, grew remarkably. The oil digested by these microbes does not build up in the microbes. No, the degraded oil hydrocarbons beome smaller carbon compounds that the organisms use to make the sugars, fats, and proteins needed for their growth and energy needs, and of course, to make more microbes.

The question rightly tumbling around in your brain may be, how did those microbes come to live on crude oil? A reasonable answer appears to be that much of the earth's crude oil is trapped in underground reservoirs, but some leak to the surface and has been doing so for hundreds of millions of years, along with these microbes that have learned to metabolize, dine on, crude oil. These oil-degrading organisms use oxygen and 'burn' oil hydrocarbons just as we use oxygen and 'burn' food for energy.

Prince William Sound

Shortly after midnight on March 24th, 1989, the supertanker, Exxon Valdez, bound for Long Beach,

California, struck Bligh Reef, in Alaska's Prince William Sound. More than eleven million gallons of crude oil from the Proudhoe oil field spilled into the sea: the largest oil spill in US waters, until the 2010 Deep Water Horizon event. Because of its remote location government and industry response was unimaginatively difficult. What did we learn from that spill? Microbes matter! That's what was learned. We learned that oil-degrading microbes are not limited to any one geographical habitat, or ecosystem. They are everywhere where there is oil, a diet they've become well familiar with. And for the future, responders to oil spills will not waste time with uncertain clean up methods. They will use the natural microbial communities as well as enhanced microbes—those that have had genes for devouring oil added to their genomes.

It was also learned that seeding the spill area with nitrogen-containing fertilizers, was useful in abetting the microbial remediation by providing an additional source of food for the gluttonous methanotrophs. Three years on, the heavily oiled shoreline was rid of its oil.

The Kuwaiti Outrage

Half-a-million tons of crude oil was deliberately released into the Persian Gulf in January 1991, by the Iraqi military pursuing a scorched-earth policy as they retreated from Kuwait; setting ablaze 613 of the 944 wells of the Rumaila oil field.

Speculations and predictions of environmental disasters ranged from a nuclear winter-type catastrophe, as the dense black smoke rose mile high, blocking the sun, to deluges of acid rain from the releases of sulfur dioxide and hydrogen sulfide, as well as forced global warming from the massive amounts of carbon dioxide released into the atmosphere by the burning oil.

None of that occurred! Recovery around the Gulf coastline was showing signs of health by 1992, driven by oil degrading indigenous microbes that played a substantial role in reducing the environmental impact. By 1995, the signs of recovery were well underway.

This unthinkable oil spill, (spill is a remarkably poor description of the deluge of oil let loose), of over 3 million gallons in a 60-mile-long slick that was the largest oil spill in history.

Savannah River Site

The Savannah River Site, SRS, a Department of Energy, and National Nuclear Security Administration Affiliate, is a 320-square mile installation located in the central Savannah River region of South Carolina, operated and managed by the Westinghouse Savannah River Company.

Over four decades, this Site has generated nuclear waste materials for defense, medical and space operations. Begun in 1950, to achieve worldwide nuclear weapons superiority for the US, it achieved its goal by 1980. In doing so, it produced tons of liquid waste including trichloroethylene, TCE, a volitile, chlorinated organic compound widely used as an organic solvent and degreasing agent. At the SRS, fuel and target elements were degreased in processing. In addition to TCE, there were huge stockpiles of perchloroethylene-PCE, trichloroethane, TCA, chlorobenzene, CB, and vinyl chloride, VC, all of which required remediation, removal, as a consequence of contaminating soil and ground water.

The Site was also heavily fouled by perchlorates, the salts of perchloric acid. The EPA has designated perchlorate, ClO_4, as "a likely human carcinogen: "disrupting the thyroid's ability to produce the hormones needed for normal growth and development, by interfering, with the uptake of iodide. Four types of perchlorates are available: ammonium, potassium, sodium and perchloric acid. Rocket and missile fuels are the heavy users of ammonium perchlorate as a propellant. Consequently there are huge amounts of waste perchlorates available to contaminate soil, air and ground water resources. But it is now evident that our specialized microbes can chew them up unsparingly.

The beauty of using indigenous microbes to eliminate these chlorinated organics is the employment of in situ bioremediation. In situ, for our Roman forebears, meant, to be used in the original or natural place, which means that environmental restoration of polluted soils and/or underground water sources need not be moved or pumped to the surface or other site for treatment. Using in situ remediation, relocation and transport of soils and water are avoided; contaminants are removed where they are. It's site specific: lowers remediation costs; lowers further contamination risks; yields shorter restoration times; increases efficiency and gains enhanced public and regulatory acceptability.[5]

Methanotrophic bacteria in sediment and ground water were chewing up TCE at a prodigious rate. TCE was becoming mineralized, that is, completely degraded to carbon dioxide and water. Evident also was the doubling and tripling of methanotrophs at the remediation sites.

The SRS had an area known as the Non Radioactive Waste Disposal Facility, which received such solid wastes as paints, thinners, solvents, batteries and rags used with organic solvents that can leach or generate hazardous organic compounds. Tests showed the presence in ground water of the pollutants, TCE, PCE, TCA, VC, and CB. Here again methanotrophic remediation resulted in undetectable levels of pollution in both ground water and soil. Also shown was that chlorobenzene could undergo microbial dechlorination, and that the benzene ring can be converted to catechol, a naturally occurring compound found in fruits and veggies, which we often see when slicing or shredding potatoes, as they turn brown from the release of the enzyme catechol oxidase. The next time you're in potato shredding mode, place a little lemon juice or vinegar in the water containing the peeled potatoes; they'll remain white.

After the loss of the chlorine atoms, the microbes go after the benzene ring. At the Site, "geochemical data confirmed that both TCE and CB levels were decreasing at a greater rate than would be expected due to ground water transport or dilution."[5]

Of course, when needed, microbial populations can be added to contamination sites where they are lacking. Recall that at Prince William Sound, where the Exxon Valdez went aground, nitrogen fertilizer was added to the water to stimulate the growth of the methanogens.

It has become evident that microbes can take on and digest a diversity of organic compounds once thought to be untouchables. If the methanotrophs, which 16S DNA sequencing has shown to include eight genera including methylococcus, methylomonas, and methylophaga, as well as Cycloclasticus and Colwella, the heretofore untouchables appear to be going the way of the Dodo. Why? Beause there is complete oxidation, destruction, of these chlorinated carbon compounds to methane, and from methane to carbon dioxide. Which means that methane, an exceptionally strong greenhouse gas, does not get into the atmosphere. That's got to be a very big plus.

Methane, the simplest of all carbon compounds, seems to have had an unusual history.

In the 16th century and 17th centuries, bulk items had to be transported by ship and it was well before the development of commercial fertilizers, so large shipments of manure were quite common. Manure was shipped dry, as dry manure weighed a good bit less than wet, but once water (at sea) contacted it, not only did it become heavier, but the process of fermentation began again, which produces methane gas as a by-product.

As the manure was stored in bundles below decks, you can see what could, and did-happen. Methane began to build up below decks and the first time a sailor came below with a lantern, boom!

Several ships were destroyed this way before it was determined what was happening. After that, the bundles of manure were always stamped with the instruction, Stow High in Transit, which meant that sailors had to stow the bundles high enough off the lower decks so that any water that entered the hold would not touch the volatile cargo, starting the production of methane. Thus evolved the term, S.H.I.T. Stow High in Transit, which has come down through the centuries and remains in use to this day. More than likely most of us never knew the history of this word. I'm one of them. I always thought it was a golf term.

Envirogen Technologies

Headquartered in the Houston suburb of Kingwood, Texas, Envirogen Technologies, with a regional office in New Jersey, twenty minutes from my home in Princeton, focuses primarily on the treatment of ground water for the provision of high quality drinking water, ground water remediation, waste water treatment, and volitile organic chemical control. But its singular contribution is the use of microbes in a fluidized bed reactor—a bioreactor. This fosters the luxuriant growth of a mix of microbes; methanogens, methanotrophs, pseudamonads, and others, depending upon the type and degree of chlorinated hydrocarbon contamination to be removed, on a hydraulically fluidized fine media of sand or carbon granules. This bed provides these microbes with remarkably huge surface areas, allowing them to grow and digest whatever chemical comes their way.

The fluidized bed concept was originally applied on an industrial scale in the 1950's for the incineration of waste, and became a standard chemical processing technology in Europe; arriving in the US, in the late 1960's.

A fluidized bed is a bed or layer of sand, carbon or other granular material depending upon the chemicals being treated in a chamber fitted with thousands of tiny holes through which compressed air is continuously forced. The air pressure lifts and separates the granules, creating a turbulent mixture of air and granules that behave as though it were a liquid, or fluid, with continuous movement. The microbial mix in the reactor chamber obtains tremendous surface area on the granules for digesting chemical contaminants rapidly, while increasing its population: microbes prosper, and contaminants are destroyed. A model of a win/win condition. It's efficient and cost effective.

Envirogen builds reactors at a site requiring remediation-a form of in situ remediation. A mix of microbes is either naturally at the site, or is grown at the site from a concentrated culture.

So, for example, a bioreactor was built at a site in the City of Rialto, California to provide high quality drinking water after removing nitrates and perchlorates from the City's ground water. This will clean up a perchlorate plume that has compromised Rialto's water supply since its detection in 1997. The end products of this microbial treatment are innocuous nitrogen gas and common table salt, sodium chloride. Any organisms in the cleaned up water are removed by the City's normal water purification system.

Envirogen has also entered into a joint venture with an Israeli company, Shikun & Binui Water Ltd., to perform a pilot-scale demonstration of its fluidizeded reactor in the city of Ramat Ha'Sharon, to remove nitrates, perchlorates, chromates, and RDX, at a former Israeli military Industrial site, north of Tel Aviv. RDX, by the way, stands for Research Department Explosive, used around the world, and is more powerful than TNT-trinitrotoluene. RDX is a white, crystalline solid whose chemical moniker is cyclotrimethylenetrinitramine. With a molecule of such Herculean proportions, it takes brave microbes to take it on. But these hearty bacteria are also quite clever. They don't go for the fences, or the goal line in one swoop. No, they take small bites, doing it piecemeal. It works beautifully. If Envirogen's microbes can enjoy an RDX meal, they can dine on anything. Envirogen and the Israeli's are confident of the outcome.

The future of bioremediation is not just bright it's sparkling, booming. Microbes are easy to work with, and they love the diets they are being fed. These single-celled creatures can and will dine on most anything on their table, which can be soil, air, ground water, rivers, and seas. They are everywhere, and always ready to dine.

To participate in this princely dinning, the Kroger Supermarket chain is using bacteria at its Compton, California large distribution Center to convert 150 tons-a-day of damaged produce, bread and other organic waste to biogas that is burned on site to produce 20 percent of the electricity the facility uses. In so doing, the Company removes itself from the utilities power grid, saving itself well over ten thousand dollars a year. Nothing more than Bacteria doing what they do best.

Which brings us to cleaning up nuclear waste, and *Geobacter sulfurreducens*, which is doing it nicely. But how? A team of researchers at Michigan State University, East Lansing, led by Prof. Gemma Reguera, asked that question and pursued it, to determine just how Geobacter was able to get rid of nuclear waste left behind in ground water of Colorado mines.

It appears that the Geobacters have short, nanometer thin hair-like structures, called pili around their outer membrane. OK, but how do these pili interact with deadly uranium, precipitating it out of ground water? The MSU researchers, forced Geobacter to grow pili in their lab, which others were unable to do, finding that the pili added electrons to the Uranium ions, which makes the uranium more water soluble, dropping the metal out of solution,to be easily handled; cleaned up. Furthermore, the pili grew so abundantly that they formed a protective barrier around the bacteria allowing them to thrive in the neighborhood of otherwise killing Uranium.[6]

Biofuels

Energy independence is our country's goal. Energy independence means getting us off fossil fuels that have brought us global warming, climate change, polluted the air we breathe with fine particulate matter, and made us dependent upon Middle East oil which creates foreign relations problems. Energy independence would change that by substituting energy derived from biofuels.

Biofuels are fuels that use the energy stored in living things-trees, grasses, crop residues, wood chips, food waste, animal waste (manure from cattle, poultry, and hogs) and microbes-biomass-with the energy inherent in the carbohydrate, fats, and proteins that constitute all organic matter. Even the methane emanating from landfills can be used as a bioenergy source.

Biomass has been used for energy since fire was discovered and people used wood to cook food and keep warm. Although wood currently remains the largest biomass energy source, the entire surface of the earth is covered with biomass and, because it is renewable, its potential for energy is nothing less than tremendous–at least ten times the total amount of energy consumed worldwide annually from all sources.

Biomass can be used for fuel, power production, and commercial and consumer products that would otherwise be made from fossil fuels, providing an array of benefits. Bioenergy can reduce greenhouse gas emissions. Burning biomass releases about the same amount of carbon dioxide as burning coal or oil. But, and this cannot be taken lightly, fossil fuels release CO_2 captured by photosynthesis millions of years ago— an essentially "new" and additional greenhouse gas. Burning biomass releases the carbon dioxide used in the photosynthetic process that recently created it.

Furthermore, use of biofuels reduces our dependence on imported oil. Consequently biomass offers an alternative to foreign oil, providing national energy security, economic growth, and environmental benefits. Yet another benefit is its renewability. Utilizing the energy of sunlight in photosynthesis, plants metabolize atmospheric carbon dioxide (pulling it from the air) and water, creating new biomass, producing some 140 billion metric tons annually. Combustion of biomass forms carbon dioxide which plants use to form more biomass, and around and around it goes. The overall process is referred to as the carbon cycle, which will be discussed in greater detail in Chapter SEVEN.

From an energy viewpoint, the net effect of the carbon cycle is to convert solar energy into thermal energy that can be converted to more useful forms, such as electricity and fuels. Recall too, that coal and oil were originally created from biomass deep in the earth millions of years ago and, because of the millenia needed for their formation they are not renewable.

Biomass is a complex mix of carbohydrates, fats, proteins and minerals. However, it's the carbs that are the center of attention. They are primarily the long-chain cellulose and hemicellulose fibers that impart structural strength, along with lignin, which holds the fibers together. Plants also store starch, another long-chain polymer. These carbohydrates lead directly to its use as a biofuel as they can be converted in a two-step microbial process, in which one set of microbes converts starch to sugar, and another set of microbes converts the sugar to alcohol—ethanol. Sounds simple. It should be, but isn't. It's too simple and too direct to overcome political issues, while obtaining the immense quantities of alcohol needed to make energy independence a realistic goal.

There is the domestic political conundrum created by the rising price of flour for bread and other corn-based foodstuffs, as farmers sell their corn for the higher prices offered by the alcohol producers. Then there is the fraught issue of competition for land to grow the needed corn crops. Will there be sufficient cropland for corn and its flour for bread, or cropland for corn and its alcohol?

To circumvent these controversial issues, researchers around the country and world have taken another tack: forget corn. Let's use cellulosic, non-food biomass to obtain the yields of alcohol needed. The earth is bursting with cellulosic biomass. However, it will be more difficult, as the microbes normally available, have great difficulty digesting cellulose. Nevertheless, the race is on using a potpourri of approaches to grab the pot of gold at the end of the alcoholic rainbow.

In fact, there is no such thing as the one perfect method, or fuel: no one will develop one. A diversity of approaches and products will be needed to make us energy independent. So, although many experiments leading to alcohol production have used common microbes to convert cornstarch to sugar, and on to ethanol, a new generation of scientists seek to enhance, reengineer certain microbes by giving them genes from other organisms. These genes encode directions to create enzymes that can split the celluloses of the multiplicity of non-food plants and waste products. At least, that's the concept.

What's the problem here? Cellulose is the stumbling block. It's a tough chemical, and the most abundant natural polymer on earth. It is a long chain of tightly linked glucose sugars, and as such is the primary structural component of all plant cell walls. The length of the sugar links can vary up to hundreds, to over six thousand in cotton! Along with cellulose there is lignin with its own chain of phenolic rings that provides additional structure to many plants. These twin structural components have proven all but impregnable to most microbes. That's why another level of attack is required if huge amounts of alcohol are to be obtained.

Switchgrass, Panicum virgatum, a cereal grain, member of the Millet family, currently used for fodder for cattle, horses, sheep and goats, is being touted as a sure-fire crop for ethanol production. This perennial grows abundantly on the prairies of our great plains. Considering that there is so much of it, and that it is easy to grow, it may be the cellulosic biomass to provide the ethanol as a sustainable fuel.

Similarly, Miscanthus giganteus, aka, Elephant grass, another cellulosic perennial growing profusely throughout Asia and Africa, is a leading candidate. Miscanthus is extremely efficient in converting sunlight to biomass, producing some 25 tons per acre; five times more than Switchgrass. Studies have shown it to yield 3,250 gallons of ethanol per acre, 130 gallons per ton. A ton of Miscanthus has been shown to produce 18 megawatts of electricity, enough to power 18,000 homes for an hour.

To be sure, there are numerous non-food grasses, along with Willows, Salix nigra, of North America that can attain heights of 60-70 feet, and others that may lead the way to energy independence if microbes can be sufficiently enhanced to dine upon them. They'll need to use their new enzymes, their new hardware, their protein scissors, to slice the glucose bonds linking the polymeric cellulose chains. If they can do this, there may be much alcohol at the end of this grassy tunnel.

Jay Keasling, Prof. of Bioengineering, at University of California, Berkeley, and CEO of the US Department of Energy's Joint Bioenergy Institute, Emeryville, California, has inserted new genes in the common gut bacterium, E. coli, making it possible for it to digest cellulose, which it certainly could not do before its surgery. And guess what; Keasling's E.coli was dinning in Switchgrass. He also used different strains of E. coli that were given genes allowing them to take metabolic pathways producing chemical precursors for gasoline, diesel or jet fuel. Unfortunately his coliforms didn't perform all that well, making only small amounts of fuel. Prof. Keasling will be trying to up production by inserting new genes in yeasts. However, Keasling has a different view of biofuel production. He is shooting for reengineered microbes to produce, not ethanol, but a direct replacement for gasoline. He has shown that his enhanced coliforms can produce diesel fuel. It remains only for his organisms to produce this fuel in commercial quantities. It's a wait and see.

Then there is the bacterium *Zymomonas mirabilis*, which produces far more ethanol from simple sugars than yeasts. Zymomonas was originally isolated from African Palm Wine and Mexican Pulque (a light alcoholic beverage fermented from the Agave plant which is primarily known for its sisal fibers) and has produced 2.5 times greater amounts of ethanol than yeasts. It also has a greater tolerance for ethanol and is easily manipulated genetically. Recently it has been shown to produce substantial quantities of ethanol from sweet potatoes.

Although Zymomonas has a certain celebrity status among biofuel scientists seeking to increase yields of ethanol, it has never been featured or reported upon in newspapers or popular magazines. Nevertheless, it has been modified and can breakdown the 5-carbon sugars, Xylose and arabinose, which are uncommonly difficult for most organisms. Most importantly, it can dine on cellulose with comparative ease. Expect to hear more about Zymomonas in the years ahead.

Dr. Michelle A. O'Malley shocked and surprised the scientists gathered at the American Chemical Society's annual meeting in New Orleans, in April 2013.

Prof. O'Malley, a Chemical Engineer at the University of California, Santa Barbara, collaborating with scientists at MIT's Broad Institute, let it be known that she had isolated a fungus from horse feces and their intestinal tracts that can release the energy locked away in the lignocellulose feeds that ruminants dine on. Most microbes lack the enzymes, the scissors, that can slice cellulose's tightly linked sugar chains. But Piromyces, the fungus she identified, has phenomenal cellulolytic capability. It has the enzymes, and has also been thriving on lignan for thousands of years, turning it into the sugars that horses and other ruminants, cows, sheep and buffalo, require; As Dr. O'Malley puts it, this fungus, which other scientists had simply overlooked, missed, in their single-minded pursuit of a bacterium, "is a potential treasure trove of enzymes for solving the biomass to ethanol problem." Her idea is to remove Piromyce's genes for the enzymes needed, and deftly insert them into yeast cells that have had eons of time to perfect the conversion of sugar to alcohol.[7]

Because fungi are present in low numbers in the ruminant gut, they had been misinterpreted as being of little to no consequence. She and her collaborators at the Broad Institute, experts in genetic manipulation, have identified literally hundreds of enzymes capable of digesting the cellulose/lignan duo. The next step will more than likely be the insertion of one or more of these enzymes into yeast cells. This could be a game changer, and should theory support practice, they could be swimming in alcohol, and the country could be on its way to saying farewell to oil.

Just as Prof. O'Malley tumbled upon the fungus Piromyces, so Prof. Michael Cohen, at Sonoma State University, Rehart Park, California, surprisingly fished out Cellulomonas, of all organisms, from a high alkaline spring, in a valley tucked away from casual wanderers. His Cellulomonas can of course dine happily on cellulose, and thrive in high alkaline conditions.

Just what sent Prof. Cohen into the Cedars, Sonoma County's hidden treasure, is not all that clear, but how that spring became alkaline, which most natural bodies of water are not, is clear.

The Cedars, located inland from the state's Outer Coast Range, is stamped with deep canyons, rocky serpentine barrens, and travertine springs, formed from calcium carbonate from the eroding serpentine rock. The spring's water has a pH of 11-remarkably high. pH is a scale of acid/alkaline conditions, running from 1 to 14, with 1 being the most acidic, as for example the hydrochloric acid in our stomach's, to 14, the most basic or alkaline, such as sodium hydroxide, lye, which is extremely corrosive. Distilled water at pH 7, is neutral, neither acidic or basic. Our blood is near neutral at pH 6.8.

At the Cedars, nature was at work, soaking woody material from fallen tree and shrubs in a highly alkaline water bath and breaking down the lignocellulosic material with the aid of on-site Cellulomonas bacteria that can readily make a meal of cellulose.

Prof. Cohen got lucky and may just lead the way to that pot of gold at the rainbow's nib. He has aligned himself with highly experienced researchers at the Lawrence Berkeley National Lab, a US Department of Energy Facility managed by the University of California, Berkeley, where Cellulomonas will undergo surgery to provide it with genes needed to produce and tolerate high levels of ethanol. That's the kicker, getting a normally alkaline thriving bacterium to thrive at a pH below 6. Surgery could do it.[8]

We appear to be confronted with a two-edged sword, in that we have a number of potentially suitable microbes capable of producing alcohol, but the feedstocks holding out the greatest promise of supplying alcohol at commercial amounts, are lignocellulosic, requiring specialized microbes to degrade, which also adds to production costs. Nothing is simple.

Seaweed avoids all that. Why? Because seaweed is lignin-free; does not compete for arable land, or scarce resources, and does not need fertilizers. But seaweed's biopolymer is alginate, which has proved difficult for microbes to digest. Can that be overcome?

A team of researchers at the relatively new BioArchitecture Lab, BAL, Berkeley, California, believe that seaweed, specifically Brown macroalgae are the feed stocks of the future, able to provide ethanol in commercial quantities.

So, to unlock the sugars, and other valuable organic biochemicals from seaweed, they designed a strain of E.coli that can attack the normally locked away alginate, mannitol (a sugar alcohol) and glucose. Although seaweed does contain cellulose as a structural component of its cells, it doesn't contain lignin, which makes the treatment of seaweed, much simpler. About sixty percent of its biomass is alginate sugars. It doesn't get much better.

To free these sugars, the BAL team designed an E.coli to do the heavy lifting. E.coli naturally metabolizes glucose and mannitol. But it can't get a grip on alginate. To give it that ability they inserted genes from bacteria that can: Vibrio splendidus, Sphingomonas, Pseudoalteromonas, and yes, Zymomonas mirabilis, for those interested.[9]

These insertions gave E.coli the scissors it needed to split alginates tightly linked sugar chain. By the way, alginate is not unlike the polymer pectin, found in many fruits and used to solidify jams and jellies.

Having re-designed their E.coli, they set it to dine on seaweed, and found that it produced ethanol rapidly and in large quantities. Their results may lead the way forward providing much of the ethanol the country requires. It remains to be seen what their unique E.coli will do when they scale up their reaction vessels to multigallons.

Prof. Hiroyuki Takeda and his research group at the Graduate School of Agriculture, Kyoto University, Japan, also working with seaweed, developed an "alginate-assimilating "Sphingomonas species, along with what they referred to as an "over expression" Zymomonas mobilis strain, and obtained a remarkable conversion of 54 percent of alginate to alcohol. Furthermore, their modified organisms did not require expensive enzymes for pretreatment of the alginate. They concluded that, "alginate to ethanol conversion by bacteria opens up new possibilities for high-efficiency, low cost marine biomass usage for biofuel production with little environmental disruption."[10]

J. Craig Ventor has long thought along these lines. Ventor, CEO of Synthetic Genomics of La Jolla, California, was the first to sequence the human genome, and also designed the first synthetic cell. He too, favors the use of seaweed and believes that commercial conditions must be applied to microbial fermentations. His team believes that if a microbe is to lead the way to an ethanol universe, it will be necessary to re-write an organisms genetic code, and test it under real commercial conditions. Accordingly, to accomplish this, they joined with, Exxon Mobil, moving their algae growing project from their lab to a large greenhouse where they could test their algae under more real world conditions. This large greenhouse will test whether algae can produce large-scale quantities of alcohol. In this greenhouse, open ponds and closed photobioreactors are being used to determine algae's optimal growth conditions. Should the greenhouse goals be met, Exxon Mobil expects to support Ventor's biofuels endeavor to the tune of 600 hundred million dollars.

Most recently, Synthetic Genomics purchased an 81-acre site in California's Imperial Valley, near the Salton sea, to scale up and test newly identified and engineered algal strains. To Ventor, it's a ten-year plan to achieve real results. He says, "Algae are a bigger challenge than the genome."[11]

Prof. John Love of the University of Exeter, England, has taken a different approach to solving the world's energy needs. He and his team began with the belief that "the ideal biofuels would be structurally and chemically identical to the fossil fuels they seek to replace." So, rather than making the biofuel ethanol, they have engineered an E.coli strain to convert sugar directly to an oil that is almost identical to conventional diesel fuel; a substitute for fossil fuel. Prof. Love maintains that, "we won't even notice the difference." If he can pull that off, that would really be the game changer the transportation industry is longing for.

What Love and his team have managed to do is get their E.coli to produce a fuel with the exact long-chain length required of an oil, for the current generation of car engines, and, is exactly the composition required. Now that is remarkable, and very cool. How did they do that? They inserted specific genes from the luminescent bacteria *Photorabdus lumescens*, (normally lethal to insects) along with specific genes from the Cyanobacterium, Nostoc, a blue-green algae, as well as genes from the common soil bacterium Bacillus subtilus, and added additional genes from the Camphor tree, Cinnamonium camphora. Manifestly, that took an enormous effort to search out existing data bases for specific DNA strips of these four hugely different organisms to move their E.coli down the metabolic pathway that would produce a long-chain oil. Each set of genes contributed directions for producing specific pieces of the hydrocarbon chain that has the same petroleum-based molecules in current fuels at our gas pumps.

By altering E.coli's genetic code to such an extent, they transformed the bacterium into a fuel-producing factory: an astounding accomplishment. However, and nevertheless, at this stage their made-over E.coli didn't make much diesel fuel. Their next trick will be to scale-up yields, which they believe will take three to five years. During that time they will be weaning their E.coli off its diet of sugar and yeast, and on to a more mundane set of victuals consisting of agricultural waste and sewage. Three to five years is not all that long of a wait to get to the rainbow's end.[12] Stay tuned.

Solazyme, a relatively new company pursuing the holy grail of a substitute for fossil fuel, is based in Palo Alto, California, and has set its sights on producing oil from algae. Moreover, as they tinker with the genes of various algal strains, they are doing what other companies failed to do: remain financially afloat until their tinkering hits pay dirt.

How do they stay afloat? By having their algae produce many other kinds of oil, oils with the mouth-feel of cocoa butter in chocolate, and another that mimics palm oil for soap. Their algae, wondrously inventive creatures, also produce oils for cosmetics: Alginist, their skin care product has been a hit on QVC, and also sells well at Sephora.

Almagine is their powdered fat and protein supplement used to replace eggs and saturated fats. In the works are oils for salad dressings, Alfredo sauce for pasta, brioches, short bread, cookies and ice cream, all in low saturated fats and calories-a far cry from ethanol, but a wider glimpse at the versatility of microbes. Nevertheless, Solazyme's founders, Harrison F. Dillon and Jonathon Wolfson, say they'll get to the fuel business eventually. Although their many specialty products keep them in business, their future is geared to oil to move our cars. Will they remain in business; it sure looks that way.

Recently Solazyme hooked up with Unilever, the international soap products giant to provide alge-produced oil for its widely used Lux soap. They also tied up with Ecover, a Belgium company that makes so-called "green" household products. Ecover will now be trading its palm oil for alge oil to save palm trees and reduce deforestation, which has got to be a plus. Of course the specific algal oil is the result of a gene transfer that provides the alge with the instructions, the code to produce an oil not normally found in its DNA repertoire.

Solazyme, with its unique business acumen has gotten Nordstrom, the department store chain to feature its Alginist as a skin care product in their many stores.[13] More than likely Solazyme's business model has put them on the road to success.

Clearly, there is no lack of creativity and determination by scientists around the country and the world to solve the problem of non-fossil fuels by modifying microbes that will do the job. You can bet the farm on it.

It never ceases to amaze, but when least expected, along comes a creative piece of research that no one had thought of, that takes us down an entirely different path to solving the biofuel problem.

Taking a cue from nature, Prof. Gary Strobel, a plant microbiologist at Montana State University, Bozeman, Montana, thought, why not do what nature did to make oil. After all, buried plants and leaves, under great pressure from soil and mud for 70 to 100 million years, along with fungi living and dinning symbiotically on those plants and leaves, produced hydrocarbons, oil. So Prof. Strobel jerried-together a contraption that simulated conditions existing millions of years ago on a Cretaceous-era rainforest floor. He combined leaves from Maple, Sycamore and Aspen trees, his biomass, with a fungus that grows inside semitropical Key Lime trees, then sandwiched the leaves and fungus between two layers of bentonite shale for pressure, poured water into his tank, and gave the mélange time to incubate. It took the fungus about a month to digest the sugars, starches and cellulose, converting them into a variety of hydrocarbons resembling the oil-rich Montana shale. His hydrocarbons contained molecules of each of the major classes of natural hydrocarbons. If that isn't proof of principle, what is! Not allowing grass to grow under his discovery, Endophytics, LLC, of Wilmington, Delaware, was founded to pursue this encouraging enterprise to the generation of huge gallons of oil at the end of this rainbow. If it works, we'll all profit. Let's cheer them on.[14]

With the daily mean concentration of atmospheric concentration of carbon dioxide having reached four hundred parts per million-ppm's- for the first time in human history, the need for alternatives to fossil fuels has never been greater. The efforts currently underway should get us off fossil fuels and help reduce those four hundred ppm's to more livable levels. The window of opportunity is still open, but closing faster than expected. A sense of urgency is called for. The race will be to the swift.

The use of microbes, although they weren't known, is as old as history. They have been used to bake bread, make cheese, breed food crops and domestic animals, brew alcoholic beverages, and as we shall see, much more.

As we have seen, recent developments in molecular biology gave biotechnology new prominence and vast potential that is beginning to have dramatic effects on world economies and society generally. An outstanding example is recombinant DNA technology, or as is commonly known, genetic engineering, the transferring of individual genes between organisms or modifying the genes in one organism to add or remove a desired trait or characteristic that will be expressed as an entirely new characteristic, and of course, passed on to offspring.

Genetically Modified Food: Genetically Modified Organisms

"As for the future, your task is not to foresee it, but to enable it." – Antoine de Saint-Exupery, The Wisdom of the Sands, 1948

In his chapter on Orthobiosis, (living in accordance with proper hygienic principles) Ilya Metchnikoff, the Russian Nobelist, lauds Luther Burbank an outstanding American botanist, for his improvement of useful plants. "Burbank," he tells us "cultivated great numbers of fruit trees, flowers, and all kinds of plants, with the object of increasing their utility." He goes on to say that:" He has modified the nature of plants to such an extent that he has cactus plants and branches without thorns. The succulent leaves of the former provide an excellent food for cattle…and to obtain such results much knowledge and a long period of time were necessary. To frame the new ideal of the plant it was necessary not only to have an exact conception of what was wanted, but to find out if the qualities of the plants in question furnished any hope of realizing it. Indeed, results could never be predicted; only hoped for."[15]

Random genetic variation occurs naturally in all living things and is the basis of evolution via natural selection. Well before its scientific basis was understood, farmers took advantage of natural variation by selectively breeding wild plants and animals to produce variants better suited to their needs. But this selected breeding involved the transfer of unknown numbers and types of genes between organisms of the same species that rendered outcomes haphazard and unpredictable, and could take decades. Specificity, predictability, assurance, and timeliness had to await recombinant DNA technology. An era of directed genetic change had arrived.

Scientists are simply using DNA, the same chemical in all living things, from viruses to humans, from frogs to fireflies and foxes, and inserting it into the DNA of another, which means that the only things being transferred are four nitrogenous bases: adenine, guanine, cytosine and thymine, which are the same four bases in fleas, flowers, those frogs and foxes, and my friend Fred, which translates to a base, is a base, is a base: adenine is adenine no matter where it is found. Understand this, and genetic modification becomes a no brainer. Am I preaching to the converted?

The total and complete four-letter alphabet rendered by adenine, guanine, cytosine and thymine, a, g, c, and t, in different sequences, repeated over and over, constitutes the astonishing "alphabet" in which the genetic code is written. The words of the code, the instructions, govern and direct how and when the hundreds, or thousands, or tens of thousands of proteins depending upon the complexity of the organism, will be made. The "words" are determined by the order of the bases along the DNA molecule. Remember that all our body's cells–except red blood cells, which do not have a nucleus and no DNA–and all cells in plants and animal tissue contain their specific DNA sequences that make each organism unique. Each with their own genomes.

Each sequence of bases describes an amino acid. The code specifying an amino acid consists of three bases. These three-letter words, these codons, 64 in all, can spell the twenty essential amino acids. So, for example, TTT, codes for lysine; CAT, for methionine; GCC, for alanine, and ACC, for tryptophane. Thus the arrangement of the bases in their codons, delineates all the amino acid sequences. Amino acids then join to form polypeptide chains, which join to form proteins. The various combinations of the 20 amino acids can literally spawn hundreds of thousands of proteins. Again, the takeaway message in all this is a chemical is a chemical, is a chemical, no matter what its initial origin. That's the indispensable reality. Know that, and genetic transfers become emotionally impotent. Since all living things have the same four-letter alphabet, A, G, C, and T, they share the same genetic language and thus any sequence of bases can be "read" and understood as an instruction to make something. That's why inserting a gene from a camphor tree, or a gene from a fungus from a horses intestine into E.coli, the common gut bacterium, will be understood and acted upon by E.coli, and will proceed to produce the chemicals written in the code. It's reasonable. Makes sense. The organism receiving the new instructions in effect becomes a facility for producing a desired substance. Nothing otherworldly about it. And avoids all the uncertainties Metchnikoff remarked upon.

Similarly a set, or sets of bases, can be inserted into plants that can prevent freezing, permit growth under low moisture conditions, or tolerate high salt levels in soil, prevent formation of toxic chemicals, prevent specific microbes from initiating plant disease, increase the size of fish, permit more rapid growth, and increase vitamin content. Another unadulterated verity informs us that it is impossible to identify a gene as belonging to a turkey, tomato, trout or tomcat. A gene, is a gene, is a gene.

With these fundamentals as prelude, the question before us is, why genetically modified foods? What are their potential benefits? Changes to food by gene transfer are no different from those occurring from selective breeding, except that in gene transfer, a selected gene or genes, drastically reduce the time to achieve a desired new trait. That a gene from a fish may be inserted into a plant, gives the Luddites the shivers, and raises the specter of "Frankenfoods" which immediately tells us that these, Anti's, have not a scintilla of understanding of the four letters of the genetic code. If they did, we would not be having this discussion.

Gene transfers are truly revolutionary and bring with them the potential for a range of benefits, but they have also brought such bones of contention as safety, ethics, environmental impact and consumer choice. Given these concerns, it is essential to inquire how it all began, how gene transfers are made, and what safety issues are involved.

It was 1901, in Japan, and the silk worms were dying. Shigatone Ishiwata, a microbiologist/entomologist at the Japanese Institute of Sericultural and Entomological Science, isolated the bacterium that was infecting, softening and killing the silk worm's larvae. He called the silkworm disease Sotto, and the culprit, Bacillus sotto.[16] In 1915 Ernst Berliner, in Germany, was investigating a disease of the Mediterranean flour moth, Angasta kueniella, which he obtained from a flour mill in Thuringia. In his published report he described the isolation of a spore-forming pathogenic bacterium from the dead and dying insects, which he dubbed Bacillus thuringiensis.[17] As it turned out, B.sotto, and *B.thuringiensis*, were the same soil bacterium. B.thuringiensis persevered.

This bacterium possess the unique ability to produce a crystalline protein during sporulation that is not only insecticidal but exquisitely selective, with double-digit strains found in soils around the world, with the ability to selectively infect different insects, and produce several insect destroying proteins. Insects are not all that different from we humans in their susceptibility to microbial infection and death. Microbes are one of nature's ways of limiting harmful insect populations, and B.thuringiensis has been performing this function for eons.

From 1915 to the 1960's, the number of insect orders that B.thuringensis was found to infect and destroy jumped from the single Lepidoptera to nine additional orders, that now encompasses flies, beetles, mosquitoes, protozoa, worms, flatworms, mites and ants. The delta-endotoxin of the crystalline protein, possess the impressive attributes of an ideal biopesticide:

Easily grown and made

Petrochemicals are unnecessary

Nontoxic to vertebrates: mammals, birds and fish

B.thuringiensis (Bt)'s insecticidal promise took off in 1981 when H. Ernest Schnepf and H.R. Whitely of the University of Washington, Seattle, sequenced the Bt toxin gene: its composition of amino acids was revealed. In 1987 scientists inserted Bt genes in cotton plants. A year later the first cotton plants containing Bt genes, with its insecticidal crystalline protein expressed, were harvested. In 1995, the Bollgard gene, a Monsanto product, became commercially available throughout all cotton-producing US states as well as worldwide. For the first time in human history there was a crop that could defend itself against the voracious bollweevil. The cotton plants defend themselves the way all crops containing the Bt crystal do. Ingestion of the CRY toxin (CRY for crystal) results in paralysis of the gut and mouthparts. When swallowed, the protein is released at specific receptor sites in the insect's stomach. The protein opens a channel in the insect's stomach, flows in, and dissolves the intracellular cement. As the gut liquid diffuses between the deteriorating epithelial cells, paralysis occurs, followed by bacterial invasion and subsequent death. The key here is that Bt protein is alkaline, functioning effectively only at the higher pH ranges. Receptor sites for this protein are lacking in acidic environments, meaning that Bt is harmless to all but insects: a point to retrieve when the Luddites raise the specter of safety.

Another good question is, where do we get a gene, any gene, or the gene we're interested in? The world is fortunate in having a bank,whose name is Genbank, and is an integral part of the National Center for Biotechnology Information, NCBI, established in 1988 at the National Library of Medicine, Bethesda, Maryland.

GenBank contains an annotated collection of all publicly available DNA sequences. As of August 2013, as noted earlier, it had on deposit 154 million-plus bases in 167-plus sequences which are freely available to anyone, having been deposited by our public-spirited academic scientists as well as scientists the world over. When it began, there were 680,338 bases and 606 sequences. Over the ensuing three-plus decades the deposits have been astonishing, or is it astounding. GenBank can be accessed at: www.ncbinlm.gov/Web/GenBankOverview.htm

The question that follows would be, how is a gene delivered? One of the available ways is by blasting DNA-coated pellets or beads into a plant's tissues via a gene gun, a modified air pistol, invented by scientists at Cornell University. The DNA shot into tissue then migrates to the plant's nucleous, and the cell regenerates into a new plant with its new genome, which will express the newly acquired traits. With the new gene now inserted, it is copied, literally copied millions of times over, and the original DNA in the new genome is trifling. The newly inserted genetic material is now present in miniscule amounts. Yet another safety consideration.

Writing in the Atlantic Monthly, Jonathon Rauch, a guest scholar at the Brookings Institution, made a significant case for genetic modification of foods.

Rauch affirms the United Nations estimates that global population will rise from its current 7.5 billion, to approximately nine billion by midcentury, 2050. He also notes that across the world people must have their pet dogs and cats to the tune of another billion mouths that not only must be fed, but when people move beyond a subsistence lifestyle, they will want to be provided with "the increasingly protein-rich diets that an increasingly rich world will expect-doing all that will require food output to at least double, and possibly triple."[18] And he continued:

"If in 2050 crop yields are still increasing, if most of the world is economically developed, and if population pressures are declining, or even reversing, than the human species may at long last be able to feed itself, year in and year out, without putting any additional net stress on the environment. We might even be able to grow everything we need returning cropland to wilderness, repairing damaged soils, restoring ecosystems. In other words human agriculture might be placed on a sustainable footing forever. The great problem then, is to get through the next four or five decades with as little environmental damage as possible."

And that, he maintains, is where genetically modified food comes in. Given pest pressure and current crop protection, the largest yield gains are expected in South and Southeast Asia and Sub-Saharan Africa.

"South and Southeast Asia and Sub-Saharan Africa are also the regions with highest population growth, so increases in agricultural output per unit area are vital for poverty alleviation and food security. Bt [Bacillus thuringiensis] cotton, Bt maize, and Bt potatoes, which have already been commercialized in some countries, have direct relevance to the developing world. Bt rice, Bt sweet potatoes and a number of other food crops with other pest-resistance mechanisms will further broaden the portfolio in the near future."

Pest resistance, while a substantial benefit, is but one among others. So, for example, GM holds out such advantages as:

1. Allowing a wide selection of traits for improvement such as nutritional, taste, and visual improvements.

2. Results obtained rapidly and at a lower cost.

3. Greater precision in selecting traits.

These advantages can lead to such benefits as:

1. Improved yields with less labor and overall costs.

2. Reduced use of herbicides and pesticides.

3. Benefits to the soil by no-til farming, which foregoes plowing and allows underground ecosystems to return which reduces erosion and runoff. Worms do the plowing, which saves the farmer fuel, which in turn saves energy, reducing pollution. But no-til farming depends on GM crops.

4. Crops can grow and flourish in previously inhospitable environments—drought, saline, flooding, temperature extremes, which translates to increased yields. Genes to overcome each of these are currently available.

5. Improved flavor and texture.

6. Removal of allergens and toxic components such as cyanide in cassava.

Pertinent and apropos examples are readily at hand. A more nutritious version of golden rice offers a practical solution to vitamin A deficiency. Initially golden rice was genetically modified to produce ß-carotene in its seeds, but low levels of ß-carotene in the kernels of this transgenic crop raised questions about its nutritional value. Biotechnology changed that by inserting a gene from the Daffodil (Narcissus pseudonarnissus) to convert geranyl diphosphate to phytoene, and a second gene from the soil bacterium Erwinia to further convert phytoene to lycopene, which itself is converted to carotene by enzymes in rice. Quite a testament to, and evidence of, transgenic legerdemain. But the level of ß-carotene was insufficient to make a difference. Another upgrade was needed. Researchers at Syngenta took up the challenge, and found a gene, phytoene synthase, psy, in maize, that substantially increased carotenoid accumulation and developed Golden Rice 2, which increased the carotenoid level 23-fold. A child given 60-70 grams of this rice, less than a quarter of a pound, per day, now obtains their full daily requirement of vitamin A. A splendid accomplishment for science, agriculture and humanity. Is this something to be against?

Mastitis in dairy cows has been, and is an unwanted consequence of selection for improved milk production. Dairy cows are quintessential examples of hundreds of years of imbreeding for increased yield and quality of milk. But this has had unintended consequences: mammary gland susceptibility to a staphylococcal infection that is refractory to cure, and is the dairy industry's most costly veterinary condition the world over, as well as a major cause of premature animal death.

Staphylococci in the milk of infected cows can cause human illness. To deal with this stubborn problem, researchers at the US Department of Agriculture's Bovine Functional Genomics Laboratory, Beltsville, Maryland, sought to make cows resistant to Staph. aureus by inducing mammary gland cells to produce the enzyme lysostaphin, an antistaphylococcal protein:obtaining the lysostaphin-producing gene from another staphylococcal strain. The transgenic cows they created now secrete an antibiotic of bacterial origin in their milk, and staphylococci can no longer be found in milk, and the USDA researchers clearly demonstrated the feasibility of introducing disease-resistant genes in cattle to confer protection against a specific disorder.

Before delving into the safety of GM foods, let's hear from Stewart Brand, the quintessence of environmental activism and founder of the Whole Earth Catalog. Musing out loud, so to speak, in an article in MIT's Technology Review, Brand informs his acolytes, to their chagrin, of four environmental heresies: reversals of fortune, that they will not only have to accept but also support; population growth, urbanization, genetically modified organisms, and nuclear power. Heresies indeed! Here we deal solely with genetic modification of microbes.

Brand maintains that, "The success of the environmental movement is driven by two powerful forces; romanticism and science—often in opposition." He compares the two this way, "The romantics are moralistic, rebellious against the perceived dominant power, and combative against any who appear to stray from the true path. They hate to admit mistakes or change direction." As for scientists, "They are ethicalistic, rebellious against any perceived dominant paradigm, and combative against each other. For them, admitting mistakes is what science is." He is quite correct in stating that there are more romantics, environmentalists, than scientists, which translates into environmentalists having their say and way. Listen to this, "It means that scientific perceptions are always a minority view easily ignored, suppressed, or demonized if they don't fit the consensus story line." Brand is honest and has the self-confidence to say this out loud, even though his environmentalists have held us all in thrall these many contentious years. When they are good and ready to change things, they'll change. Not before; because they own the catbird seat. It's galling, but he does have the troops. Why else would government agencies refer to them, acquiesce to them; request their romantic views?

His approach to biotechnology is brazen. One area of biotech, he informs his cohorts "with huge promise and some drawbacks is genetic engineering, so far rejected by the environmentalist movement."

Environmentalist leaders and their organizations have led an unrelenting and vicious crusade against genetic engineering. Those rejections, he writes, is a mistake. One could expect the heavens to open and a bolt of lightening to strike. These are the people who have impeded GM crop development for decades in the most needy countries, simply because GM crops were the off spring of corporations, and environmentalists would rather swallow hemlock than approve anything corporate. Brand has the temerity to tell his fellows to ignore the corporate and fix on the technology, given the facts that GM crops are more efficient, produce higher yields on less, and often hard-scrabble land, with less pesticide use, facts that the Amish have clearly seen, understand, and hue to,their traditional avoidance of technology notwithstanding.

Possibly the most shocking of his pronouncements, pertain to the "scare stories that go around have as much substance as urban legends about toxic rat urine on coke can lids." But this is not the end of it. He is quite forthright in telling readers that many leading biologists who double as environmentalists, have no concerns about genetically engineered organisms, but they don't say so publicly because,"they feel that entering the GM debate would strain relations with allies and would distract from their main focus which is to research and defend biodiversity."[19] A pox on both their houses, for deep-sixing the public—the people.

The biotech brouhaha is a political contretemps, not a scientific or safety issue. For the public, this cloak of invisibility would be better removed and the real case made on its merits—which appear to be considerable. Little is to be gained by frightening the public with fraudulent horror stories about our food supply. In fact, what does the public know about GM foods?

For several years the Rutgers University Food Policy Institute, New Brunswick, New Jersey, sought to take the pulse of the American public's knowledge of GM foods. Sample surveys were conducted in 2001,

2003 and 2004. Here is a summary of their findings.[20]

Most Americans have heard or read little about it, are not aware of its prevalence in their lives, and are confused as to which types of GM products are available. Respondents struggled with the factual questions related to GM food and the science behind it; could not recall news stories related to the topic, and were not very knowledgeable about the laws regarding the labeling and testing of GM food. Americans are also unsure of their opinions about GM good and split in their assessment of the technology when forced to take a position.

Not an encouraging scenario. Furthermore, we learn that the responses changed little between 2003 and 2004, although there has been a small but signifiant increase in awareness since 2001. The numbers are dismaying: 44% of respondents had heard or read nothing about GM foods, while another 42% had read something, which suggests that 86% are poorly informed. This relates to the fact that 79% believed that GM tomatoes were available for purchasing in supermarkets. Of course, the first and only GM tomatoes, the Flarsavr, were taken off the market in 1997. Yet the belief continues. More disturbing was the fact that 32% believed that, or were uncertain whether eating a GM fruit, a person's genes could also become modified. 40% either believed or were unsure if tomatoes modified by a catfish gene would taste fishy. No, not at all encouraging.[20]

If the Rutgers survey is representative of the nation generally, it is obvious why environmentalist groups have such success purveying their brand of nonsense. It would be further illuminating to know, now a decade on, if awareness has improved beyond the 2004 numbers.

We now turn to the safety of GM foods.

As the WHO tells it, the safety assessment of GM foods generally investigates direct health effects (toxicity); tendencies to provoke allergic reactions (allergenicity); specific components thought to have nutritional or toxic properties; the stability of the inserted gene; nutritional effects associated with genetic modification, and any unintentional effects which could result from gene insertion. "Thus far no allergic effects have been found relative to GM foods currently on the market." Moreover, "GM foods currently available on the international market have passed risk assessments and are not likely to present risks for human health. In addition, no adverse effects on human health have been shown as a result of the consumption of such foods by the general population in the countries where they have been approved." WHO also informs us that, "GM products currently on the international market have all passed risk assessments conducted by national authorities. These different assessments generally follow the same basic principles, including an assessment of environmental and human health risks; they are thorough, and have not indicated any risk to human health." This information is freely available for anyone to obtain and consider. Do the nay-saying activists know something the World Health Organization doesn't?

The most recent news provides yet another pat on the back for GM crops: soybean and cotton are the preferred choice of US farmers, according to newly released data from the USDA.

In their Economic Research Service's report, July 10, 2013, of all the soybeans grown in the US, 93 percent are genetically engineered; of all corn grown in the US, 90 percent are GM:up from 88 percent in 2012. As for cotton, 90 percent is genetically modified. Doesn't this indicate that US farmers clearly prefer seeds improved via biotechnology? It would surely seem so.

Scientific innovation allows growers to produce the most reliable and abundant yields with less tilling of the soil, and fewer applications of insecticides and fertilizers, that reduce fuel costs, increase profit margins, and keep our food costs affordable.

Genetic engineering, or more to the point, recombinant DNA biotechnology, the insertion of a gene into a cell, and nothing more, is now more important than ever given the increasing need to provide the food, fuel and fibers for the nine billion people estimated to populate our earth by 2050–not all that far away; more than likely within the lifetimes of most of us.

USDA scientists also tell us that 40 percent of corn farmers had adapted Bt (insect resistant) corn by 2005; and in some states it was 66-100 percent. They note too, "that corn borer infestations have decreased considerably," and that corn rootworms and corn earworms have also decreased due to the insertion of the Bt gene into the corn genome.

These Bt adaptors now obtain, higher corn yields: some 17 bushels higher per acre, along with increased profits. How can anyone be against that? Why would anyone be opposed to transferring a gene?

In May 2012, Cynthia La Pier, 44, made the front page of the New York Times. She and her anti-GM activists were caught plastering Kellog's Mini wheat cereal with stickers—"warning may contain GMO's," at the Big Y grocery store in Great Barrington, MA.[21]

Defacing food labels is a state and federal offense, a criminal offense, but meaningless to them. She and her Luddite activists were telling shoppers that the WHO, FAO, FDA, and the EPA were not to be believed, and that consumers should boycott GM foods.

Just what were they warning against? As noted earlier, the only change in a modified food is the addition of a gene, a harmless bit of protein. Genes, we continue to say, are nothing more than sequences of the A's, T's, C's and G's. The position of these four bases directs the plant or animal to make a specific protein. That's it. There's nothing more. It's that straight forward. Changes in the position of these nitrogen-containing bases changes the plant or animal's characteristics. Plants and animals whose genome contains a gene with DNA foreign to it, are referred to as transgenic.

To deal with these transgenic organisms, the FDA treats them as drugs, which means the new "product" must undergo the entire gambit of tests for safety that all drugs undergo. Consider that food supplements offered for sale in our supermarkets, on TV, radio, and in magazines and newspapers, get a free pass: no FDA testing for either safety or effectiveness. There's a major disconnect somewhere.

Where does Ms. La Pier and her gang of activists get their information, and chutzpa, to decide that GM foods are hazardous, and need re-labeling, and get away with it? Why weren't they arrested and fined? They were not above mangling the truth for their self-interests, and worse, yet, no federal or state agency appeared to give a hoot!

In his new book, Something to Chew On: challenging controversies in food and health, July 2013, Prof. Mike Gibney, University College, Dublin, Ireland, a leading Irish scientist and authority on food and nutrition, claims that "unfortunately most of us don't know what we're talking about when it comes to food and health." He goes on to say that, "apparently all we have to do is eat to proselytize on all matters food and nutrition."

When it comes to GM foods, he writes, "Angola, Mali, Mozambique, Nigeria, Zimbabwe and Sudan, have all rejected food aid shipments on the grounds that they might contain GM grains, because European AID groups fund anti-GM initiatives in those countries. After all, Africans just want to be as safe as Europeans." In that case, however, he maintains, "Africans risk blindness from vitamin A deficiency by following Europe's metaphorical blindness over the benefits of GM crops. "As a citizen of Europe," Gibney says, "I feel utterly ashamed."

He goes goes on, "So great is the level of confusion, that a staggering one in three European citizens agree with the statement that, "ordinary tomatoes don't have genes but genetically modified ones do."[22] That's even more confusing than what the Rutgers survey learned about American confusion over GM foods. Is it confusion or bald ignorance? My Oxford American Writers Thesaurus informs me that confusion means uncertainty, doubt; but ignorance is incomprehension, beyond one's grasp. Would I be wrong to believe that you'd choose ignorance? To believe that activists call the tune to which the countries dance, is itself incomprehensible.

As Emily Anthes writes in her lively and engaging new book, Frankenstein's Cat: cuddling up to biotech's brave new beasts, July 2013, "In the United States, the debate over genetic engineering has been dominated by loud anti-technology activists, and a stamp of government approval (of GM foods) may not be enough to overcome pervasive fears about safety–or ethics–of GM products."[23] But federal and state agencies avoid the fray, which may be why the Cynthia La Piers of this world get away with their felonies and will doubtlessly engage in repeated performances.

Echoing Prof. Gibney, a group of scientists from Madrid, Barcelona and the UK, spoke out in May 2013, on the GM food issue, stating that, "If the European Union is to have any hope of feeding its population in the future, it must end its illogical aversion to genetic modification." They added that, "EU politicians will not come off the fence on the subject of GM crops for fear of upsetting a small but vocal minority." They weren't finished. "It's hard to see," they maintained, "any technology gets adopted when faced with the constraints applied to GM agriculture in Europe. Despite the fact that GM crops have illustrated their safety, opponents demand cast iron proof of zero risk—proof that has never been demonstrated for any product or technology in history and that cannot be demonstrated because it is impossible to prove a negative." Their hackles were up. They were resolute. "The time has come," they declared, "to fight against this insidious attack on the progress of European science. It is fair to ask questions, demand answers, and ask for evidence of safety. But it is not fair to continue an aggressive campaign of Luddite opposition when all the evidence supports a positive role for GM agriculture in Europe."[24] Wouldn't it be lovely if American scientists entered the lists with similar gravitas. We dare not hold our breathe for that, as Stewart Brand has them wrapped up. Nevertheless, the times cry out for the participation of informed citizens. It's never too late for that. Or is it?

At the University of Florida's Institute for Plant Innovation, Gainesville, Florida, researchers are trying to develop a more flavorful tomato. But they are using traditional breeding techniques, "to avoid potential consumer backlash, along with the cost to obtain regulatory approval to sell a genetically engineered tomato."

Let's hear from Emily Anthes again. She writes that, "Rejecting genetic engineering wholesale, means that we'll lose the good along with the bad. And when it comes right down to it, I don't think anybody in the world will turn down a drug from a transgenic animal if they need it or their loved ones need it. Or a transplant, if they need it." She went on to say, "It's easy to oppose biotechnology in the abstract, but when that technology can save your life, grand pronouncements about scientific evils tend to dissolve. Most of us would do a lot more than drink transgenic goat milk to have even one more day with our loved ones, or in some cases to spend more time with our beloved pets." Who would disagree with those sentiments?

In early August 2013, protestors tore down fences surrounding a field of genetically modified rice in the Philippines, and tore out the growing Golden Rice; rice with a high level of beta-Carotene, the precursor of Vitamin A. The protesters were outraged that such rice could be a risk to people's health. "We do not want our people, especially our children, to be used in these experiments."[25] Hard to believe? Of course it is. It reminds me of a dandy experiment done by a young boy.

Nathan Zohner, a fourteen-year-old, and at the time, a freshman at Eagle Rock Junior High, won top prize at the Greater Idaho Falls Science Fair. His award-winning project had two parts to it. First, he explained the scientifically proven dangers of dihydrogen monoxide:

It can cause excessive sweating and vomiting.

It is a major component of acid rain.

It causes severe burns when in gaseous form.

Accidental inhalation can kill you.

It has been found in the tumors of terminal cancer patients.

Nathan then asked fifty people at the Fair whether they would support a ban on dihydrogen monoxide. The result: 43 favored a ban, 6 were unsure, and 1 person was opposed. Why was he opposed? He knew that dihydrogen monoxide is also H_2O-water. Zohner's project was titled, "How Gullible Are We?" His conclusion: "I'd say they're extremely gullible. They need to pay more attention." The moral: scary-sounding names can turn everyday phenomena into bogeymen for the uninformed.

And then there was Steve Allen, of blessed memory, a very funny guy, who had been making us laugh for decades. PBS, the Public Broadcasting System, celebrated his seventy-fifth birthday with an hour of clips from a number of his past TV shows. They were howlers. On one, he took a microphone out to Broadway and 42nd Street, stopping men and women, shoving a mike under their noses and asking the question: "If a man running for President goes on TV and openly admitted that he was a practicing heterosexual, would you vote for him?" "Good God, no." "Well, I believe a person's private life is his own. It shouldn't disqualify him from office." "A what! Oh, no, never." And on and on. The audience was doubled over laughing. So was I. Hilarious, yes, but sad, too, very sad. The Zohner Effect again. On a summer's day, are Broadway and 42nd Streets, or Idaho Falls, cross-sections of America?

There is yet another factor at work here: natural vs. man-made.

It is worth recalling that the many cross breedings, cuttings, and hybridizations Luther Burbank made were man-made: not at all natural. This natural vs man-made is a major sticking point for anti GM activists. The anti-GM'ers, are violently opposed to anything man-made. So,we recall that it was Burbank who crossed a plum with an apricot and got us the delicious Plumcot. He also gave us the Flaming Gold nectarine, a fuzzless peach. Of course the Russet Burbank Potato, we now know as the Idaho, was due to his handiwork. Need I mention the Shasta Daisy? Burbank believed and proved that man could improve on nature, and we have. He also received patents for his manipulations.

Let us not forget the Yukon Gold potato, a cross between the Peruvian Yema de huevo and the Norgleam, which was developed at Canada's University of Guelph.

With cross breeding, farmer's and Horticulturalists have no idea what they are going to obtain after waiting many years for the result to appear. Nor do they have any idea what other characteristics of the plant they are changing. It's a hit or miss process. With genetic recombination, a specific gene for a single specific trait is inserted which is the only modification that occurs. Gene transfer is of course, a man-made process, not at all natural. But neither are any of the cross breedings, cuttings, or hybridizations, natural. They too are man-made! So, why the ranting about gene transfers as unnatural or man-made! Something's very wrong here.

We conclude with two current issues demonstrating the ongoing resistance to inserting a gene in a plant and an animal.

The headline on the front page of the New York Times read, "A Race to Save the Orange by Altering its DNA–Contagion Raging, Florida Industry Tries to Build a Better Tree." That was in July 2013, and the story recounted the on-going struggle to defeat Citrus Greening, a disease that had been devastating orange, grapefruit and lemon crops around the world, and was now attacking orange groves in all 32 of Florida's orange growing counties. It had attacked similar groves in California. If not defeated, Citrus Greening could absolutely wipe out Florida's nine billion dollar orange industry, which would mean farewell to OJ. It's that serious. Citrus Greening, causes sourness in oranges, fruits fail to mature, and trees slowly die. Currently, over seven hundred thousand trees, and counting, have been destroyed. The race is on to develop trees resistant to the disease.[26]

Citrus Greening is the work of a nasty duo; an insect, the jumping plant louse, *Diaphorina citri,* a true bug, a Hemiptera that includes Aphids, Leafhoppers, and Cicadas. Diaphorina moves from tree to tree, sucking up sap and injecting *Candidatus liberibacter asiaticus*, a bacterium so devilish that it has been declared a bioterror weapon!

Candidatus, which in Latin means candidate, and refers to the white togas worn by Roman Senators, is a provisional name, a candidate for a more permanent one, as this awful organism cannot be grown in laboratory media. Its identification comes via 16SrRNA sequencing of its nitrogenous bases and thus far resists all attempts to kill it off.

The only way to stop the devastation of the oranges is to create resistance to the bacterium, which can only be done by inserting a gene for resistance into its genome. And therein hangs the tale.

To fight C.lieberibacter, several approaches were considered: plant pathologists at the University of Florida suggested taking a gene from a virus that destroys bacteria, a bacteriaphage-harmless to humans, but orange growers believed that the idea of a virus gene in an orange that attacked bacteria would face public resistance. That idea was short lived.

A second suggestion came from Texas A & M, where Dr. Eric Mirkov had inserted a resistance gene from spinach, into trees he was growing, that produce a protein deadly for invading bacteria. That idea faced skepticism from many growers who knew that people would ask, will the orange become green, and would it taste like spinach, and would the public stop drinking OJ, believing it no longer pure and natural? Would a transgenic orange be rejected?

For Florida Orange growers it was either, lose our oranges completely, or go forward with a transgenic orange hoping that people would get used to the idea and continue drinking orange juice. Here we are in mid 21st century America, with a major industry's future seemingly in the hands of ignorance. Does that boggle the mind!?

The growers opted to experiment with the spinach gene, and tests showed conclusively that the gene protected their experimental orange trees, which remained healthy. Furthermore, they now believe that their trees would pass all of EPA's and FDA's safety tests. If they win regulatory approval, they will be planting thousands of trees that would be ready to produce oranges and juice in five years.

Plant pathologists at Washington State University have undertaken a 9 million dollar, five-year project, to develop a genetically modified Diaphorina citri that cannot transmit Citrus Greening's Candidatus bacterium. And the Coca Cola Company, owners of Minute Maid orange juice, plan to invest two billion dollars to plant 25,000 new orange trees.

Rick Kress, President of Southern Gardens Citrus, believes the only way to save Florida's entire citrus industry is to alter the tree's DNA. With the positive results provided by the spinach gene, he has been musing out loud, "Maybe we can use the technology to improve orange juice, and maybe we can find a way to have oranges grow year-round, or get two for every one we get now on a tree."

Answers will come soon enough. However, if anti-GM activists persist in their war against anything GM, none of us will ever drink OJ again—unless it comes from Brazil.

There is also the conundrum; will the Florida orange growers face the same protracted regulatory process that has hog-tied Aqua Bounty? It remains an open and troubling question. So, what is the Aqua Bounty story, and how does it impinge on citrus greening and orange juice?

Aqua Bounty Technologies of Maynard, Massachusetts, developed its AquAdvantage salmon by injecting fertilized Atlantic salmon (Salmo salar) eggs with a gene from the Ocean Pout (Zoares americanus), anti-freeze gene that expresses a protein preventing the salmon's freezing in extremely cold conditions. This gene was coupled with a growth-stimulating hormone gene from the Pacific Chinook salmon (Onchorhynchus tshawytscha) that accelerates the Atlantic salmon's growth. Recall that a gene is a stretch of DNA containing the information to code for a specific protein. This piece of DNA, this gene, is spliced into the salmon's DNA, and nothing more.

AquAdvangtage salmon can now grow to market size and weight in 18 months rather than the 24 to 30 months normally required. For fish farmers, this means raising fish faster and cheaper. For the world generally, it means a far greater supply of high quality protein at lower prices. That's the long and short of it: or what it was supposed to be.

Furthermore, the newly fertilized eggs are subjected to high pressures that create triploid cells. Triploidy is a means of making a population sterile: unable to reproduce. Most cells in animal bodies, including ours, are diploid; having two sets of chromosomes, one from each parent. Triploid cells have three sets of chromosomes. Consequently, triploid fish can no longer produce sperm or eggs, as they cannot attain sexual maturity. For the modified salmon this means they cannot mate with wild salmon. Ergo, any modified salmon that might slip away from its farmed pool will be unable to mate and develop new populations of larger fish; a major level of security.

However, slip away, for these farmed salmon is impossible as their growing site in Panama is seventy-two miles from the Pacific Ocean. Additionally, these aqua-cultured fish are confined in physical containment barriers, and a natural thermal barrier of lethally high water temperature (for Atlantic salmon) downstream of the facility effectively precludes any live AquAdvantage salmon from going anywhere: unless they grow wheels.

In 2012, the FDA published its environmental assessment, finding that these modified salmon neither presented an environmental, nor health risk. There would be no harm in eating it. Shortly after, Environmental Canada, and Health Canada, the two Canadian government agencies mandated to protect the peoples health and the health of the environment, weighed in with the same evaluations: not harmful to human health or the environment.

Some two years has now passed since the FDA issued its initial findings. Public comments, however, by anti-genetic engineering activists has so bullied the FDA that they have withheld final approval for the AquAdvantage salmon which could contribute to increasing aqua culture productivity to meet the demand for these fish and their protein. As of July 2014, silence prevailed, two decades of regulatory rigmarole.

Dithering. Clearly this has become another political can to be kicked around.

As these activists have managed to block commercial production of all genetically modified crops and animals, it is more than worrisome that orange trees with an inserted gene preventing citrus greening, will meet the same fate. No more Florida orange juice would be a national disaster. Therefore, it is reasonable to wonder about the fate of our OJ once the genetically modified orange is in the hands of the FDA. Do not even think of holding your breath as dely is a recurring theme at this agency.

At this juncture, activists might consider Mark Twain's pithy remark: "It aint what you know that gets you in trouble, it's what you know for sure that just aint so." A powerful myth has taken root: that GM or GE foods are harmful to health and the environment. False, false, false, as a hundred studies from the world over have shown. It is for good reason that the World Health Organization, The Royal Society of Health, the FDA, and Health Canada have given their backing unreservedly to GM and GE foods. Unfortunately this vital issue has become a political ballgame to the detriment of us all.

As September 2013, came in view, orange juice prices jumped almost five percent following forecasts of a still smaller harvest in 2014. The squeeze is on.

Negative activism notwithstanding, over the past 30-plus years, there has not been a documented instance of harm from any transgenic plant or animal. Scare tactics. Loads. Anti GMO activists march to their own drummer, no matter how hungry millions of people around the world remain.

A Bit More to Wrap Up

Although the word synthetic derives from synthesis, which translates as combination, union, or amalgam, synthetic has the pejorative connotation of fake, mock, or ersatz, which for me does not evoke what is being accomplished by genetic modification. I'm (of course) partial to combination and union as in synthesis. There is nothing fake or ersatz about the placement of a gene or genes from one living species into another living species. As we've been saying, an amino acid, is an amino acid, is an amino acid, no matter where it originates, and where it ends up. And Guanine, Cytosine, Adenine and Tyrosine are the same nitrogenous bases that spell out every amino acid whether in a frog, fly, flower, fox or my neighbor Francine.

And so, Prof. Jay D. Keasling of the University of California, Berkeley, who we met earlier, and is now, the co-founder of Amyris, a company also based in Emeryville, California, that refers to itself "as a company that applies its industrial synthetic biology platform to convert plant sugars into a variety of molecules–flexible building blocks that can be used in a wide range of products." And, they go on to say that, "We use our engineered microorganisms to convert sugar into renewable hydrocarbon molecules from fuels, to plastics, to cosmetics."

Keasling has pioneered the use of re-engineered microbes, yeasts and bacteria, to produce a potpourri of products including flavorings such as Vanillin, for vanilla flavor, Saffron powder, Valencene, the biochemical responsible for oranges orangy aroma, and Nootkatone, the natural organic chemical that gives grapefruit its fruity aroma, which is also used as an insect repellent against deer ticks. Amyris also produces Patchouli, a fragrant oil, spices, and moisturizers for cosmetics, as well as Stevia, a sweetener, and Cammomile, that has made Italy the calmest of nations.[27] And they are now producing Squalene, an essential oil (a hydrocarbon) previously obtained from shark liver and olives. Surely a benefit to the shark population. A half-dozen other companies in Europe and the US have jumped in to supply a demanding market. Microbial produced products are closer to the original plant derived product than those synthesized chemically. They are also cheaper to produce, are available year'round, and their concentrations are reliable. It is also believed that wide usage of recombinant products will reshape how land is used globally.

Along with the products noted, interest is also in producing rubber for tires, Cannabis (Marijuana) and Morphine (Opium) for the medical market, and goats with a spider's genes that produce super-strength silk, in their milk. Indications are that microbes can produce almost anything desired for commercial and industrial use.

On the negative side, critics are concerned that genetic recombinant products would take the bread out of the mouths of small farmers in Africa and Asia that supply the original plant produced products for food and cosmetics manufacturers.

We appear to be on the horns of a dilemma just as mass production took over from master craftsmen, and the steam engine and motorcar made horses obsolete, and the computer is reshaping just about everything we do, and people lacking computer literacy are clearly disadvantaged in the job market.

Activists against genetically modified products are already ranting against these new recombinant products. If history is any guide, recombinant products will have as rocky a road ahead as genetically modified crops.

Microbes in Industry: Masters at Making Complex Molecules

In its broadest sense, biotechnology dates from antiquity, having a proud lineage and pedigree beginning with the Sumerians and Babylonians who discovered the use of Yeasts in making beer around 6000 bce. Not to be outdone, the Egyptians and Chinese followed about 4000 bce, with the Egyptians using yeasts to make bread, and the Chinese using bacteria to make yogurt.

The term biotechnology, was coined in 1919, by a Hungarian scientist, Karl Ereky, to mean "any product produced from raw materials with the aid of living organisms."

Currently, recombinant DNA technology has made it possible to conceive of virtually unlimited new products made by re-engineered microbes, creating desirable products with economic gain, or to prevent economic loss. It has also made possible large-scale developments in bioprocessing of complex natural compounds that otherwise would be difficult to obtain. Consequently we can think of microbes as nicely packaged chemical factories for converting almost any raw material into new products.

So, for example, Citric Acid and its salts are so widely used, and produced in such quantity, some 1.7 million tons annually, that we give it pride of place, as no other fermented product is produced in such quantity. Before 1918, all citric Acid was extracted from culled fruits. Today, all of it comes from the growth of the fungus Aspergillus niger or the yeasts, Candida.

Citric acid is used widely in foods and beverages, in pharmaceuticals, cosmetics, anticoagulants, candies, medications, household cleaners, inks and dyes. Curiously enough, the Aspergillus lacks an enzyme permitting Citric Acid to accumulate, rather than be metabolized to carbon dioxide. It doesn't seem to mind being relieved of its burden.

Another important fungal produced product is Amylase, from Aspergillus oryzae, used widely by bakers, for its ability to break down starches to sugars, allowing yeasts to dine, producing the carbon dioxide needed for dough to rise. Amylase is also used in beer fermentations to digest the starches in grains, and it is used as a spot remover in laundry detergents.

Pectinase, another enzyme, obtained from a Clostridial bacterium, is used to clarify fruit juices by digesting the proteins that cause the cloudiness, decreasing the filtration time by as much as 50 percent. It also releases fibers from flax that are then spun to make linen. Retting is the use of microbes to separate cellulose fibers. Pectinase decomposes the pectin that holds the fibers together. And it is used to remove sizing agents from cotton, replacing corrosive lye, sodium hydroxide.

Proteases, also obtained from Aspergillus oryzae, are used to tenderize meats, and as spot removers on materials containing egg, blood, and milk proteins; also providing improved cleansing of laundry, dishes and cutlery. Perhaps its most important use is in baking bread to adjust the amount of gluten in wheat.

Synthetic Insulin obtained from E.coli and/or yeasts is based wholly on recombinant technology. Millions of diabetics worldwide use synthetic Insulin to regulate their blood sugar levels.

Human growth hormones are also obtained from a modified E. coli to treat several types of dwarfism. These products are much safer than the products they replaced as the older products were purified from cadavers and could transmit disease.

Streptokinase, an enzyme obtained from Streptococci, is used to dissolve blood clots in individuals with coronary blockages, while the Hyaluronidases' contributed by both Strep and Staph, are used to enhance a group of enzymes that lower viscosity, increasing tissue permeability speeding drug dispersion and delivery ensuring absorbtion of injected fluids.

Invertase, produced by several strains of yeasts and the fungus *Aspergillus niger*, is used to make liquid centers and invert sugar in candy making. When Invertase is added to sugar candies, such as fondant fillings (a sugar-water paste) it gradually liquifies the fondant. Think chocolate cherry cordials, and think microbes.

For those interested, invert sugar is called invert because sucrose rotates polarized light to the right, but when it is split into its component monosaccharides, glucose and fructose, light is rotated to the left-it is inverted!

Using the short-chain 3-carbon based pyruvic acid as its primary metabolite, the streptococci and lactobacilli produce copious quantities of lactic acid, used as an acidulent in many foods for its flavor. The Clostridia use it to produce butyric acid, often used as a fishing bait, the Carp love it. It is also used in foods, perfumes and animal feedstuffs.

Propionibacteria use pyruvate to give us acetic acid and propionic acids. Acetic acid is, as many know, the primary ingredient of vinegar, and is used as a food preservative, and also used to make rayon. Of course, the Acetobacter are also major producers of acetic acid. Propionic acid is a widely used hay preservative, preventing mold growth, and is used as a food supplement in animal feedstuffs.

The Enterobacter's use pyruvic acid to yield formic acid, the simplest organic acid used as an antibacterial in livestock feed, and is applied to hay to promote the fermentation of lactic acid. By the way, it's the formic acid from ants that is the irritant causing itching.

Vitamin B_{12}–Cyanocobalamin–required to prevent pernicious anemia, is produced by the Pseudamonads, Propionibacteria, and the fungus, Streptomyces.

Vitamin B-2, riboflavin, is excreted by yet another mold, Ashbya gossypii, which pumps it out in huge quantities.

Without the altruism of a re-engineered E.coli, that normally excretes the amino acid tryptophane, whose molecule is similar to that of indigo, re-engineering got us indigo's blue dye, used for Denim jeans. How can anyone think ill of E.coli?

Although Glutamic acid, rendered by Corynebacteria, is a non-essential amino acid, it is the most common excitatory neurotransmitter in our central nervous system, and is essential for memory and learning. It's also the acid used to make MSG, monosodium glutamate, the flavoring agent in soy sauces and other Asian sauces. It was named after the wheat gluten in which it was first discovered.

Gluconic acid, another metabolite of Aspergillus niger, is used to clean bottles as a pre-treatment prior to filing with beer and soft drinks. Nor can we overlook its use in dishwashing detergents to prevent mineral deposits on tubs and sinks. Calcium gluconate is also added to chicken feed to strengthen egg shells.

What about bacterial batteries? Geobacter and Desulfuramonas, two recently identified microbes oxidize organic compounds in underwater sediments or sewage, transferring a current of electrons to graphite electrodes. These bacteria are acting as parts of batteries that use mud or sewage as fuel to produce sufficient electricity to power a small calculator.

Currently, (no pun intended) this is far from practical for large-scale energy production, nevertheless, scientists are working to develop microbial electricity as inexpensive batteries. And, as these microbes use sediments as their source of energy, they could be useful in removing pollutants on the sea floor by metabolizing them to electricity. This is far from a stretch.

Gibberella fujikuro, a mold that excretes Gibberellins, plant hormones used by Botanists to speed up seed germination and flowering, is also used for setting blooms in plants.

Silage

Cows, pigs, horses and goats adore silage, which comes from a Silo, which can be thought of as a multistory fermentation tank for the microbial conversion of cellulosic grasses to digestible cattle food. In these concrete or wood tanks, hay, corn, and waste vegetables are packed away and allowed to ferment over months, giving a complex of microbes an opportunity to feed, digest and excrete in an environment lacking oxygen. During their banquet time, lactobacilli, enterococci, pediococci, streptococci, clostridia, candida, and half-a-dozen others all playing their specific roles, producing juicy fodder for the animals so that they continue to produce milk during the winter. That's the name of the Silo game.

To improve the production of lactic acid, an enzyme from Bacillus amyoliquifaciens has been spliced into Lactobacillus plantarum which is added to the tightly packed silage to ensure conversion of the huge amounts of starch to ever greater levels of lactic acid: while the menagerie of microbes are digesting carbohydrates, producing a number of acids that preserve the silage, rendering it a tasty porridge for the animals; an inexpensive but nutritious diet.

Although invisible, the bevy of microbes in our lives become visible in the shower of vital products they contribute to benefit our lives in countless ways.

Wine

The juice of the Gods seems a realistic point of departure. We are of course treating with wine,"oinos" from the Greek, and which the quaffing of, harkens back to antiquity: to southern Armenia where archeologists from UCLA recently found grape seeds from the same grapes, Vitus vinifera, used today. Also found were dry grape vines, a wine press, and a clay fermentation vat. The site dates to approximately 4100 bce, which tells us that those Armenians were imbibing wine over 6,000 years ago.[28]

Indeed, wine does have an ancient history. In the days when the earliest Egyptian pyramids were being built, vintners knew nothing about microbes, but they knew that crushed grapes left in the open produced a drink that relaxed them, and kept them drinking until they dropped. Wine was produced in Egypt about 3200 bce, over five thousand years ago, and may have tasted like today's Greek Retsina. As Thanksgiving, 2013, was upon us, news arrived out of Israel of the discovery of a 3,700 year old wine cellar containing forty amphorae, unearthed in Tel Kabri, an ancient Canaanite city in northern Israel.

According to Archeologists there, chemical analysis of the tall ceramic jars revealed calcium tartrate residues on their inner surfaces. The salt of tartaric acid speaks directly to the presence of wine or grape juice having been present. The Archeologists also believe the Wine's ingredients consisted of honey, mint, cinnamon bark, and juniper berries, to smooth the harsh and intense wine. Resins were used to prevent the alcohol from turning into cider. These resins were obtained from pine, cedar and terebinth trees, according to the Roman writer, Pliny the Elder, who also noted that terebinth resin was the least harsh and with the best aroma. Pine resin from Aleppo, Syria, was a widely used ingredient but was awfully harsh. Terebinth resin, from the so-called turpentine tree, a sumac, has a rewarding aromatic aroma. With all these ingredients the wine could easily have tasted like 1930's cough syrup, which by the way, early wine was supposed to be—medicinal.

Furthermore, wild grapes didn't grow in Egypt. Grapes for their wine came from extensive trade with ancient Palestine and its Canaanite towns.[29]

Wine does have a remarkable lineage, and the microbes involved just keep on doing what comes naturally. But it was Louis Pasteur, who we recall, demonstrated that wine, was the product of an alcoholic fermentation of grapes by yeasts. Unquestionably, microbes are fundamental to wine making. The large number of organic compounds synthesized or modified by wine yeasts during fermentation make a significant impact on wine quality and style.

When grapes are crushed, to begin wine making, any type or color of grape, yields a white juice—the must. Red wine requires that red or purple skins remain in contact with the must, before fermentation to release their anthocyanin (purple/red) pigments. Fermentation begins either naturally or after inoculation with specific yeasts and /or bacteria. The specific grapes used, Vitus vinifera, Cabernet, Merlot, Pinot noir, to note but a few, contribute their distinctive fruity character.

White wines, with their grapes, Chadonnay, Semillon, Traminer, and Sauvignon Blanc, take a different pathway. Their white must is rapidly drained away from their skins to avoid the contact that would darken the must. Rosés, the pinkish/red wines, from red or purple grapes, allow their white juice a brief contact with their skins.

Grape juice contains high levels of malic and tartaric acids, which need to be decreased during fermentation or the wines will be far too acidic. In addition to the Saccharomyes yeasts, the fermentation will also consist of a diverse collection of lactobacilli that metabolize the malic and tartaric acids to lactic acid and carbon dioxide, which lowers the acidity.

Facts on the ground suggest that each wine region is different, unique. But the unanswered question hovering about has been, why? What is it that sets each one apart? An answer appears to have arrived.

Researchers at the University of California, Davis, believe they know why, and have supporting evidence: fungi and bacteria growing on the surface of grapes.

When grapes are crushed, these microbes become an integral part of the liquid, the must, that is the beginning of the wine making process. These microbes play a lead role in the ensuing fermentation. Most importantly, these organisms, the microbial communities of each region, are sufficiently stable, that's the key, so that one set of microbes is closely associated with Chardonnay, while another distinctive set contributes to

Cabernet Sauvignon. Prof. Mills and Bokulich of the Department of Oenology, inform us that this can explain why one regions Zinfandel tastes different from another regions. They also tell us that there may be genetic affinities between particular microbial species and each grape variety. Now that's got to be a head spinner. The next question to be investigated is whether wine quality can be predicted from the types of microbes on the grapes![30] Stay tuned.

Distilling wine produces a higher alcohol content yielding an explosive brandy. With the addition of the bacteria Acetobacter or Gluconobacter, alcohol is further oxidized to acetic acid, producing wine vinegar. Then there is wine royalty—Champagne, a sparkling wine. To give this wine its high level of carbination, white wine, or Rose´ is fermented a second time by adding more yeast and sugar when the wine is bottled, corked and wired. The extra carbon dioxide generated becomes trapped in the bottle, giving Champagne it delightful bubbles. The wiring keeps the corks from flying out, bullet-like, propelled by the irresistible pressure of the carbon dioxide.

Furthermore, the same grapes from different sections of a vineyard can be different because they harbor different species of yeasts on their skins. Conventional wine growers can use pesticides and fungicides to protect their grapes, but in doing so, they kill off many of the yeasts that would be in the natural fermentation. These wine growers then rely on commercial yeasts strains for their fermentation, attaining less diversity and complexity in the taste and style of the wine, compared to wines with the full complement of natural yeasts. With attention to the folks at UC Davis, growers can make the changes needed to deliver more captivating wines.

Beer

There's good reason for Ben Franklin to have said, "Beer is our best proof that God loves us, and wants us to be happy." And two hundred years on, Dave Barry raised his Stein observing that, "Without question, the greatest invention in the history of mankind is beer, oh, I grant you that the wheel was also a fine invention, but the wheel does not go as well with pizza." Furthermore, no human microbial pathogen has ever been associated, connected, to beer, as its level of acidity is totally inhospitable.

Any substance containing sugar can be fermented by wild yeasts in air. Consequently, it's reasonable to assume that people everywhere had their beers, accidentally arrived at.

Chemical tests of ancient pottery jars indicate that beer was produced some 7,000 years ago. In Mesopotamia, today's Syria, evidence of beer drinking was depicted on six thousand-year-old Sumerian clay tablets showing a group of people drinking a beverage through reed straws: a recipe for making beer from barley was also found.

Beer is made from grain—barley, wheat, and rice, and by law in most countries beer consists of only four ingredients:hops, yeast, water and malt. For the past five hundred years, hops, the dried flowers of the perennial female plant, Humulus lupulis, resembling small, light green pine combs, were originally added for flavor and to inhibit spoilage organisms.

Apparently medieval brewers realized that hopped beer maintained its quality longer than unhopped beer. But although hops are bitter, it provides a balance for the sweetness of the malt sugars, as well as flavors and resins that act as antibiotics, retarding spoilage by wild yeasts and bacteria.

To make a well-received, drinkable beer, the complex carbohydrates in grain must first be transformed into fermentable carbohydrates. Five stages are universal: malting, in which barley is moistened, germinated and able to sprout, as if it was a plant in soil, releasing its enzymes that solubilize its carbohydrates, converting the starch into the sugar, maltose; hence malting.

Drying and grinding stops the germination. Washing combines the malt and other carbohydrates with warm water allowing the enzymes released during malting to produce additional sugars. This sugary liquid is the Wort.

Hops are now added and the wort mixture is boiled to stop enzymatic action, extract flavor from the hops, kill any extraneous microbes, and concentrate the mixture.

At this juncture, Yeasts are added to the wort to produce alcohol. Most often the yeasts are strains of Saccharomyes carlsbergensis or S.cerevisiae. Cerevisiae, comes from the Latin, cervisia, from Ceres, the goddess of agriculture, and from the Spanish and Portuguese, cerversa. Of course our word, cereal is connected to the goddess.

Beer flavor is also dependent upon small amounts of acetic acid and sweet gylcerol. This final brew is then pasteurized at 140°F, filtered, bottled, or canned and aged.

Let us not forget that bacteria closely associated with the yeast fermentation produce the diacetyl (2,3,butanedione) that imparts a buttery, butter-scotchy flavor, generated as a by-product of amino acid metabolism. Microbes and biochemicals are joined at the hip...forever.

The current rise of microbrewries, seek to satisfy cravings for different tastes. To achieve that, contemporary brewers use Brittanomyces, a so-called wild yeast that has become the darling of microbrewers. This wild yeast was found in beers before the advent of strict sanitary controls, and has been resurrected. In these new foodie beers various strains can impart spicy, fruity, earthy, funky, flavors that satisfy local imbibers. For the home brew folks, there are dozens of yeast strains for sale that people swear by. And why not?

No microbes, no beer, and there'd be no
Oktoberfest, that annual 16-day downing of hundreds
of thousands of gallons, in Munich, Germany. Nor would
there be the Great British Beer Festival in early August,
called the biggest Pub in the world. And what would
Denver do without its Great American Beer Festival,
in late September, where judges evaluate 3 thousand
different beers. It's unimaginable! So, Drink up!
And a toast to our microbes!

Whiskey

Ah, the Devil's Spirit, or the Poet's inspiration.
Whiskey, from the Gaelic, usige, (pronounced, wishge
ba), the water of life, or as the Romans had it, Aqua
vitae.

Until the 1490's, distilling alcohol to make whiskey
was the concern of pharmacists, Apothecaries, (the Guild
of Surgeon Barbers) and Monks in Monasteries, for use
as medicine, as treatment for Smallpox, and colic, as well
as an antibiotic and anesthetic.

American history buffs will recall the Whiskey
Rebellion of 1794, when Scottish and Irish immigrant
farmers in Pennsylvania, referred to as "western
moonshiners", got their noses bent out of shape when
Alexander Hamilton, and Congress, called "federal
revenooers," placed an excise tax of seven cents a gallon
on whiskey in 1791, to help pay off the debt incurred by
the Revolutionary war. There was so much corn whiskey
being made, it was used as currency.

These Westerner's became an unruly mob and
began ruffing up government officials, and signed a
covenant never to pay the tax. When the Governor of
Pennsylvania refused to intervene to put down the
rebellion, President Washington called out fifteen
thousand men from militias in four states, and with
Hamilton at his side, both in uniform, marched at the
head of this army over the Allegheny mountains to

confront the moonshiners. The rebels fled and the rebellion was over.

Where beer required four ingredients, whiskey requires only three: barley (or corn) water (this is significant) and strains of yeasts. Again, five stages are involved to obtain smooth, velvety spirits: malting; mashing; fermentation, distilling and maturing.

The barley is malted, germinated to convert the starches in the grain to simple sugars. Distillers prefer plump, ripe barley with lots of starch and not too much nitrogen from protein and amino acids.

After germination the malt is dried, and flavor is imparted by the furnace's peat smoke; mashing occurs, producing a, sweet sugary wort. Water quality plays an essential role, as water differs in mineral content. Soft, acidic water is preferred, as it doesn't have the saltiness of hard water, which would precipitate out when heated forming scale in the copper kettles.

After mashing, yeasts are added for the fermentation of the wort, which is cooled quickly to get the yeast fermenting the sugars to alcohol. With the production of alcohol, distillation occurs to increase the alcohol level, which takes place in large copper pot stills with swan necks.

The heat of distillation turns the liquid to vapor, followed by condensation by cooling of the vapor back to liquid, raising the alcohol volume to 40-50 percent. This alcohol cannot be called Scotch whiskey until it has been aged for a minimum of three years. However, if Scotch whiskey is to be sold as a single malt whiskey, it must be aged for 8-12 years. Single malt Scotch whiskey is made from a mash of a single grain, most often barley, and aged in oak casks. Some few Irish Whiskies are distilled three times to achieve a smoother finish, by removing congeners, the by-products of fermentation, the fusel alcohols-ethyl acetate, acetone, propanol and other chemicals that contribute sharp tastes as well as, it is believed, the well known hangover.

So, while these five stages are essential for the changes they produce, without our microbes, there would be no whiskey. It was ever thus.

So, heat a fermented liquid and the lighter, more volatile alcohols, ketones, and esters, evaporate. That vapor, cooled down and condensed, is a spirit. Distill wine, and we get Brandy, with a far higher alcohol content. Distill beer and yes whiskey, is our libation. Continue to distill, and Vodka comes into being.

Checking my supply of spirits, I found that my Irish Bushmills, has an alcohol level of 43 percent; much the same as my Talisker and 16-year old Lagavulin, Scotch whiskies. The label on my yet unopened Belvedere Vodka tells me the alcohol level is 40 percent. Way down at 17-20 percent, are my dry and cream Spanish Sherries.

Gin is much the same as Vodka, but for the addition of Juniper berries that provide aroma and flavor.

Yeasts and bacteria must be credited with building huge worldwide alcoholic beverage industries. Cheers! Salud! Slancha! L'Chaim! Skol! Alla Salute! Prost!

Bread: The Staff of Life

We've been consuming bread in some form for thousands of years. Up to the mid 19th century most people obtained the bulk of their calories from bread. "The social contract was written in flour, water and leavening, and breaking bread together is considered the central act of sociability."[31]

For all that, bread is nothing more than flour, water and yeast. The earliest breads were more like flat cakes. More than likely leavened breads were discovered accidentally some seven thousand years ago. About eight thousand bce, the first grinding stone, called a quern, was developed in Egypt, and the first grain was crushed. The early breads resembled today's Chapatis of India, and Mexico's Tortillas, made from corn. In Rome, around

100 bce, well-to-do Romans insisted on the more exclusive and expensive white breads made of refined flour. The darker, whole grain wheat and bran breads were for the masses, but they got the more nutritious breads. This dichotomy has persisted into the 21st century.

Some clever baker kept a piece of the leavened dough, placing it in other loaves, continuing the process, and leavened bread was invented. Yeast dough production, done under aerobic conditions, results in greater levels of carbon dioxide that makes a dense mass of dough rise.

Bread making also requires a number of steps. As water is added to the ground grain, the flour, amylase enzymes released in the moistened dough produce the sugars, maltose and sucrose, from the starch. Strains of the yeast Saccharomyces, are added which contribute additional enzymes that split the sugars into carbon dioxide and ethanol. Carbon dioxide trapped in the pockets of dough, developed by the kneading, cause the dough to rise, producing, a lighter texture, while the ethanol and other end-products of fermentation contribute to the final flavor.

Yeasts contribute more than leavening: fermentation helps to strengthen and develop gluten, which itself is the result of two proteins glutenin and gliaden which, when combined with water, form gluten. Yeasts are also the producers of the biochemicals that contribute flavor chemicals along with the ethanol.

By using a mixture of yeast strains, including Saccharomyces exiquus, combined with lactic acid producing bacteria, along with a hint of acetic acid, sour doughs are produced. San Francisco sour dough uses wild yeast gathered from the air and the skins of fruits and veggies, along with *Lactobacillus sanfrancisensis*, and *Lactobacillus brevis*. Folks in San Francisco noted that their sour dough stays fresh longer than other breads, which prompted a study of the dough and found that it also contained Lactobacillus hammesii that produces an antifungal compound inhibiting mold contamination.

Sour dough was the primary bread made in northern California during the gold rush, and continues to be an integral part of California's culture.

Sour dough appears to have arisen in Egypt about 1500 bce and was likely the first leavened bread available.

Challah is the bread Jewish people serve at their Sabbath meals in which the twelve ancient tribes are represented by twelve braids on each loaf. For leavening, there's nothing fancy, just active-dry yeast, baker's yeast and, for its pleasing shine, an egg wash is used unsparingly.

Of course Bagels, a small ring of dough, was originally made of white flour, water and yeast. First mention of it appears to be in the 1610 statutes of the Jewish community of Krakow, Poland. The round shape symbolized the cycle of life.

Legend has it that a baker alerted the Viennese of the approach of the Turks in 1683. After the victory over the Turks, the bakers commemorated the Viennese victory with a crescent shaped roll that evolved into our Croissants, as the Turkish symbol was the crescent moon.

And the take away message is—nowhere in the world is there any type of alcoholic beverage, bread, or pastry that is not the consequence of microbial intervention. No microbe, no alcohol: no microbes, no dough rising.

Cheese It! Fermented Milk Products

No one really knows who made the first cheese or when, but recent evidence suggests that farmers around Poland's Vistula river, were using cows milk to make cheese 7,200 years ago. Scientists at the University of

Bristol, England, tested ancient perforated clay pots finding fatty acids that had soaked into the ceramic sieves. They surmised that these perforated clay pots were used to separate the liquid whey from semi-solid curds, and that the first cheese was likely a watery concoction resembling a cottage cheese or a fromage frais.[32]

But why make cheese? In the beginning, a good place to start, people tucked away in mountain hamlets and wide-open savannah's needing to preserve the nutrients milk provides, as well as ensuring their food supply, discovered cheese; perhaps as an ancient legend suggests: Accidently. An Arab merchant put his supply of milk into a pouch made of a sheep's stomach as he set out on a day's journey across the desert. The rennin, an enzyme, in the lining of the pouch, combined with the heat of the sun, caused the milk to separate into curd and whey. That night he found that the whey satisfied his thirst, and the curd, the cheese, had a delightful flavor that satisfied his hunger. A reasonable notion.

The cheeses discovered in diverse parts of the world, were (are) as different from one another as their local terrain, culture, climate and resources–the availability of animals supplying milk: horses, cows, sheep, Yaks, water buffalo, goats, and camels, which also connects terrain; grassy, hilly, rocky, watery, and sandy soils.

All milk, no matter the animal providing, contains water, lactose, fats, minerals and protein-casein and whey. And all cheese makers, what should we call them, cheesers, perhaps, follow similar paths, as they have much the same objectives: expel water, demineralize the casein using acids provided by a medley of bacteria, and add salt.

The specific goal of these objectives is, however, different for each type of cheese: each has its own water, salt and acid content which will affect the cheese's ripening, and most important, which microbes will be involved to impart flavor, aroma and texture. By the way, currently more than one-third of all milk produced in the US is used to make cheese.

Types of Cheese and Their Microbes

In a word, all cheese, all 1,400 different kinds, can be grouped by type; five of them: soft, unripened; soft, ripened; semisoft; hard, ripened, and very hard, ripened. And each of the cheeses within each type has its own community of microbes. It would be the odd cheese, very odd indeed, that claimed to be fermented by a single bacterium or fungus. Furthermore, cows, sheep and goats produce volumes of volitile fatty acids, acetic, propionic, and butyric, that enter their blood streams. The fat and flavor of fresh cow's sheep or goat's milk comes from their mammary glands synthesis of fats from these acids. Each of these animals, as well as horses (mares), camels, and buffalos, as would be expected, produce a different number of fats from these volitiles, in collaboration with microbial enzymes, which make for the unique flavors of the cheeses made from the milk of these animals.

Let's have a look at each type of cheese to become familiar with the microbes giving us the enjoyment we've come to expect.

We begin with Cottage and Cream cheese, Mozzarella, and Feta, examples of soft, unripened cheese. Cream cheese, fresh, non-aged and unripened, was an American invention from upstate, New York, made from pasteurized non-skim milk and is similar to the French Neufchatel and the Italian Mascarpone, made from cow's milk and fermented by Lactococcus lactis. Cream cheese has a high fat content, over 30-plus percent, is also high in calcium, and its fairly high acidity is masked by its high fat content. High fat and low moisture act as a preservative, as few if any microbes have the temerity to dine upon it.

Cottage cheese, originally made in cottages by women using milk left over from butter making, is also the handiwork of Lactococcus lactis. The cheese is drained but not pressed, which obtains the large pieces of curd, and removes the acidity. Little Miss Muffet who sat on a tuffet was in fact eating cottage cheese, before the spider who sat down beside her, frightened Miss Muffet away.

Mozzarella, from southern Italy, was originally made with milk from water buffalo's, then cow's milk, and currently is often a mixture of the two. Sometimes pasteurized, sometimes not. To achieve its mildly acidic taste and smooth texture requires a triumvirate of microbes: *lactobacillus bulgaricus, lactobacillus helveticus*, and *streptococcus thermophilus*, each contributing flavor components. With its high moisture content, it spreads easily, but needs to be eaten soon after it's made.

Feta, from the Greek, meaning slice, is rich, creamy and crumbly, and most often kept in a brine solution. Feta is made from a mixture of sheep and goat's milk, and has a 40-50 percent fat content, and 3-4 percent salt. That milk combination garners microbes galore: lactobacillus plantarum, brevis, coryneformis, and fermentum, along with the fungi, Pichia, and Kluyveromyes, which have been identified in different feta cheeses. However, the brine's high salt concentrations, rapidly stops the microbial action.

Feta cheeses also come from Bulgaria, Albania, Turkey, France, Finland, and a number of others, as it makes great salads, anywhere.

The soft, ripened cheeses include the well respected Cammembert and Brie from France, both requiring the distinguishing intervention of lactococcus lactis, lactococcus cremoris and Penicillium cammemberti in combination with Penicillium candidum and completed with Brevibacterium linens. An outstanding quintet and community of players if ever there was one. Both Brie and Cammembert are sprayed with P.cammemberti that forms a soft, white mossy surface, giving the cheeses their characteristic flavor and texture. For Camembert devotees, the luscious rind, habitat of a clutch of microbes, is the best part. Moreover, the rind protects the cheese from unwanted microbes that would like a taste, but would also impart nasty flavors. Brevibacterium linens breaks down proteins into organic compounds having fishy, garlicky, oniony, and sweaty aromas. And yes, it is the same organism that resides between our toes creating the very aroma we equate with sweaty socks. We pay top dollar for the cheese, but turn up our noses at the socks. Go figure.

The realm of Semisoft cheeses includes Blue, and Roquefort from France, Muenster from the US, and Limberger from Belgium. Blue cheese is inoculated with P.roqueforti that quickly germinates into fungal threads that run along veins in the cheese. The fungus is abetted by two lactococci bacteria, that together, create the compelling bounty.

Roquefort, mentioned in the dusty records of the Monastery at Conques, France, as early as 1070, is made from the milk of ewes which is fermented by the trio, lactococus lactis, l.cremoris, and finished off by the addition of P.roqueforti.

Brevibacterium linens did it again, making Limburger cheese, truly distinctive—among the top ten worst smelling cheeses ever produced. With an aroma (odor?) only the brave can savior, or is it endure.

This semisoft cheese, made of cow's milk, and often of pasteurized goat's milk, has a buttery texture and nutty flavor, but you'll be hard pressed to penetrate the notorious odor required to get to the cheese. It takes three months to mature to its full bloom. It is often said that Limburger smells so awful that it makes sweaty socks smell like perfume.

Limburger was originally made in Limburg, an area between Belgium, the Netherlands, and Germany. Currently, it is made in Germany, and Wisconsin, where it remains in favor with the older folks. The younger generation appears to have given it a pass. Not too difficult to comprehend.

Other semisoft cheeses include Gorgonzola from Italy, Stilton from England, Niva, from Czech, and Mycella from Denmark. Microbes know no borders, performing exotic manipulations wherever nutrients lead them.

Swiss, Edam, Gouda, Colby, Chedder, Emmenthaler, and Gruyere, are among the hard-ripened cheeses, a highly popular group that the world has embraced. Unlike Edam, Colby and Chedder, Swiss cheese gets it singular flavor from the addition of *Propionibacterium shermanii*, coupling with two lactococci and Strep.thermophilis, another dandy quartet. However, Swiss' sharp bouquet and trademark holes are the work of Propionibacterium that metabolizes acetic acid to sweaty smelling propionic acid and carbon dioxide that can only punch the required holes in the cheese if it is sufficiently elastic. This widely consumed cheese was originally made in Switzerland's Emmenthal Valley in the fifteenth century, and shows no sign of letting up.

Chedder, Colby, Edam, and Gouda, each have their complex communities of strains of lactococci and lactobacilli. Chedder, is a pale yellow to off-white cheese with a sharp to pungent flavor that originated in the southwest Somerset village of Chedder, England, where it has been produced since the 12th century. Barber's 1833 English Vintage Chedder, is aged for two years to give the wee ones time to do their best work, producing the characteristic intense flavors. It does come with a cost; almost as much as Kobe beef: double digit dollars per pound. If you can afford it, it's well worth it. That 1833, by the way, is the year the Barber family began producing their distinct Chedder.

Lactococcus lactis, Wisconsin's state microbe is vital to the production of Chedder in the US. It can be combined with strains of lactobacilli, but it is most often used alone to produce the over three billion pounds produced annually.

Any discussion of cheese, as far as I'm concerned, must include that Spanish delicacy, Manchego; the tangy, earthy, cheese from La Mancha, that "The Man of La Mancha" surely carried in his saddlebags, and sank his teeth into, between jousting with windmills.

This semi-hard cheese made from unpasteurized ewe's milk is nothing less than a catalog of microbes. It may just be that its passle of seven that are known:a lactococcus; two lactobacilli;an enterococcus;two leuconostocs; a micrococci and a pediococcus, come together to produce tasty biochemicals. And to be authentic, Manchego must be made from ewe's milk, and come from La Mancha. Aging is also essential. Manchego fresco is aged for a few weeks; Manchego curado, for six months, and Manchego viejo, the oldest and hardest, for a year or more. With side-by-side slices, the great differences in taste and aroma become evident.

Hard ripened cheeses are also referred to as firm, grating, or grana. These cheeses have long ageing periods that affect their flavor and texture and prolong their edible life. Included here are Romano, Parmasan, Pecorino,and Gran Padano. Pecorino, made in Sardinia, from sheep's milk requires a quartet of microbes to obtain its exceptional flavor and texture: *Enterococcous fecalis*, leuconostoc mesenteroides, lactococcus lactis, and Strep.thermophilis work together to make it possible. They can be counted on to do this year in and year out. Team work that's hard to beat.

Romano and Parmasan require three: two lactobacilli, and a *streptococcus*. Gran Padano, Gran, or Grana, comes from the Italian for grain, that refers to its grainy-texture, and Padano refers to the valley in northern Italy where it was first made by Cistercian monks some nine hundred years ago, as there way of using ripened cheese to preserve milk. Gran Padano owes its delicate flavor to *Lactobacilius helveticus*, and *L.fermentum*, along with *Strep.thermophilis*.

Recently a team of researchers, led by those from Newcastle University, Newcastle, England, identified a new group of bacteria that could not be grown in artificial culture media, but were identified by DNA fingerprinting. They came up with eight organisms that add flavor to some of the world's most exclusive cheese.

Reblochon is one of France's great mountain-made cheeses. Like Limburger and Port de Salut, Reblochon is a smear-ripened cheese that washes the surface of the cheese with a salt solution containing bacteria. It is soft and creamy, like Brie.

Reblochon begins with a starter culture of, whew, Brevibacterum linens. But now a new group of organisms has been found that surely makes a difference. The Newcastle University scientists named one of the new bacteria Mycetocola reblochoni. The smear-ripening process helps to spread the bacterium across the surface of the cheese, ripening it from the outside in. New molecular fingerprinting techniques may just provide a world of new organisms that contribute mightily to our gustatory delights.

Cheese makers, those cheesers, or mongers, exert great effort and experience into creating the complex microbial communities that exist on and in all cheeses, seeking to control each step of the way to the finished cheese. The various milks must be colonized by the exact microbes at the appropriate time. However, with the microbes accounted for, Affinage may just be the final and crucial phase of cheese production. Affinage deals with aging, and far beyond placing a wheel of cheese on a shelf in a cave.

Aging is a skill developed by Affineurs, the go to guy's responsible for ensuring that the prior steps and the appropriate microbes are cared for, such that year after year, after year, the cheese will be exactly what it's expected to be. No mean feat!

Ergo, no microbes, no cheese.

Fermented Milk: Drink It or Spoon It

Fermented milks, Yogurt, buttermilk, Kefir, Koumiss, Liben, sour cream, Matzoon, Creme fraiche, Ayran, sour and clabbered milk, and Acidophilis Milk, and many others around the world, owe their tastes, textures and nutrients to their microbes. All european countries, along with African, the Middle and FarEast, have their fermented milks. You'd be hard pressed to name a country without a fermented milk-for all the same reasons.

Here we consider a dozen and begin with Koumiss (Kumis) which comes to us from Central Asia, and is made from the milk of mares (horses) and Camels. Koumiss was originally fermented in a horsehide bag, which contained the microflora from a previous batch. It has a higher alcohol content, about 2 percent, than Kefir's one percent, as Mare's milk has a higher sugar content than cow or goat milk. With the high demand for Koumiss, cow's milk with added sugar is currently used.

To produce alcohol from milk sugars, yeasts begin the fermentation, which is taken over by the acid producers: lactobacilli, and Enterococcus fecalis.

Kefir, also from Central Asia, and Russia, derives its acidic tastes and buttery smooth texture and flavor, produced by diacetyl, a metabolite of the diverse Lactobacilli including L.kefir, yeasts and a complex mixture of fungi of the genus, Kazachstania. These delightful organisms ferment cow, goat, and sheep milk used by different populations. The Lactobacilli also produce sufficient carbon dioxide to give Kefir its bubbly sensation as well as its alcohol level.

Originally, traditional buttermilk was the creamy liquid remaining in the churn after making butter from fermented cream. Currently, real cultured buttermilk, made by a few purist farmers, and hard to come by, is a fermented milk with a piquant tartness contributed by either Lactobacillus bulgaricus, or Strep. lactis. L.bulgaricus provides greater lactic acid, greater acidity, which means increased tartness. This increased acidity lowers the pH, clumping the casein, the primary milk protein, making the buttermilk thicker.

Today's so-called cultured buttermilk is a far cry from its ancestor, being made from low-fat, or skim milk, inoculated with bacteria to make it acidic, then thickened with locust bean gum and/or carageenan, and Annatto added for light yellow color. The result is a poor facsimile of real cultured buttermilk.

In the Middle East, Leban (Laban) is their buttermilk, a slightly sour product, low in fat, as the fat is left behind in the butter. Streptococci, Leuconostoc and Lactobacilli do the fermenting. Ayran, is a Turkish yogurt, similar in tartness to Leban, usually made in summer to spoon or drink cold. Apparently many Turks prefer to add cold water and salt to it. Furthermore, Yogurt is a Turkish word, meaning thicken, which it does nicely.

Yogurt made from cow's milk is fermented by, *L.bulgaricus* and *Strep.thermophilis.* At times, *Bifidobacterium* is added. These work together to produce the acid and aroma we've come to enjoy. Currently, a riot of fruits are added for those who can't abide plain vanilla. The newer Greek yogurt that has become all the rage is somewhat tangier, less sweet, and thicker, achieved by squeezing out the whey, and lactose sugar, which results in a higher protein content, and lower sugar. As for health benefits of all yogurts, that has yet to be determined. Don't shoot! The jury is still out on that.

Acidophilis milk is the handiwork of, yes, *L.acidophilis*, and acidophilis means, acid loving bacteria, often referred to as a probiotic, as it is advertised as being beneficial for our intestinal and

343

immune heath. Unfortunately the marketing and PR has outpaced the science, which has yet to obtain clinical evidence to support such claims. But it does taste good, as the casein is curdled to a custardy-like consistency.

Matzoon, similar to Kefir, comes from Armenia and Georgia, the country, not the state, where cows, goats or water buffalo milk is fermented by several strains of yeast, a micrococcus, and *L.lactis*, providing a fruity, acidic, smooth curd that can be eaten with a spoon.

Sour cream is also eaten, and is acidified by Strep. lactis, giving it a subtle, tangy flavor, but is a much thicker, smoother product, that I can't get enough of.

Creme frais, fresh cream, is only slightly acidic, but smooth and thick, acidified by Strep.lactis, but is a fatter version of sour cream.

Sour milk, or cultured milk, can be made at home by adding a tablespoon of sour cream or cultured buttermilk to whole milk in a bowl, setting it aside with a sheet of wax paper or gauze loosely covering it. Three to four days later you will be able to eat a smooth, custardy-like tangy pudding. For best results, do this in the warmer months between May and September. Vegetarian restaurants offer this by the glass, along with a spoon. Of course the delicate taste is due to the mix of organism in the buttermilk and/or sour cream. I've made it using a bit of both. But care must be taken to avoid wild yeasts or bacteria in the neighborhood from gaining admission to your bowl, delivering an ugly tasting affair.

Then there are those mouth-watering fermented veggies, sauerkraut, Kosher dill pickles, olives and vinegar.

Sauerkraut (sour cabbage) is a pickling via lactic fermentation that involves numerous players. Klebsiella and Enterobacter initiate the fermentation, producing an acidic environment from the sugar in the cabbage, favoring lactobacilli. When the acid level gets too high for them, the leuconostocs and pediococci take over. When the fermentation is complete, the Sauerkraut has far greater nutrient content than the original cabbage. It is now high in Vitamins C, B, and K, low in calories, and a good source of fiber.

Kosher dill pickles arrive via a natural fermentation as the cucumbers bring with them the lactic acid-producing bacteria, picked up in the field. As the cucumbers ferment, garlic, dill and mustard seeds are added to the brine. With the production of carbon dioxide, the "cukes" turn from bright green to brownish green, ready for joining corned, roast beef or pastrami. I'm salivating worse than Pavlov's dogs.

You can do this at home. Purchase a jar of bright green half-sour cucumbers. At home, open the lid, but leave it on. Set the jar aside for 3-4 days. You'll see the bubbles of carbon dioxide rising to the top. Tighten the lid and place the jar in the refrigerator for another 3-4 days. Now you and they are ready. The aroma itself is worth the wait. For me, the pickle juice beats any wine.

Olives, the fruit of the Olive tree, some call it a vegetable, native to the Mediterranean, Africa, and Asia, also undergoes a natural fermentation having picked up microbes as they grow. This spontaneous fermentation in brine is promoted by Candida yeasts *lactobacillus pentosus* and *l.plantarum*; which rids the olives of their naturally bitter taste while the yeasts produce biochemicals from the high fat content, providing the compelling flavor. The high salt concentration of the brine prevents salt-sensitive unwanted bacteria from joining in. The enterobacters, lactic acid bacteria and yeasts, play a dominant role.

To preserve their nutrients, improve their digestibility, and develop flavor, aroma and texture, many vegetables are fermented. Lactic acid bacteria and yeasts are the primary fermenters in the US and Europe, while fungi are preferred in Asia. Carrots, cauliflower, celery, artichokes, cucumbers, eggplant, tomatoes, peppers, and beans, often mixed together, providing leuconostoc mesenteroides and lactobacillus plantarum with the sugars needed for conversion to acid and addition of flavoring biochemicals.

Vinegar, widely used in salads, sauces and gravies, is made from wine, beer, and/or cider, which means grapes, grains, apples, and other fruits that Acetobacter aceti, and Acetobacter pasteurianus metabolize to acetic acid by way of ethanol.

Again, it's microbes, microbes, microbes, that we're consuming every day. It's the microbes that feed us, and it's the microbes that provide enjoyment. That's the essential message.

Coffee, Tea and Cocoa

Have you thought about the connection of microbes to coffee, tea and cocoa?

Before that can of your favorite coffee is placed on a shelf in your favorite supermarket, coffee beans must be fermented to prepare the fruit for your cup. The goal of coffee fermentation is the breaking down of the pulp surrounding the beans.

Coffee cherries, the beans, grow grape-like in bunches in a tree-like plant of the genus Coffea. Coffea arabica, a widely used species, is one of the five commercially important species. The coffee fruit is a berry about the size of common cherries. A ripe coffee cherry consists of two green beans surrounded by pulp, which must be removed to obtain the beans.

For the most part, ripe coffee fruit is harvested and part of the pulp is removed mechanically. Fermentation, the next step, converts the pulpy mucilage-like layer to a water soluble substance that can be removed by washing.

Fermentation occurs in concrete tanks where the mucilage is digested by a complex of microbes. Because the mucilage is primarily pectin, the bacteria must be able to produce the enzyme pectinase. Enterobacter and Escherichia do this nicely, as do the fungi Aspergillus and Fusarium. From here, it's on to drying, grinding, roasting, canning and, your cup.

Moreover, bacteria are the dominant group in soils surrounding coffee plants. The Pseudamonads and Bacillus provide nutrients for the plant and are essential for improving plant growth and productivity, as well as building a healthy coffee farm. Enjoy.

Now consider this. Prof. Jeffrey Barrick of the University of Texas, Austin, reengineered an E.coli to become addicted to coffee; it now depends on coffee for its growth. But this addiction offers us great benefits as this E.coli can now be used to measure caffeine in pharmaceuticals, a diversity of beverages, and breast milk. Commercial companies are looking to use this coffee-crazed organism to decaffeinate tea and coffee, a more environmentally friendly method than the current methylene chloride extraction process. Furthermore, the processing of coffee beans yields nutrient-rich waste that could be used as animal feed and fertilizer, but for the caffeine content. Ergo, this reengineered organism could be used to decaffeinate this waste. Another plus for reengineering our friendly, and beneficial, microbes.

Tea, from the Theaceae family, and the shrub, Camellia sinensis, is an evergreen of tropical and subtropical Asia, with fragrant, tender, white flowers. Its hand-picked leaves are dried and used to make an infusion in boiling water.

When mature, tea leaves are tough. Young leaves are the ones picked for tea. After picking, they are rolled under pressure and broken into pieces to rupture the leaf's cells, releasing their juices, then twisted and coated with those juices. The leaf changes to a copper color, and its characteristic aroma develops.

Fermentation and bacterial enzymatic digestion occurs as leaf pieces are spread on fermenting beds and held under high humidity. The strength or body of the tea depends entirely on this fermentation.

Tannins, a bitter tasting polyphenolic organic compound, plays an important role. When it is split, digested by the enzyme polyphenol oxidase, supplied by the molds Aspergillus niger, and *A.glaucum*, along with Penicillium strains, the bitterness is lost and flavoring chemicals, the flavins, are produced. Drying of the fermented leaf pieces follows, as it then makes its way to our cups of hot water.

Without any added ingredients, there are only four calories per cup, and we get the benefit of Vitamins B-2, and Niacin, B-3. An additional benefit is the fact that tea is basic, while coffee is acidic, which translates as easier on our stomachs.

Cocoa is another hot beverage that must be fermented for flavor development. Chocolate/Cocoa, comes from the seeds of the plant Theobroma cocoa. Theos, means God in Greek, and broma means food, ergo, food of the Gods. As a chocolate lover, I heartily concur.

It was the Spanish, in the 17th century, who added sugar and vanilla to the bitter Mayan drink, which was enough to set off the chocolate explosion and on to the world's stage.

The cocoa tree bears pods some four inches long and three wide, weighing over a pound. These pods ripen into a rich, golden-orange, and within each pod are from 3-40 inch-long purple beans or seeds, covered in a white mucilagy pulp.

The chocolate/cocoa story really begins with the harvesting of the pods, their splitting open, releasing the seeds, and their fermentation. Once the seeds are released, fermentation begins by microbes naturally present on the pods surface. Additional microbial contributions arrive via worker's hand's, the baskets in which the pods are transported, and insects flying about;

almost anything in the neighborhood of the ripe seeds contribute organisms.

Fermentation goes on for about a week, releasing the seeds' aromatic biochemicals including the fruity esters, ethyl benzoate and ethyl octanoate along with dozens of alchols, aldehydes, and ketones that convert bitter cocoa to finger-licking chocolate. During that week, there are yeasts, lactic acid bacteria, acetic acid bacteria, Bacillus, and fungi actively digesting. The beans are turned over allowing air (oxygen) to oxidize polyphenols, providing the flavanols that give chocolate and cocoa its brown color.

The number of organisms isolated from fermenting seeds is upwards of a hundred, and the succession appears to be-yeasts to lactic acid bacteria, to acetic acid bacteria, to fungi. The numbers and diversity of microbes dinning on cocoa seeds varies by country. So, for example, Ghana's cocoa seeds are fermented by a quartet of lactic acid bacteria–a trio of acetic acid bacteria and a team of nine yeasts. By comparison, a dozen lactic acid bacteria, and two dozen yeasts appear to do the heavy lifting in Belize, Central America.

These dozens of microbial types grow almost immediately, but rise and fall as biochemical compounds are produced along with changes in the acidic environment. The high sugar content of the pulp favors the growth of yeasts that produce ethanol. They also digest the pulp's pectin. The alcohol level kills off the yeasts (self destruction) allowing the lactic's to rise, until the acid level becomes too much for them, which brings on the acetic acid organisms, such as *Acetobacter* and *Gluconobacter*. This complex fermentation procession produces a great diversity of biochemicals that become chocolate's prominent flavor and aroma components.

Roasting the seeds kills off all the microbes and adds to the characteristic color of chocolate. After roasting, it's on to the fabricators who process the finished seeds into the powered cocoa, and on to our markets.

Recall that microbes are used in the production of finished chocolate products. The enzyme amylase from *Aspergillus niger*, splits starch for chocolate syrup, and the enzyme invertase, from yeast, splits sucrose for soft-centered chocolates.

Life without chocolate would be a catastrophe for my wife and the chocoholics the world over. Is chocolate addictive? Are chocoholics addicts? It sure seems so. Chocoholics are everywhere. No country is free of them. How did this happen?

The history books tell us that when the Spanish Conquistadors arrived in Mexico expressly to haul away gold and silver, the Indians were drinking cocoa. In 1519, Montezuma, the Aztec king, served it to Hernon Cortes, which he was keen enough to bring to Spain in 1529. He was also clever enough to add copious amounts of sugar and spices to this naturally bitter beverage, and they loved it. In 1580, Spain opened the first cocoa processing plant. Someone spilled the beans and the secret was out. Cocoa,"the food of the gods," spread across Europe like a virus in winter. Cocoa butter, cocoa powder and bars of chocolate were all the rage.

In Europe, liquid chocolate "was promoted in medical and scientific treatises as a stimulant, love potion, cure for impotence, and an aid to conception." The Spanish physician "Antonio Colmenero de Ledesma, wrote in the 17th century that chocolate, "vehemently incites to Venus, and causeth Conception in women, hastens and facilitates their delivery." Such potency was believed to affect men as well. The English doctor Henry Stubbs, writing in the same era, extolled his countrymen's great use of chocolate in venery and for supplying the testicles with balm and sap."[33] Currently, venery appears to be surging as we are informed in 2014 that cocoa planters worldwide are hard pressed to keep up with the demand for chocolate. Love is in the air, and chocolate along with it, thanks to our microbes.

"Shrimpers and rice, they're very nice . . ."

To the question, can Shrimp become the new chicken of the sea, without damaging the ocean, the answer appears to be, yes, if..if microbes are deployed appropriately. How's that? In aerated shrimp ponds, beneficial marine bacteria flouirish, helping to supplement the Shrimp's diet by recycling nutrients already in the pond. Lovely. With the addition of a source of carbon, such as wheat flour, these bacteria convert ammonium (NH_3) from Shrimp waste, into protein. The bacteria latch onto the floating particles, creating nutritious masses of biofloc that the Shrimp gobble-up, sharply reducing the need for costly protein supplements. Consequently, microbes are leading the way to Shrimp as cheap as chicken, and less polluting.[34] A round of applause, please!

Meats, Fowl, and Fish: The World Over

Is there a country in the world that doesn't have its distinctive fermented meats? These meats, the result of inoculating specific microbes into a variety of meats, offers a basket of benefits: available nutrients, distinctive flavors, textures, color, taste, tenderness, and extended shelf life, freedom from spoilage. Now there's a tidy basketful.

Fermentation produces safe and marketable products by increasing acidity, lowering moisture content, and drying.

Cold-loving pseudamonads, enterobacters, along with several lactic acid producers, are naturally present in meats and participate in fermentation along with the inoculated starter cultures of *Lactobacillus plantarum*, and *L.casei*, and *Pediococcus*, to obtain the higher acid levels. In Europe, the most common starters are *Staph.xylosu* and *Staph.carnosuss* and Mirococci which produce different tastes and flavors than meats fermented in the US and Asia.

As these organisms dine on their sausages and hams, producing flavorful metabolites, alcohols, volatile acids, amines, and peptides, they impart the desired tastes and textures. Using these specific cultures assures little product variation year after year.

In the US, mold cultures deliver the white mold on Salamis. In addition, Penicilliuim spores, and the yeast Dabaryomyces are sprayed on fermenting Sausages to impart flavor and prevent the growth of mycotoxin-producing fungi.

Clearly, the greater the mix of microbes, the better the end product with their sharp, tangy tastes. Color is also the province of the inoculated bacteria. The changes occurring in raw meats are induced by a pride of microbes doing what comes naturally.

Sausages are by far the most widely fermented meat products; whether they are prepared in Argentina, Denmark, Hungary, Italy, The US, Germany, Mexico, Poland, Thailand, or Norway, they use beef, pork, veal, lamb, goat, reindeer or horse, or any combination of meats; or are smoked or unsmoked. The finished product is chopped or ground, mixed with sugar, spices, and seasonings. These comminuted meats are stuffed into a semi-permeable casing to limit contact with oxygen, and heated to kill off both the fermenting organisms as well as any lurking pathogens.

With their different meats, spices, seasonings, and fermenting organisms, German Thuringer is a world of difference from Italian Cappicola, Belgium Ardenner, Argentinian Cervalet, and France's cervallas de Lyon.

The term sausage, comes from the Latin, Salsus, meaning salted. Of course, they had no idea that the compelling tastes and textures were the work of a mix of microbes, which was not known until the 20th century was well underway. As the 20th century aged, it was learned that many of these products were, are, excellent sources of Vitamin C, (Ascorbic Acid), Thiamin, Vitamin B-2, and Niacin, B-3. The 21st century may bring metabolically engineered bacteria that will provide greater acid levels, increased fat and protein metabolizers, and the sausages will only become more delectable.

Fish and Shrimp

Because fish and shrimp can spoil rapidly, fermentation has had a long tradition around the world, as it stops spoilage in its tracks. Fermented fish and fish sauces have been a well-received delicacy for at least two thousand years. Garum, a fermented fish sauce made of tuna intestines and Morray Eel, was a frequent choice around the Iberian peninsula and Mediterranean towns where Garum was in high demand to make otherwise bland food, tasty. One of the major Garum sauce producers of Pompeii, Italy, circa 60-70 ce, made a huge fortune as his Garum was considered top of the line. With the sudden, and total destruction of Pompeii, his recipe was lost forever.

Lactic acid bacteria are the major players, producing antimicrobial lactic and acetic acids, as well as hydrogen peroxide.

Most fermented fish are made from fatty fish and are usually highly salted and fermented until the flesh proteins, fats, and complex sugars are transformed into simpler compounds. During the lengthy fermentations, which can be a year or more, fish muscle can turn into a paste, or become sauce-like. So, for example, Bagoong, a traditional fish paste of the Philippines, is made of either fish or shrimp, as are Vietnam's Nuoc-nam, and Thailand's Nam Prik Nam-pla. All are allowed to ferment for at least a year. Their protein content ranges from 10 to 15 percent, and for many, is their main source of protein. Here too, the Bacillus, and micrococci, along with other salt-loving halophiles predominate in the fermenting products, and the fish or shrimp are no longer raw as the proteins have been denatured by the acids.

On the other hand, as some have been quick to note, the line between a well fermented and preserved fish product, and a spoiled one, with obnoxious odors, can be palpably thin. However, Icelander's, mostly the elderly, enjoy Harkal, a concoction whose microbial content remains to be determined, is a wild fermentation of Greenland shark heads that are buried in the ground for a month or two, cut into strips and hung out to dry. Some say its ammoniacal, fishy odor is the most disgusting and awful thing that anyone would ever want to place in their mouths. But then, there's the Inuit's Igunaq, a wild fermentation of whale meat that takes great courage to even be near. It is usually saved for the winter as the meat contains high levels of vitamins, protein and iron. Nevertheless, people have died from eating over-aged, over fermented, Igunaq. The cause of these deaths has yet to be determined. Then there are the Swedes who come close to winning the prize for the nasal bending odor of their Surströmming, a fermented Baltic herring.

After all, in their natural aquatic environment, fish have their own microbiota in the slime on their surface, in their guts, and in their gills. When they are caught and die, these indigenous, wild-flora begin their proteolytic activity, which can mean the production of horribly smelling amines, residues of proteins. For too many of these fish pastes, sauces and pieces of fermented fish muscle, it is necessary to grow up with these products to be able to get beyond the awesome odors, that, after years, may smell like perfume...to them. Perhaps it's best that few, if any of these products are available beyond their countries borders.

Then again, if you haven't had the good fortune to taste cured Anchovies, a delicacy in Spain, Portugal, and North Africa, there's a lip-smacking gustatory experience waiting for you. The best are those with a high fat content that have been salted under pressure for half-a-year.

Mushrooms

The answer is yes. A very definite yes. We've been eating fungi cooked, uncooked, and/or marinated for a thousand years: those mushroom aficionados among us.

Mushrooms, the edible varieties, of course, are in scientific parlance, fungal fruiting bodies, multicellular reproductive structures that generate spores.

Mushrooms of the genus Agaricus, and species campestris, the common white button fungus, the button mushroom, or field or meadow mushroom, give us flavored protein as well as minerals from the compost they are commercially reared on. The protein content of edible mushrooms based on their dry weight runs as high as 20-25 percent. Hard to beat in a food.

Truffles, Tuber melanosporum, the black truffle, has a puffy cap, from whence cometh its name Tuber, which in Latin means swelling.

It was the renowned French Chef, Jean Anthelme Brillat-Savarin who referred to it as "the diamond in the kitchen." And a French maxim maintains that "your wife, your truffles, and your garden; guard them well from your neighbor." Hey, after all, with their pungent taste, black truffles, tartufo nero in Italian, go for as much as $400 per pound, and white, or winter truffles, tartufo bianco, up the bar to $1,500-2,000, per pound. So, indeed, guard them well. But remember, truffles are not ripe until you can smell them, or more to the point, until a dog or pig can smell them. That's why dogs especially, are almost a necessity when you're out truffle gathering. Pigs are great sniffers of truffles, but they also devour them, so with them it's a losing game.

Shiitake mushrooms, *Lentinula edades*, comes to us from a number of Asian countries, and is the second most cultivated mushroom in the world. It's also referred to as the Golden Oak mushroom, and was originally in demand for its medicinal qualities. Today, its soft, fleshy caps are in great demand for their smokey flavor, which fresh or fried, are often sauteed in vegetarian dishes. These mushrooms have huge potassium and Vitamin D levels, as well as high levels of Vitamin B-9, folate.

Agaricus prunnescens bisporus, the Portobello, can grow half-a-foot wide, is often used as a meat substitute, supplying high levels of Vitamin B-6, pyridoxine.

Chanterelle's, *Cantharellus cibarices,* the vase-shaped, bright yellow to orange mushroom that can't be missed, has a compelling peachy, nutty flavor, and fruity aroma, that brings an extra zest to salads and vegetable dishes.

Not to be dismissed out-of-hand, fungi are central to terrestrial ecosystems, playing a crucial role in decomposition, nutrient cycling and symbiotic relationships with plants and animals. Fungi engineer soils, allowing plants to grow by forming beneficial relationships with tree roots. Many animals dine on mushrooms for their diverse nutrients, and, of course, we all know of the antimicrobial properties possessed by several fungal genera.

After Many a Summer

Arriving in Hollywood in 1937, Aldous Leonard Huxley, the eminent British author of Brave New World, Point Counter Point, and Heaven and Hell, among others, took no time at all to see the cynicism, narcissism, and obsession with youth in American culture. Heavens! Doesn't that describe our country today!? In 1939, he published, After Many a Summer Dies the Swan, a title taken from a figure in Greek mythology to whom Zeus gave eternal life, but not eternal youth. That's the key.

The action in, After Many a Summer, revolves around a Hollywood millionaire in his sixties who fears impending death. To try to increase his life span, he hires Dr. Obispo, who has been researching the lives of animals with exceptionally long life spans, to try to increase his.

Dr. Obispo believes he is on to something as Carp have exceptionally long lives and the microbes in their gut may be the answer. He wonders if the fact that we eat cooked Carp loses the possible benefits the microbes may provide. He also wondered if the intestinal flora of a Carp could be transferred to a mammal-a human, with similar life extending possibilities. Huxley thought that preposterous and sardonic. At the time he was right. But time changes things.

Going to England, Dr. Obispo and his millionaire patron learn that the Fifth Earl of Gonster, is still alive after two hundred years. Apparently the Earl had managed to eat, after great revulsion, the raw guts of Carp daily. As time passed, he became healthier and more vigorous. However, when they saw him, two hundred-plus years on, behind a barred door, deep down in the mansion's cellar, the Earl was shrunken and covered with hair, a lá our primate cousins. Of course this was Huxley at his cleverest. But that was 1937, seventy-seven years ago. Much has been learned since then, including genetic manipulation.

If gut microbes are the basis for longevity, they might just work for us. I was titillated by the idea when I recently re-read After Many a Summer. However, I was also reminded of St. Augustine of Hippo's (354-430, ce) pithy request: "Make me chaste oh, Lord, but not quite yet." Not quite yet, is a normal human response, and more than likely the hope of millions not ready to slip into the long dark night. That microbes may hold the answer may be coming into focus. But what about eternal youth? Will that be part of the package?

Ashes to Ashes

Municipal sewage, household and industrial waste water require treatment before discharge into rivers and oceans. Waste water treatment plants provide the primary, secondary and tertiary treatments that will polish waste streams to drinking water quality.

The usual first step is referred to as physical or primary treatment that screens out large, floating objects, particulates, along with precipitation of smaller insoluble particles, and finally, the settling of fine solids in tanks or basins. This collection of final sludge, as it is called, is dried and removed for use as fertilizer or landfills, as it has a high level of nitrogen and other nutrients. The liquid now moves on for secondary treatment that is a microbial process in which a mix of bacteria combine to digest the soluble organics in the waste water.

Trickling filters or activated sludge plants, are called "activated" as a consequence of their microbial activity, where Zooglea, filamentous Nocardia, pseudamonads, Flavobacters and Methanogens breakdown the organics, generating methane in quantities that can be recovered for fuel.

At this point, what was waste water is no longer so, and goes onto tertiary treatment for final purification, by chlorination and/or activated carbon filtration, prior to discharge into a flowing river or ocean. However, because of its added expense, tertiary treatment may be limited to areas where discharge of secondary effluents could upset the ecological balance of lakes or wetlands.

The take away message here is that the action of microbes converts human waste into safe drinking water, which is a mighty plus. Given the onset of global warming, climate change, many areas of our country will be sorely pressed to provide clean, drinkable water, as their normal water supplies will be severely diminished. Microbially polished waste water will be critical to their survival.

Quite obviously our lives would be unlivable without the great diversity of microbes working for us 24/7 in so many beneficial ways.

As this chapter flows to the next, we must sing the praises and applaud the work of Dr. Daniel P. Molloy, of the New York State Museum, Albany, New York, who recently discovered the bacterium *Pseudamonas fluorescens* CL145A in lake mud, that kills Zebra and Quagga mussels, two uninvited, destructive pests.

Pseudamonas fluorescens is a common rod-shaped, non-pathogenic bacterium inhabiting soil, water, plant surfaces and roots. But there are so many strains of this organism that it took Dr. Molloy and his team years to discover CL145A.

With its arrival in the US in the 1990's, the striped Zebra mussel, no bigger than a thumbnail, and with no predators, simply took over lakes and water intake pipes, blocking water flow into power plants and homes. This tiny critter, along with its cousin the Quagga, both of the genus Dreissena, have hairs projecting from one end of their shells. It's these hairs that no other mussels have, that allow the Zebras to literally glue themselves to surfaces: any surfaces. Rocks, docks, pipes, ships and clams are fair game. These minuscule marauders can clog three-foot diameter pipes. Clams with dozens of Zebras attached become an easy meal. And with their unimaginable fecundity, their tremendous numbers gobble up plant and animal marine life, leaving little for the fish. With their voracious appetites, lake water becomes clear; so transparent that sunlight can penetrate to the bottom exploding the growth of marine plants, clogging lakes. The ecological distortions are unsustainable! And these insidious invaders had escaped all attempts to eliminate or control their numbers until Molloy and his team uncovered his Pseudamonas.

The next step was to work with Marrone BioInnovations, a pest management company, in Davis, California, to pursue a biological solution, rather than a chemical one, for controlling these pests. Over several years he was instrumental in developing Zequanox (Ze for Zebra, and qua, for Quagga) an environmentally friendly formulation of dead pseudamonads that carries a toxin into the mussels destroying their digestive systems, but does no harm to fish, shrimp or other species.

With large-scale field tests successfully done, and with a 90 to 95 percent kill rate, the next test will be in open water. How to spread Zequanox so that it continues killing these dreadful mussels, but isn't so costly to be prohibitive, is the challenge.

With Dr. Molloy's years of experience in pest management there is every reason to believe success is only a short way away.[35]

Moreover, it's evident that microbes are with us every step of the way, filling every need. Chapter SEVEN makes that clearer still.

SEVEN

Lots More Good Guys

"The capacity of life to master even the most inhospitable environments is remarkable." – Theo. Dobzhansky, *Evolution, Genetics and Man. 1965*

We begin with the biogeochemical cycles of life.

That microbes are everywhere, from the clouds, to the deepest ocean floors; from boiling hot springs to acid mine drainage, brings us to the realization that microbes are also the engines driving the earths phenomenal and invisible biogeochemical carbon, nitrogen and sulfur cycles, along with, photosynthesis. Each requires a modicum of elucidation, as together they make all life possible.

Life is based on the carbon atom. All living things are composed of carbon-containing biochemicals. Life as we know it could not exist without them. The major source of carbon for all living things is our atmosphere, and the principle way carbon moves from that sphere to our living biosphere is via the carbon cycle and its handmaiden, photosynthesis.

Without our nitrogen-fixing microbes, there would be no human or animal life on earth as nitrogen gas in our air, an inert and highly stable gas, 78 percent of the air we breathe, is unavailable to us oxygen breathers. As we must have nitrogen to make the protein we require, it remains for our indigenous nitrogen-using microbes to convert nitrogen gas (N_2) to forms we can use for growth and development.

Furthermore, our proteins need sulfur and the only way for sulfur to be incorporated into proteins is for it to become part of amino acids. Our sulfur bacteria perform this function admirably.

Simply put, microbial activity is the driving force for cycling these elements that make our lives possible.

The earth is a closed system with limited amounts of carbon, nitrogen and sulfur. Microbes have that rare ability to transform C, N, and S to the chemical compounds we can use. By no means are these transformations haphazard. It doesn't just happen.

It's precisely driven by our friends and co-inhabitants cycling the three simultaneously, endlessly, forever. However, our recent intrusion into these cycles is producing unwholesome disturbances, consequences, which requires additional commentary, a bit further on.

We now consider each of these cycles, beginning with carbon. Carbon, the fourth most abundant element exists in our atmosphere primarily as the gas carbon dioxide.

The carbon atoms in the atmosphere and in our bodies have been circulating since the earth cooled; microbes, the first forms of life developed, and humans came down from the trees. Ergo, carbon has been cycling and re-cycling for billions of years. How does it work? Two ways: plants and photosynthetic microbes.

Green is the color of photosynthesis, and through photosynthesis, plants, grasses, and trees absorb and convert carbon dioxide in combination with, water and the sun's energy into sugars, starches and cellulose.

In the early years of the 17th century, naturalists believed that plants derived their nutrients, and hence their growth, from the soil–a not unreasonable concept given the location of the roots. In a simple but elegant experiment, a Flemish physician, Jan Baptista van Helmont, (1577-1644) sank that notion. He planted a five pound willow tree in a box containing 200 pounds of oven-dried soil. After five years on a diet limited to rainwater as needed, the tree had gained 164 pounds and the soil was 2.2 ounces shy of its original 200 pounds. Given that water was the only substance added, van Helmont could hardly be faulted for concluding that it was the water, not the soil, from which the tree drew sustenance. Of course he was mostly wrong, but not totally. Minerals in the soil, conveyed by water to the roots, play a vital role. It would take another 300 hundred years before scientists demonstrated that the primary plant nutrient was inorganic carbon dioxide, which plants obtain from the air, and is the essence of photosynthesis, on which most life on earth depends. Carbon dioxide is probably the earth's most important element. Without it, most living things would die. Plants could not produce more of themselves, and without plants, animals and insects and other species along the food chain would perish with them. Without plants and animals there'd be no us. Ergo, the importance of carbon dioxide and its precursor elemental carbon, simply cannot be overstated.

In its most elemental form, the process of photosynthesis can be stated as, carbon dioxide plus water yields a sugar plus oxygen which means that the inorganic gas carbon dioxide, together with water, produces an organic compound:in this instance the six-carbon sugar glucose and oxygen. Its simplicity raises more questions than it answers. An improved statement would be that sunlight plus CO_2 and H_2O yield glucose plus oxygen plus heat energy. Indeed, light energy must drive the chemical reaction. But this too, is far from satisfying for plant biochemists. For them, a fifteen-step chemical transformation occurs that ultimately results in the sugars, starches cellulose and oxygen. Simple it's not.

Along with the obvious importance of CO_2, it is essential to recall that oxygen, the stuff we breathe, without which there'd be no life for us, is another vital product of photosynthesis, which by the way, means "joining together with light"-a complex set of chemical reactions that produces food for all.

The certainty of plants exhuding invisible oxygen can be made visible and certain by submerging plants in water and observing oxygen-rich bubbles floating off the leaves.

The remarkable photosynthetic process is constantly occurring within plant leaves, where cells containing chloroplasts, harbor chlorophyll, a green pigment. The leaf, acting as a solar collector shunts light to the chlorophyll where it reacts with CO_2 that enter the stomata via tiny holes. During the day, stomata open in response to solar radiation. Although we see sunlight as white light, it's a blend of six colors: red, orange, yellow, green, blue and violet. Chlorophyll absorbs red, orange and blue, allowing only the green to reflect, which is why all plants appear green.

Photosynthesis produces biomass, vegetation, food for animals and us. We humans and animals eat the plants, produce waste that ends up on the ground or in waterways where it is degraded by microbes that release CO_2 into the air and the cycle goes round and round forever.

We humans and animals also respire: taking in oxygen for our cells, and exhaling waste carbon dioxide. And of course, CO_2 is the end product of the burning of all organic matter–oil, coal, wood, and food waste. It does add up. No, it multiplies: especially as population increases along with commerce and industry, with their huge fleets of cars, trucks, busses, planes, and trains adding immense tonnages of CO_2 from burning gasoline and oil. Add to these the towering office buildings, hotels, restaurants, homes, supermarkets, sport venues, houses of worship, libraries, museums, and schools, all pouring tons of carbon dioxide daily into the atmosphere. In fact, fourty-four percent of our greenhouse gas emissions come from transportation and buildings. Our colleges and universities are especially culpable consumers of monumental kilowatts of electricity, as students lug bevies of electricity consuming devices to their dorm rooms, ratcheting up the level of CO_2 beyond anything since the last ice age. These are the same people who rail feverishly against the oil and coal producers who they rightly see as prime producers of carbon dioxide, and with it, climate change. But they too, are calling the kettle black.

The CO_2 level in our atmosphere has doubled from its 200 parts per million after the last ice age to over 400 ppm's currently. More about that further on.

All plants use one of three metabolic pathways to produce their carbohydrates and cellulose. Photosynthetically, plants are classified as C^3, C^4, and CAM. For those interested in the details, the enzyme ribulose diphosphate carboxylase catalyzes the insertion of CO_2 into the metabolic pathway early in the process to form the three-carbon compound 3-phosphoglycerate, hence the designation C^3 for all those plants-crops-that use this pathway to carbohydrate and biomass formation. Included here are wheat, barley, rice, soybeans, alfalfa, cassava, cotton, potatoes, sweet potatoes, rye, oats, sugar beets, tomatoes, bananas, oranges, grapes, mangoes, onions, eggplant watermelon, cucumbers, carrots, and all trees, and many others.

Another smaller group inserts CO_2 into a metabolic pathway via the enzyme phosphoenolpyruvate (PEP), which yields the four-carbon intermediate oxalacetate: thus the designation C^4. Corn, sorghum, millet, and sugar cane are members of this specialized group.

CAM, or crassulacean acid metabolism, is limited to desert plants, succulents such as cactus and agave that have evolved in arid conditions. They have adapted to extremely low moisture levels by being able to keep their stomata closed in the hot, dry daytime when water loss would normally be great. Their stomata open at night, taking in CO_2 when it's cooler. It's often referred to as "working the night shift." Of the major plant crops, only pineapple follows the CAM pathway. CAM is named after the plant family Crassulaceae, to which the Jade plant, Crassula ovata, belongs. Some Orchids and Bromeliads are also members. The importance of the C^3 and C^4 response to CO_2 enrichment underlines the current concern for world food supplies.

I use enrichment here rather than excess, as it is not certain that climate change, which has already kicked in, and is a vexing addition to the carbon cycle, will have a negative or positive effect on growth of food crops equally the world over.

This brings us to the oceans of the world with their Brobdingnabian concentrations of microbes, but especially the colossal numbers of photosynthetic microbes that convert sunlight energy to organic compounds that play key roles in those multi-step chemical reactions producing more microbial cells and biomass that feed fish, seafood, and we humans, while sending large amounts of oxygen into our air, and storing great amounts of carbon that would otherwise rise into the atmosphere. Indeed, the oceans of the world are carbon sinks. Let us hope they don't give up their carbon.

In the world's seas, Cyanobacteria, also known as blue-green bacteria, along with Prochlorococcus and green algae, are the primary photosynthesizers.

The Cyanobacters reside in the photic zone, from the surface down to some 300-plus feet, the region reached by sunlight. Not only are they the oldest forms of life on earth, encompassing 3.5 billion years to be somewhat exact, but the chloroplasts land plants use for their photosynthetic activities, were once Cyanobacters. That's similar to the fact that the mitochondria in our cells were also microbes in the long ago. These Cyanobacters obtain their energy by capturing sunlight

via phycocyanin a bluish pigment, and chlorophyll;
the same chlorophyll land plants use.They take in hugh
amounts of CO_2 from air and store immense amounts of
carbon.

Cyanobacters are among the most successful and
diverse forms of life on earth and not just microbial. First
discovered in 1988, by Sallie W. Chisholm, of MIT's
Department of Civil and Environmental Engineering, she
found more than a hundred million of these tiny creatures
in a liter of seawater.[1] Doubtless they are the most
abundant photosynthetic organisms on earth, accounting
for more than sixty percent of all the oceans chlorophyll,
and are the oceans primary producers, responsible for at
least fifty percent of the oxygen we breathe. For that
alone they are deserving of a hearty round of applause.
Without them we would not be breathing, and you know
what that means. Is it any wonder that it is considered the
most important microbe most of us have never heard of?
By the way, Prochlorococcus, a Cyanobactrerium,
means, "Little round progenitors of chloroplasts." After
Prof. Chisholm named this miniscule creature, she had
second thoughts—believing she could have done better.
Any suggestions? Imagine! These critters produce life
from sunlight, water and the CO_2 in air. In doing so, they
control the biogeochemistry and productivity of the
oceans, which drives atmospheric chemistry, contributing
substaintially to global photosynthesis.[2] Not only
remarkable dynamics, but consider that we're dealing
with microbes. Dwell upon that. Our world is controlled
by microbes. Is that understood!? That has to be mind-
blowing. It means microbes do rule!

Between Prochlorococcus, and the larger
Cyanobacteria, over fifty percent of the photosynthesis
occurring on our planet is their doing. Clearly, they are
doing the heavy lifting. Of course they are prominent
players in the Carbon cycle and climate stability—
as small as they are!

As we humans have insinuated ourselves directly
into the carbon cycle with the potential to destabilize our

planet's climate, it is incumbent upon us to consider the possibility of global warming, or climate change.

Climate change is the preferred idea among climate scientists as changes in climate are expected to affect different parts of the world differently. Some regions will be hit harder than others. Some, as we shall see, will even profit. Therefore, global warming does not mean that the troubling changes increased CO_2 and temperature must bring will occur equally over the planet.

Why then, is there such pyrexic concern about excessive levels of carbon dioxide building in the atmosphere? Let's have a look.

Some three hundred miles above the earth's surface, a blanket of gases girdles the earth; a veritable protective cocoon. This gaseous cloak, consisting of water vapor, CO_2, methane (CH_4), nitrous oxide (N_2O), chloroflurocarbons (CFC's), and ozone (O_3), are the so-called greenhouse gases that trap heat in the atmosphere.

Global warming, or climate change, refers to the rise in global temperature near the earth's surface caused by increasing concentrations of these greenhouse gases. (GHG's)

It works this way. As light waves from the sun, transparent white light, pass into the atmosphere, a portion is scattered as the waves bounce off molecules of air, water, and dust. Another portion is scattered and re-reflected by clouds, and a substantial portion reaches the earth, striking everything in its path—trees, homes, people, animals, cars, lakes and hills—to be absorbed and reflected, depending on the type of surface. Much of this short-wave radiation is transformed by the cool earth into the longer wave infrared, which is reflected back into the atmosphere striking the greenhouse gases that are both strong infrared absorbers and emitters.

These GHG's then re-reflect a portion of this heat energy back to earth, while another portion of this infrared energy continues on through the GHG's into outer space where it dissipates. This reflection and re-reflection has maintained our planet's balmy, comfortable, and stable average temperature at 15°C (59°F) for the 10-12 thousand years since the last ice age.

Over the past six decades, inordinate amounts of CO_2, CH_4, N_2O, CFC's and water vapor have been added to the greenhouse that the window allowing IR energy, heat, to pass through, has been closing, meaning that rather than escaping into outer space, the IR continues to be absorbed by the ever increasing number of greenhouse molecules, which bounces heat back to earth, warming it beyond its clement 59°F. That's the issue, and it's continuing and increasing. The evidence is on the ground, around us.

It's essential to understand that the natural "greenhouse" effect is, was, a highly salutary condition found only on planet earth. Rather than a greenhouse, Venus is a hot house, a very hot house, and Mars is a veritable icehouse. We are, unfortunately, on the way to upending the delicate balance that has served us so well over these 10-12 thousand years.

During the 19th century the level of CO_2 in the atmosphere was about 200-220 parts per million- (.002%). By 1950, it was pushing 280 ppm's. Currently, it is a very worrisome 405, and rising by one percent per year. Some areas of the earth get more heat than others, causing as we see in our west and southwest, drought and blazing fires. Other areas are getting torrential rains flooding, and sea level rises as glaciers melt.

On a more subtle level, here is a cautionary tale The New York Times offered its readers in October 2013.

"Moose are dying off across North America for a number of reasons, most of which can be linked to a warming climate and an eroding winter. Long, warm autumns and early, wet springs benefit winter ticks, which can cluster on moose in unbelievable numbers, causing anemia, loss of appetite, hair loss from rubbing—weakening the animals at the onset of winter, just when they need their strength most."

In the upper Midwest, moose are at risk from liver fluke, a parasitic disease, and brain worm, which can afflict the nervous system. In British Columbia, they have lost protective cover thanks to the die-back of white pine forests caused by an epidemic of pine bark beetles. The epidemic, largely attributed to climate change, has also robbed grizzly bears of the seeds they depend on for winter food.

The collapse in moose numbers–one Minnesota population has fallen from 4,000 animals to fewer than 100–is something scientists can track but otherwise can do nothing about. It is typical of the kind of shifts that a warming climate is causing, tipping the balance in ways that favor some species and do grievous harm to others. It is the sign of an entire ecosystem caught up in changes largely brought about by human activity."

Such disruptions have been documented in many areas. As for example, the Polar bears in the arctic, that are on the verge of extinction as their food supply vanishes.

Temperatures may rise three to five degrees by the end of the 21st century, and with that sea levels are expected to rise three to five feet, which will inundate many coastal areas, dislocating literally millions of people, with the profound problems that will bring. The general perception is that climate change is most serious at the poles, in the arctic and antarctic,but a new analysis indicates that the greatest risks to human society may actually be in the tropics, and will take hold by 2047, if not sooner, if emissions continue at their present pace.

Given the fact that there is yet no decrease in burning fossil fuels, additional greenhouse gasses will continue to be trapped in the atmosphere and bounced back to earth, continuing the excessive warming. We may even see a tripling or quadrupling of CO_2 levels before necessity stares us in the face. We humans dislike change; which means little will be done to alleviate this warming before it's too late. Curiously enough, warming may bring benefits. With more sunlight C^4 plants will grow faster than $C^{3'}$s, so that corn should produce higher per acre yields. As should sugar cane. Both should tolerate drought better than many $C^{3'}$s. But rising temperatures and rising carbon dioxide have different effects. Wheat and rice, both $C^{3'}$s are expected to fare far better than $C^{4'}$s in a high CO_2 world. Interestingly, weeds are primarily $C^{4'}$s. With rising CO_2, the many C^3 crops would outgrow the weeds, which would keep farmers happy. But corn farmers based primarily in the droughty Midwest, may well suffer from lack of water. The predicted benefits may be more ephemeral than real. On the other hand, with the new re-combinant genetics readily available, C^4 corn and sugar cane would get a huge boost in yield by the addition of C^3 genes to their genomes. But these are all in the realm of great expectations. How it will all play out is a wait and see. Fortunately, or unfortunately, too few of us will be around to see how it turns out. Nevertheless, unintended consequences may just come back to haunt our children and grandchildren.

Yet another aspect of this warming conundrum is the unvarnished fact that our political officials (I had used the word leaders, but the lamentable lack of leadership, suggests officials is appropriate), whose terms of office are two, four and six years, could care less about what is predicted to occur 20, 30 years down the line. That's another reason there is so little action to reverse the trend. Dwell upon that also.

As 2013 was reaching its demise, a frontpage article in the New York Times shouted, "Climate Change Seen Posing Risk to Food Supplies."[3] An IPCC (Intergovernmental Panel on Climate Change) scientific panel had indicated that food output could drop two-percent each decade for the remainder of the 21st century as demand rises. Demand could easily rise 14 percent per decade, as population rises to over nine billion by 2050, from our current seven billion.

A portion of the fifth major UN report on climate change was published in September 2013. The final document arrived in June 2014, dealing with possible ways to mitigate the rise of greenhouse gasses. Hope does spring.

The Nitrogen Cycle

Closely related to the carbon cycle, and a contributor to it, is the nitrogen cycle, which transforms nitrogen gas, (N_2), in the atmosphere to usable forms of nitrogen. This inert, highly stable gas is converted from its inorganic form to a useful organic compound. Nitrogen exists in the air to the tune of approximately 78 percent, but we oxygen inhalers cannot use it, but must have nitrogen for our amino acids and proteins. So, how do we get it?

Nitrogen gas cannot be used by our body's cells until it is converted by nitrogen-fixing microbes, which play a major role in the nitrogen cycle and our lives.

The nitrogen cycle is a four-step process that includes fixation, nitrification, ammonification, and denitrification.

Nitrogen is a natural by-product of waste: dead organic matter–plants, animals and us, along with all the organic waste we create. This, of course, provides nutrients for plant growth and is a core building block for amino acids and on to proteins.

Plants require more nitrogen than any other nutrient. But plants can only take in nitrogen as inorganic nitrate or ammonium ions (NH_4). However, most nitrogen in soil is bound to organic molecules from the decayed plant and animal tissue. The release of this organically bound nitrogen is referred to as ammonification, also called deamination, the degrading of amino acids, in which the nitrogen containing molecule (NH_2) is removed by bacteria as they produce ammonia, hence, ammonification. But let's back up a moment.

Nitrogen gas must be converted by nitrogen-fixing microbes, before our cells can use it. To break the strong triple bond between the two nitrogen atoms that constitute the nitrogen molecule, requires a great deal of energy. But it must be split if it is to be "fixed," converted, to a useable nitrogenous compound. Only a few brave bacteria can take on and accomplish this formidable breakup. It remained for Martinius Willem Beijerinck, another clever soul from Delft, Holland, to discover the microbial nitrogen fixers, in 1888. Who were the nitrogen fixers? Beggiatoa, Azotobacter, Rhizobium, and of course, Biejerinckia, are among the most notable. These soil microorganisms have an enzyme, nitrogenase, that has the ability to crack the triple bond and "fixes" the nitrogen atoms by adding hydrogen atoms to each of the nitrogen atoms, producing ammonia (NH_3), which is taken up by plants for the production of biomass.

This is followed by nitrification, a two-step process in which nitrosomonas bacteria convert the ammonia to nitrite (NO_2), which is then converted to nitrate (NO_3) that adds a third oxygen atom to nitrite. Plants and microbes in the soil readily use nitrate as their source of nitrogen by converting it back to ammonia, a conversion performed in plant root nodules: large, bump-like knots on roots that can often be as large as grapes or apricots. It is here in the root nodules that amino acids and proteins are made, producing the plant biomass we and animals need. In the process, the plants provide the microbes with the sugars they need for their energy. It's a win/win cycle. It is essential that the ammonia be converted to nitrates as nitrites are toxic for plants. And nitrate must be converted to ammonia before it can be converted to an organic compound. Groups of specialized microbes orchestrate these conversions symphony-like, season after season, forever.

Ammonification, is the scheme in which organic nitrogen compounds from decomposed plants, animals and us, are returned to the soil and converted to ammonia, by yet another clutch of microbes, the Geobacters, Clostridia, and Desulfovibrios.

Denitification, the final step in the cycle reverses the process. The denitrifying organisms, *Pseudamonas denitrificans*, *Thiobacillus denitrificans*, Bacillus, and Micrococci in alkaline soils, and fungi in acid soils, convert ammonia to nitrates and nitrites, along with the liberation of N_2O, nitrous oxide, a potent greenhouse gas, as well as elemental nitrogen gas, back to the atmosphere, completing the nitrogen cycle.

To sum up, microbes in soil assimilate airborne nitrogen gas, fixing it, and moving it through several biochemical reactions, producing biomass, then returning gaseous nitrogen to the atmosphere, completing and continuing the cycle.

In this cycle, plants grow, providing us with the food, the nitrogen we require for our amino acids, protein and vitamins. The diverse microbes make for the smooth transition of one form of nitrogen to another. Without these many microbial types, grazing animals would have no food—no food for them—no steaks, no milk, and no cheese for us. No plants, no veggies. It's complex, but straight forward: the nitrogen cycle is nothing less than vital for our well being, which translates to microbes being essential players for life on this planet.

Here too, we humans have jolted the nitrogen cycle by contributing unprecedented amounts of nitrogen to the biosphere by burning fossil fuels and using monumental tonnages of nitrogen fertilizers on farms, fields, and gardens around the globe. Denitrification, the re-conversion of nitrates back to nitrogen gas, also produces immense levels of nitrous oxide, which is no laughing matter as you now know that it's a greenhouse gas, a strong absorber of CO_2 as well as an anesthetic used by dentists. Consequently, although not given the media attention devoted to CO_2, the nitrogen cycle is being knocked off kilter, with consequences yet to unfold.

The Sulfur Cycle

We now consider the sulfur cycle, an element of paramount importance for animal, plant and human life. Sulfur is a vital component of amino acids, proteins and vitamins, and sulfur bacteria are the prime movers of the sulfur cycle. And here again, we get our sulfur from the plants and animals we consume.

Sulfur is a major component of three essential amino acids; methionine, cystine, and cysteine, and is an essential part of glutathionine, a peptide, necessary for a number of biochemical reactions and several coenzymes. A coenzyme is a protein with a non-protein attachment usually a vitamin, that act as catalysts for biochemical reactions.

Volcanic eruptions, hot sulfur springs, and combustion of coal and oil emit elemental sulfur that rapidly combines with, atmospheric moisture forming hydrogen sulfide (H_2S), the inorganic chemical we associate with the odor of hard-boiled eggs. The burning of coal and oil with, their sulfur contaminates releases sulfates and sulfuric acid into the air.

In soil, sulfide is converted to sulfur dioxide (SO_2) and converted again to sulfate (SO_4) by the Thiobacilli and Beggiatoa, an environmentally friendly microbial/chemical transformation as it removes the sulfide which can be toxic to both plants and other bacteria. When H_2S meets up with Thiobacillus thiooxidans in an oxygen-rich environment, it dines on sulfide converting it to sulfate in an acidic environment. In its sulfate form, plant roots assimilate sulfate forming biomass in the form of amino acids and proteins, carbohydrates and cellulose.

The cycle is completed when the green and purple sulfur bacteria along with the Desulfovibrios reconvert sulfur to sulfate and sulfide gas, which enters the atmosphere, and round and round it goes.

The sulfur cycle is no exception to our meddling and disturbance of the cycle. Acid rain is the consequence of sending immense quantities of sulfur dioxide into the atmosphere via coal and oil-fired power plants, metal smelters and burning coal and oil to heat our homes. Of course this is being done the world over which makes us all culpable. The sulfur dioxide is converted to sulfate, a negatively charged ion that attracts positively charged hydrogen, calcium and/or ammonium ions which combine with water vapor to form the sulfuric acid of acid rain. Add to this acid mine drainage, the result of mining coal and metals, as well as road building. *Thibacillus ferrooxidans* loves mine-drainage environments and diet, as it can grow at a pH of 1!

Mine drainage and road building expose large quantities of sulfides (H_2S and F_eS_2, hydrogen and iron sulfides) to atmospheric oxygen, which results in the sulfides being converted to sulfates and again to sulfuric acid.

Indeed, we do have to live, but we need to do a better job of housekeeping. Of course we can. We just haven't given it much thought. We've been leaving it to the coal and oil producers who only exacerbate the problem, as housekeeping has been of little to none of their concern. Lately, however, coal processors have begun using sulfur-oxidizing bacteria to remove sulfur from coal to reduce the formation of sulfuric acid when coal is burned, preventing the production of acid rain. It's a welcome beginning, but only a beginning.

The importance of our microbes in biodegradation and biogeoengineering lies in the adage that " there is no known natural compound that cannot be degraded by some microorganism." The proof of that is that we aren't up to our noses in whatever it is that couldn't be degraded in the last 3.5 billion years." I suspect few of us have ever thought about that.

If there are any lingering doubts about the central and controlling role of microbes in our lives, our existence, they should be expunged, given the news, the revelation about to be dispensed: microbes have not only been found alive and kicking in the upper atmosphere where it had been accepted dogma that the region was devoid of microbes. Sterile. It is now well documented that microbes are responsible for clouds, rain and snow. How does that grab you?

Clouds, Rain and Snow

Prof. David J. Smith, of the University of Washington, Seattle, wants us to know that there was wide awareness of airborne microbes as people took advantage of wild airborne yeasts to obtain lighter, more desirable bread, as far back as ancient Egypt, by leaving a mixture of grain and liquids near an open window. And of course we know about Prof. Louis Pasteur's Swan-necked flask experiments finally disproving spontaneous generation, demonstrating undeniably the existence of microbes in the air around us. Furthermore, in 1862, he discovered the presence of microbes in air several hundred feet above sea level.

Since then scientists have been trying to determine if they were actively or passively involved, at the higher altitudes.

Although the rains in Spain are mostly in the plains, rains wherever they fall, are microbes in action. The sky is teaming with microbes. How do they get there, and how do they cause rain and snow to fall?

All those kids, and lots of adults, flinging snowballs left and right, would be shocked to learn that those snowballs are packed with microbes. Harmless microbes, so keep on throwing.

To produce rain or snow, clouds require microbes–bacteria, fungi, even algae, to serve as condensation nuclei, the 'seeds' around which ice particles or rain drops form: so-called ice nucleators. Water molecules in the atmosphere cluster around these nuclei making them larger and larger. Then, depending upon the temperature, these ice nuclei turn into falling rain or snow. It is now also known that bacteria grow nicely on plant leaves. Gusting winds whisk these organisms off the leaves toting them skyward where they hover in the atmosphere until they become nuclei, the tiny catalysts around which ice forms.

The ability to initiate freezing means that rain and snow-making microbes can induce torrential down pours dispersing themselves worldwide. So, without microbes, clouds would never form because water vapor droplets are far too small to form nuclei. Ergo, without clouds, there'd be no rain, and no snow, which means drought. No growth. And as important, without clouds we'd burn up from the unrelenting heat of the sun. Microbes save us from all that. But for years these microbes were invisible.

It remained for Prof. Brent Christner of the Department of Biological sciences, Louisiana State University, Baton Rouge, to discover and identify rain-making microbes. He collected fresh snow in North America, Europe and Antarctica, and filtered his snow samples, collecting the microbial particulates, while gently lowering the temperatures. Doing this, he found the ice nucleators increased as the temperature dropped to 0°C (32°F). Furthermore, the greater the number of nuclei, the greater the number of microbes.[4] Of the many snow samples obtained, all contained rain-making bacteria.

Prof. Christner wrote that in 1972, Leroy Maki, a microbiologist at the University of Wyoming identified the bacteria on plant leaves as Pseudamonas syringae. And that a year later, Steven Lindow of the University of Wisconsin, identified P.syringae as the bacterium "that actively incited freezing on plants-frost damage."

Interestingly, experiments performed when Dr. Lindow was a graduate student at the University of Wisconsin, found what others had missed:frost can form on plants because of the presence of this harmless bacterium. He engineered a mutant organism that had a single gene deleted. This ice-minus strain, as it came to be known, was no longer capable of producing the ice-nucleation protein, but in all other respects was idential to the naturally occurring Pseudamonas.

Lindow also showed that spraying an experimental field of corn with the antibiotic Streptomycin reduced frost damage. At the time, frost damage was not seen as a microbially induced condition. In fact, the presence of specific bacteria on leaf surfaces fosters ice formation. In the absence of these organisms, water super cools (super cooled water is water cooled below its freezing point, without becoming a solid. It must, however, be free of nucleation sites) but does not freeze when temperatures drop below 0°C. Widespread use of an antibiotic is hardly an environmentally sound practice. The use of an indigenous soil bacterium, however mutated, can be. Strains of P.syringae produce a protein that inhibits formation of ice crystals.

Working with scientists at Advanced Genetic Sciences, Inc., AGS, Prof. Lindow now at the University of California, Berkeley, developed a plant-protective product called Frostban.[5]

AGS conducted field trials of Frostban. The recombinant bacteria were sprayed on strawberry and potato plants, and by the way, those trials were the first ever EPA-authorized release of a recombinant microbe. The tests were successful, demonstrating that Frostban worked by keeping the plants from freezing. Just what was needed.

True to form, environmental hysteria drummed up by Luddite activists, created a public uproar about releasing an altered microbe into the environment, which doomed ice-minus and Frostban. That was a quarter-of-a-century ago in 1987/88. Little appears to have changed.

The beat goes on, as noted in Chapter SIX. The public appears to have learned little, and the scientists remain unconcerned and quiescent in their ivy-covered redoubts, offering no information, no education, to counter the braying mob.

What could be better evidence than ice-nucleating bacteria being independently discovered by scientists at the universities of Wyoming and Wisconsin!? Following that, a half-dozen other bacteria and fungi were found to be ice nucleators. It was also learned that the aerodynamic properties of P.syringae and other organisms allow them to remain suspended in the atmosphere for weeks on end. These airborne microbes provide the structure for water molecules that bind to the microbes and freeze. Growing larger and heavier, then fall to earth as snow.

As Prof. Christner tells it, it was in 1978, that Prof. David Sands of Montana State University, Bozeman, who, flying in a small plane at 7,500 feet, captured ice-plus P.syringae on agar-containing petri dishes he plunged through the open cabin window. Prof. Sands believed that these bacteria could be transported great distances by rain, and was a means whereby they moved to new plants, a process he called bioprecipitation.[6]

In 2005, Christner and Sands began a collaboration and together found that 95 percent of the ice nucleators are biological particles, and that some 40 percent are bacterial. It is now well documented that P.syringae has an active role as ice nuclei in the atmosphere. However, "P.syringae constitutes only a small fraction of the total microflora deposited in precipitation."[4] Nevertheless, P.syringae is the most common nucleator in the heavens. Moreover, and this is quite remarkable, they believe that biological particles may just play a role in the earths water and radiative balance. They also find that literally tens of billions of microbes live on leaves the world over, providing direct evidence of bacterial and fungal involvement in ice-cloud processes. Christner's concluding remarks are farsighted. Listen to him: "We now recognize that the atmosphere plays a fundamental role in dispersing microorganisms, that clouds may support cellular reproduction, and that airborne microbes and their metabolic activities could affect the global climate. Even so, the microbiota of the atmosphere remains a relatively unexplored frontier that appears ripe for further discovery." The microbial role was indeed unfolding.

It appears that we humans have affected rainfall by the radical changes in land use we've made, especially through agricultural practices and forestry that alter the composition of microbes sent into the air. And, as they have a major role in raindrop formation, the land use changes may well affect rainfall around the earth, and climate with it. Time will surely let us know.

To this end, a crack team of international scientists from Germany, Brazil, the US, and India, led by a member of the Max Planck Institute for Chemistry, Mainz, Germany, recently reported that the properties and origin of organic aerosols remain poorly understood, as are their effects on climate.

To try to fill this gap, they went to Brazil's Amazon rain forest where aerosols could be studied free of interference of polluting organic particles. Using specialized microscopy, they found that aerosols are initiated by potassium-salt -rich particles emitted by fungal spores, which act as seeds for the formation of clouds and rain.

Their conclusion is prescient. "In view of the large impact of tropical rain forests on biogeochemistry and climate," they wrote, "the biological activity and diversity of particle-emitting organisms seem likely to play important roles in Earth history and future global change."[7]

Clearly we're only at the cusp of knowing the overarching importance of microbes to our lives and the workings of our planet. Needless to say, other researchers were adding their incremental pieces to the earth-atmosphere jigsaw.

9,068 feet (2,764 meters) above sea level, in Oregon's Cascade range, sits Mount Bachelor, where Prof.David Smith, and his team used that height to sample trans-pacific winds. They're concern was for the potential biological particulates being carried aloft from Asia.They were able to collect sufficient microbial biomass to permit analysis using 16S rRNA genetic methods. They're arrays revealed some 2,800 different bacterial species, including marine organisms that had arrived from China, Korea, and Japan. Perhaps most significant were the numbers of spore-forming organisms that could survive the arduous atmospheric voyage. Here too, microbes are seen to play a role as nuclei for cloud formation and rainfall.[8]

Pierre Amato, atmospheric scientist at the Chemistry Institute, Clermont Ferrand, France, reminds us that" we are in the early stages of thinking about the atmosphere as an extension of the biosphere, in which clouds appear to play an essential role distributing microbial species around the globe." He also raises a critical question, asking, "whether humans are responsible for the eutrophication (the inordinate increase in the rate and concentration of organic matter in the atmosphere usually thought of as occurring primarily in lakes and soils, with the death of these ecosystems over time) of clouds or are rendering them more hostile to microbial growth."[9] Amato also estimates that microbes in clouds metabolize some million tons of organic carbon compounds around the world annually. We also know that yearly around the world hundreds of millions of tons of man-made pollutants rise into the atmosphere. This is not the first time such overloading of the atmosphere has been raised. Others have suggested, as noted earlier, that we have affected rainfall by the radical changes in land use practices and forestry we've made that alter the numbers and types of microbes sent into the air. Up to this point, climate scientists have not appreciated the role of microbes in rain, snow and more than likely, climate. Consequently the United Nations Intergovernmental Panel on Climate Change (IPCC) has not taken atmospheric microbes into account in its calculations and reports, including its most recent, the fifth report, noted earlier.

Perhaps this does convey the centrality of microbes in the grand plan—if there is one—of our lives on the planet.

But there is a bit more.

Led by Professors Athanasios Nenes and Konstantinos Konstantinidis, researchers at the Georgia Institute of Technology, Atlanta, sought to fill a gap in aerobiological understanding by determining the composition and prevalence of microbes in the upper troposphere, 25 to 48 thousand feet, (5-9 miles) above the Caribbean. Hitching rides on NASA's DC-8 planes, in 2010, they collected air samples (with great difficulty) in cloudy, and cloud-free air, before, during and after the two tropical storms, Earl and Karl.

From DNA sequencing of their collection, they found viable bacterial and fungal cells of close to a hundred different genera including Shewanella, Burkholderia, Ralstonia and Methylbacters, with bacteria far out numbering fungi. During the hurricanes new communities of microbes were captured. These were swept into the upper air and were able to metabolize a number of simple carbon compounds, obtaining energy and ensuring their survival at these great heights in the presence of ultraviolet radiation, severe atmospheric dryness and unremitting cold.

The Georgia Institute of Technology scientists maintain that these microbes possess the potential to modify cloud formation, the hydrologic-water-cycle, and climate.[10] Assuredly, the atmosphere is very much alive, and can be transformative, but whether microbes can initiate planetary warming or cooling remains to be determined.

Tina Santi-Temkiv, of the University of Aarhus, Roskilde, Denmark, and her team of international scientists went off to Ljubljana, Slovenia, where there is lots of open space, and no requirement for government approvals to collect precipitation samples on public sites. This Danish team was interested in learning if living microbes would be found in raging storm clouds, and in the solid ice of hailstones.[11]

From 42 large hailstones they found an assortment of microbes. Using DNA sequencing, which has become the new standard for microbial analysis and identification of unculturable organisms, they identified Sphingobacteriales, Methylobacters, Proteobacters, Actinobacters, Bacterioidetes and others–those often found on plant surfaces, leaves, and soil, and the same types found by other researchers in other parts of the world.

The Danes believed these organisms are typical cloud inhabitants. They also agree with other researchers that the violent storms suck up huge amounts of air, bringing these microbes up into the clouds. Furthermore, the moving clouds and storms surely affect the long distance transfer and geographical distribution of microbes around the earth. Several of their bacterial species produced a pinkish pigment that appears to protect them from the strong ultra-violet radiation. They too, ventured the idea that these microbes may be influencing weather patterns.

It does begin to look as though there is growing evidence and agreement among disparate scientists about the role of microbes in the atmosphere. Obviously, as numbers of scientists in different parts of the globe using different procedures, obtain similar results, the findings become incorporated into the fabric of science. Nevertheless, there remains a way to go to firmly pin down the role of microbes in this largely unexplored region. In this instance, climate change is such a potentially transformative possibility, that greater certainty is surely called for. Nontheless, these pioneers have blazed a wide trail for others to pick up and settle the issue.

These atmospheric microbes not only live, but thrive in an extreme environment, which points us in the direction of the extremophiles.

Extremophiles

Extremophiles are microbes capable of flourishing in extreme environments: from burning volcanoes, to acid mines, and the deepest oceans. For the most part our extremophiles take up residence where darkness prevails:in lake and ocean floors, in the depths of hot springs; in dank, dark caves, in the saltiest waters, and hydrothermal vents where they are barely approachable. The uncommon enzymes produced by these curious organisms are extreme from our perspective. We thrive in an oxygen environment with temperatures and pressures favorable to our existence. Many extremophiles thrive with no oxygen and at temperatures and pressures that would kill us off instantly. Actually, they'd die in what we consider normal environments. Moreover, life in uncompromising habitats requires metabolic pathways preventing water loss. For many scientists, the intriguing question is, can whatever it is that serves these extreme creatures be discovered and benefit us? Surely a worthy question and goal.

On planet earth, a wide diversity of conditions can be extreme: acidity, temperature, salinity, pressure, radiation, drought, and anoxia. Additionally, these can range from extreme acidity to extreme alkalinity. From temperatures well below zero, to those of boiling water, and above! Extreme habitats with their living microbes have been found inside active nuclear reactors, and entombed in ten-thousand-year-old ice cores, as well as the dead sea, which is not as dead as widely believed.

With a pH of 2-3, our stomachs are an extreme habitat for acid loving bacteria. Extremophiles such as *Spirocheta americana* enjoys the mud deposits of California's Lake Mono, where a pH of 10 exists. Lake mono is also highly salty and loaded with sulfides. Yet this microbe prospers under this triple threat.

Yellowstone National Park, Wyoming, is a veritable store house of heat-loving microbes, in its thousands of geysers and hot springs whose temperatures are too hot to touch. But microbes flourish there, along with the acidity and high sulfur levels.

Rio Tinto, in Spain, is chuckfull of heavy metals from the mines that have been worked for thousands of years. Iron Mountain in northern California is much the same, with water loaded with heavy metals and mine acids, but that doesn't prevent Ferroplasma acidiphilium from growing and proliferating.[12] It was Dr. Thomas D. Brock of the University of Wisconsin who discovered microbes in Yellowstone's hot springs. Thermus aquaticus was growing at temperatures approaching 212°F (100°C). Interestingly, Thermus aquaticus produced a game-changing enzyme, Taq, now used in the polymerase chain reaction (PCR) that made DNA finger printing readily accessible, and the current basis for identifying unknown organisms, as well as its use in forensic work. Pyrococcus, which grows well at even higher temperatures in deep sea thermal vents, has a polymerase -pfu-that may replace Taq as its greater heat tolerance may yet upgrade the polymerase chain reaction.[13]

In the many areas where salty brine is harvested and evaporated, Caribbean Islands, San Francisco Bay, The Great Salt Lake, Pink Lake in Senegal, the Dead Sea in Israel, the evaporation ponds can blaze with colors— oranges, purples, reds, and pinks, the light gathering and ultra-violet protecting pigments of the halophilic (salt-loving) organisms that flourish in these punishing environments. Here, the salt concentrations spiral upwards of twenty percent, along with high temperatures and high acidity, and the microbes can grow with or without oxygen and also resist drying. Can any other life forms match that bag of tricks?

Moreover, the high salt concentrations are highly selective as no potentially contaminating organisms can possibly grow there; pathogens included. Salinobacter ruber, has adapted itself to live at salt levels as high as thirty-six percent! No respectable cod or herring can match that. Great Salt Lake has its Haloferax volcanii and Halobacterium salinarum, while Halobacterium halobium resides comforably in Owens Lake, California, and Chromohalobacter beijerincki loves salted beans, herring, salted cod, and soy sauce, all highly salted goodies. Tetragenococcus halophilius lives nicely in salted anchovies and soy sauce.

Uyuni Salt flats, Solar de Uyuni, in southwestern Bolivia, are simply the world's largest, encompassing 10-thousand square miles. To top it off, the Flats are way, way up in the clouds, over eleven thousand feet above sea level, near the crest of the Andes. Halophilic bacteria and pink algae thrive in the concentrated mixed chloride brine (sodium, potassium and magnesium). The pink algae, gobbled up by the Flamingos at the Solar, give the birds their delicate pink hues.

At Owens Lake, hard by the Inyo Mountains in Owens Valley, California, the pink *Halobacterium salinarum*, one of the most prominent bacteria, grow nicely in the 20-30 percent salinity. Astronomical numbers of them not only survive but luxuriate in the blistering heat of summer along with, the concentrated brine. Just another example of microbial legerdemain providing the magic, enabling them to alter their protein enzymes and flourish in these onerous environments–that is onerous for us.

Salty, pink lakes are also found in Australia, British Columbia, Spain and Senegal. Lake Ritba, in Senegal, is not just pink, but vivid red. With its salt concentrations of up to forty percent, it is likely the saltiest and reddest in the world. It's the green algae that do it. How's that?

Yes, *Dunaliella salina*, and *Dangeardinella saltitrix* are chameleon-like, being able to shift from green to pinks to fire engine red, depending upon temperature and salt concentrations. These colors are carotenoid pigments, precursors of Vitamin A: the same pigments that color tomatoes, peppers, and pink flamingos. Spirulina, a pink algae, also contributes. These pink algae can color Flamingos with a dazzling display of reddish hues from beaks to webbed toes.

Most telling of all is the fact that these organisms can withstand unimaginable salt levels and severe temperatures, which surely suggests they have the remarkable ability to produce, as needed, proteins to resist these hostile environments. There must be a benefit for us somewhere in there.

On the high alkaline side, at pH's of 9 and 10, Natronomonas pharaomis thrives nicely in the alkaline and salty lakes of Egypt's Sinai peninsula. Not to be overlooked is Lake Untersee, in Antarctica that is so alkaline its pH is that of Chlorox: pH 12.

Acidophiles proliferate at pH's below 5, while alkalophiles like their environments above a pH of 9. These are not just differences between four units. pH's are log numbers, which means there is a factor of 10 between each number of the pH scale. Consequently between 5 and 9, the difference is ten thousand times. 9 is 10-thousand times more alkaline than a pH of 5. Bear that in mind when reading or thinking about pH. Again, a pH of 3 is 100 times more acidic than a pH of 5. High acidity means low pH, another point to remember.

Thermophiles, those heat-loving microbes grow bountifully at temperatures well over 45°C (113°F). Hyperthermophiles appreciate temperatures of 80°C (176°F), others manage favorably at 100°C (212°F), and some even higher.

Methanococcus jannaschii lives near thermal vents 2,600 meters, some eight thousand feet, below sea level where temperatures approach the boiling point of water and pressures are sufficient to crush a submarine. Then there is Pyrolobus, well named, that lives near the punishing environments of "smokers" those hydrothermal vents that can spout water as hot as 350°C (665°F). Pyrolobus wins the prize as the most heat tolerant form of life known. Surely there must be a protein here that could be of inestimable benefit for us. I'm betting on it.

Prof. Karl O. Stetter coined the term hyperthermophiles for those microbes thriving comfortably at near boiling water-207°F-(95°C). It was from one of Iceland's hot mountain lakes that he discovered and identified a new organism, Methanothermus ferridus. He followed that up with the discovery of Pyrococcus furriosus, the rushing fireball, growing at 212°F (100°C) in geothermally heated marine sediments near the beach of Porto di Levante, Vulcano, Sicily. It's an efficient consumer of the organic material found on the heated sea floor. It grows well between 70-103°C, but its optimum is 100°C.[14]

To visualize these organisms it's necessary to heat slides to 90°C, place a drop of hot culture on the slide and quickly observe the organisms at a thousand times magnification using a phase-contrast microscope. Most cellular details are undetectable by the standard light microscope as there is little to no contrast. Phase contrast provides a sharp distinction between specimen and it's background. Moreover, it allows live visualization of specimens. No heat or staining, which kills microbes. So, phase-contrast provides stark contrast between a transparent microbe and a dark background.

Thermotoga maritima, yet another new species, was discovered by Stetter's team in geothermally heated areas of the sea floor off Italy and the Azores. These Thermotoga's grow at temperatures of 55 to 90°C, but their optimum is 80°C (176°F), far too hot to touch.

Prof. Stetter, a German microbiologist, and an acknowledged leader in extremophile studies has opted for sunny California, and is now ensconced in the Department of Microbiology, at UCLA. We are lucky to have him aboard.

Recently a team of marine scientists led by Prof. Ronnie Glud of the University of Aarhus, Denmark, sank their exotic equipment seven miles, or 37 thousand feet below sea level, into the Marianas Trench in the central western Pacific, east of the Mariana Islands, where the pressure is a thousand times greater than at sea level. There in the Challenger Deep, the deepest spot in the Trench, and the deepest oceanic site on earth, where temperatures are at (-2.5°C) (28.3°F), microbes are doing well:evidence that microbes can cope with any environment on earth. They are that versatile in protecting themselves with appropriate proteins.

These organisms, which remain to be identified and characterized, are decomposing organic matter that falls to the Trench floor–organic matter that is not digested by microbes far above those in the Trench. The instruments used by the Danes showed intense microbial activity at the extreme pressure of their habitat. Because of the difficulties in bringing up samples of these organisms without killing them, at the lower pressures, it will be some time before we learn what type of organisms they are.[15]

This discussion of extremophiles must include the Xerophiles, those curious microbes that love dryness and dry places where water is lacking or unavailable. NASA scientists believe that Mars is a natural habitat for Xerophiles and are diligently searching for them. Should they be found on Mars, it would be firm evidence for life on that cold, dry, thought to be lifeless planet. But life without water? That poses vexatious problems for us humans. For microbes, maybe, but for us, Mars doesn't seem inviting. At least not yet.

Here on earth, Xerophiles are the organisms that spoil food, some food: Dry food. They have the enzymes to split organic compounds without the aid of water. Now that's a neat trick. So, stored grain, nuts-cashews and peanuts-, dried pasta, coffee, dried fruits and meats are their preferred meals. They can also degrade salty foods and highly sugary foods such as honey and molasses. It's the Xerophilic molds and yeasts such as Xeromyces bisporus and Trichosporonides nigrescens that can dilute molassēs and honey, which no other microbe would venture near, turning those viscous semi-liquids into runny puddles.

Chrysosporium fastidium and Basipetospora halophilica are colorful green and yellow-pigmented molds that often grow luxuriantly on dry bread.

Here too, the curious enzymes at work could surely be of benefit. Any number of imaginative scientists are sure to pick up on that.

The burning question is, how do the proteins in those heat, acid, salt, pressure, dryness and temperature tolerant microbes maintain their stable proteinaceous condition without curdling a lá fried or boiled eggs?

Evidence indicates that these microbes have evolved, what are referred to as extremoenzymes. How this is managed is not fully understood. Nontheless, its quite obvious that life can thrive under the most challenging conditions. And scientists have identified genes from a diverse number of extremophiles that appear to have desirable commercial and industrial value. So, for example, the pulp and paper industry is testing polymer degrading enzymes active at low temperatures, and the cold-resistant mechanisms of the psychrophiles is being studied by the food processors who need to prevent food spoilage at higher refrigeration temperatures. Thus far we have used laundry detergents that contain enzymes, proteases, amylases, and lipases that work to remove stains at cold temperatures. The halophiles can provide enzymes for detergents to be used in salty water. Heat tolerant enzymes from thermophiles can be used for chemical reactions at higher temperatures reducing the possibility of complications from microbial contamination. Similarly being able to run chemical reactions at higher temperatures provides higher reaction rates.

Not to be outdone, skin care companies are testing extreme enzymes for their ability to protect skin elasticity, prevent dehydration, radiation damage, and aging. Remarkable if possible. Let's hope for successful outcomes.

The future holds great commercial possibilities and benefits for us should those unique enzymes become available. As more is learned about their biochemistry, genetics and physiology, we'll get the benefits of turning this microbial information into practical use.

Those of us of a certain age will recall Ripley's Believe it or NOT!, hard to believe astounding accounts of people, places and phenomena, featured regularly in newspapers.

Bacterial power cords would surely have been one of his remarkable believe it or nots. This one has documented evidence to back it up.

Danish scientists at the University of Aarhus, they surely are busy beavers, discovered filamentous bacteria never before even imagined, in the sediments of the Bay around the Aarhus port. But these filamentous organisms are actually living electric cables! Don't we know, having learned the hard way that water and electricity do not mix! Nonetheless, these thin filamentous creatures were conducting electric current steadily in the sea floor. The Dane's found that a section of these filaments contained bundles of insulated wires that carried the current. Believe it or not, the structure is similar to our conventional electric cables.

These yet unnamed microbes, 100 times thinner than a human hair, function as virtual electric cables.[16] But why? That remains to be determined. They also found that individual cells join end to end forming lengthy cables that extend for centimeters, and form an electric grid—for what purpose?

Tests revealed that these bacteria are members of a family of bacteria referred to as Desulfobulbaceae, but appear to be a newly discovered species. Living electrical cables add a wholly new dimension to our understanding of natural phenomena and may well open an entirely new field of organic electronics. It tests your capacity to be shocked. No pun intended, but it fits nicely. Can you imagine these live electric filamentous cables being implanted in our bodies to charge a system or battery? The future is electrifying with its potential benefits.

The Metallurgists

That microbes are everywhere including the earth's most inhospitable environments, requires that we turn our attention to those wondrous and natural metallurgists that extract minerals in short supply from their ores; doing so without polluting the environment, and helping to make us competitive in world markets.

Microbial metallurgy, or bioleaching, is a process in which specialized microbes extract metals from ores, converting insoluble metals to readily recoverable metals. Leaching is used to recover copper, lead, zinc, gold, silver, nickel, and iron.

Microbes are used because they can lower production costs, extract metals efficiently when its concentration in its ore is low, and leaching causes far less air and water pollution than smelting and roasting. Its far more environmentally friendly.

Bioleaching is a natural process that is being adopted for commercial use, but this process has been going on since time immemorial, long before commerce reared its head.

Rio Tinto, in southwest Spain, near Seville, is considered the birthplace of the copper and Bronze Age. The blood-red river gets its name, Red River, from five thousand years of mining copper, gold, and silver, with dissolving iron that microbes, in this highly acidic (pH 2.3) river have been naturally decomposing, giving it its deep red hue. The Romans were using the available iron over two thousand years ago, and Rio Tinto continues in use today.[12] Early miners there discovered that copper ores washed with its acidic water resulted in the leaching of copper from its ore. No one had a clue that microbes were at work here. The idea that copper could be retrieved was so remarkable that it was believed that one metal could be transformed to another. Could dross be turned to gold? That was the ancient alchemist's dream. And a dream it was, as even microbes as magical as they are, could not accomplish that. Nevertheless, large-scale extractions of copper appears to have begun by the 1750's. Acidithiobacillus ferrooxidans, how's that for a formidable sobriquet, was the first bacterium discovered capable of metabolizing minerals, and thrives at pH levels of 1.5 to 2.5. Acidithiobacillus is the current name of the older Thiobacillus. Several years ago, 16SrRNA sequencing subdivided Thiobacillus, making way for the acidophiles of the genus Thiobacillus. This now also includes *Acithiooxidans,* that have been isolated from hot springs and acid mine drainage, and grow exceedingly well at these inordinately high acid levels. The most interesting aspect is that these organisms grow in biofilms that adhere to the surface of ores.

Biofilms, otherwise known as slime, or the goop your fingernail can pick up as you run it along your teeth, is a matrix of microbes. Microbes attach themselves to surfaces, become immobilized and aggregate forming a biofilm with a defined structure that provides an optimal habitat for the exchange of genetic material between cells. Biofilms can accelerate corrosion rates of metals, and digest ores, freeing their metals.

By seeding waste ore heaps with microbes, specifically Acidithiobacillus, and/or Leptospirillium along with a dollop of dilute acid, these eager eaters munch their way through the ores and as they feast, they produce muscular sulfuric acid. This spicy munching degrades the ores, freeing the desired metals. Biomining, as this is being called, for the microbially associated metal recovery, has two main types: Irrigation, which percolates leaching solutions containing specific microbes through crushed ore that has been stacked in columns, dumps or heaps. As the solution moves through the stacked ore, the microbes digest the ore, and the freed metals are collected at the bottom. In the Stirred Tank Type of biomining, crushed ores are constantly stirred and aerated as leaching solutions drench the ore mass. Free metal is then collected at the bottom of the tanks.[17]

As no other potentially contaminating organisms can grow in the highly acidic, high temperature operations, temperatures up to 70°C (158°F), there is no need for sterile procedures, which cuts the cost of extraction considerably. Rates and efficiency of extraction are far greater here, but the reactors are expensive so they are used only with high-value ores.

The future of biomining appears to be at temperatures of 70°C and above, where the reactions proceed at even more rapid rates and the organisms can still thrive. Current research focuses on identifying new microbes that can do the solubilization at the higher temperatures. As many marine microbiologists believe such organisms are there to be found, this is becoming an exciting and challenging area of research, with the potential for a rash of benefits for all of us.

Additionally, microbes are being used to clean up acid mine drainage, a legacy of still active and old abandoned mines, extracting the needed metal in the process. Desulfovibrio and Desulfotomaculum, two tenacious metallurgists, neutralize acids, creating sulfides that bond to copper, nickel, and zinc, pulling them out of the drainage, making them available for industrial use. That's got to get our microbes a few additional accolades.

Then there is gold, a precious metal, and has been for literally thousands of years. *Delfia acidovorans* converts normally toxic gold ions into harmless gold nanoparticles, forming biofilms on gold grains. For this to occur, the microbe produces a protective peptide, (a peptide is an organic compound consisting of two or more amino acids) delfibactin, which can convert soluble gold to solid gold, and delfibactin precipitates gold from iron ore where it is often found, within gold deposits. Isn't that another plus? Companies dealing in gold ore are interested in using Delfia to both detect and extract gold. A microbe-assisted gold rush may yet occur.

Prof. Frank Reith, an environmental microbiologist at the University of Adelaide, Australia, believes that the bacterium *Cupriavadus metallidurans*, which he discovered a decade ago in biofilms in gold nuggets, could one day be used to collect gold from mine waste. This bacterium detoxifies dissolved gold by accumulating it in inert nanoparticles inside their cells. At this point he and his team don't know how the bacteria do it.[18]

On the other side of the world, Nathan Magarvey a Biochemist at McMaster University, Hamilton, Ontario, Canada, and his group of investigators found Delfia acidovorans growing in the presence of a gold solution and discovered that the bacterial colonies were surrounded by dark halos of gold nanoparticles. They concluded that their bacterium was creating gold particles outside its cell wall: totally different than what C. metallidurans does. Prof. Magarvey believes the genes his team identified produce delfibactin and shunts it outside its cell. By precipitating gold, D.acidivorans appears to prevent the metal from entering its cells in solution.[19]

Both Profs. Reith and Magarvey believe their findings complement one another's. It may be that their two organisms have a symbiotic relationship with D.acidovorans using delfibactin to reduce the soluble gold to levels both organisms can cope with.

A year or two down this golden road, these two researchers may well have worked out their organisms modus vivendi, and put their bacteria to work piling up gold that has been lying about. With the price of gold as high as it currently is, these two teams could easily turn the academic world on its head, becoming fat cats.

One thing is certain, as should be evident by the diversity of reports described, creative and imaginative scientists around the world are working for the betterment of humankind. But it's the microbes, masters at making complex molecules that hold "the keys to the kingdom," as they can provide just about anything we want. They are that versatile, remarkably diverse, and generously cooperative. Moreover, our microbes can be readily coaxed into giving up their secrets for our benefit. That's why it's essential to support those scientists, allowing them to continue discovering new microbes in the most unlikeliest of places.

Approaching the terminus of this multifaceted rendering of our atypical microbial universe, there remain problems in need of attention and solution.

So, for example, dust! As in desert dust, dust storms, and the dust churned up by off-road vehicles. This, along with the onslaught of climate change in the already drought-challenged western and southwestern states, will further reduce soil crust formation and growth of essential grasses, which help hold soil grains together. Dr. Jayne Belnap predicts that by 2050, the fragility of the southwest region will be equal to that of dust bowl days.

Actually, it's the soil microbes that stabilize soil, producing the sticky, gooey stuff that holds water and soil grains together, keeping soil moist in arid areas. That gooey stuff, a kind of starch, holds nutrients as well, keeping them from leaching out. It's the Cyanobacters we can thank for initiating plant growth and keeping soil from blowing in the wind: especially Microcoleus vaginatas, filamentous organisms whose long, sticky hair-like structures bind soil particles. These Cyanobacters are also nitrogen fixers that add nutrients to nutrient-poor desert soils. They work together with fungi and green algae to do the job.

Unfortunately, cattle, off-road vehicles, bikers, drought and the titanic-sized energy-exploring vehicles, combine to disrupt the soil crust, creating dust and reducing nitrogen fixation. Without our microbes holding soil particles together, the dust problem must worsen. Undeniably, creativity and imagination are needed to sort out these pertubations, yet permit normal activities: what those are, is far from clear. Nevertheless, we're fortunate to have Dr. Jayne Belnap, a research ecologist at the U.S. Geological Survey's (USGS) Biological Resources Division, Moab, Utah, leading the charge to preserve a home, a habitat, for the microbes living in the top soil, while warning of the consequences if we fail to win this struggle.[20]

Dr. Belnap's research links soil microbes, soil nutrients, and the composition of desert vegetative communities. She and her team of scientists are alarmed about the transformations wrought by the outsize energy exploration vehicles moving immense areas of soil, and impacting soil that destroys animal burrows, tramping grass, plants and small animals, with its losses of soil fertility. By reducing vegetative cover, there is increased reflectance which dries out soil, further increasing erosion. Dark dust settling on snow pack, causes snow to melt faster, which is lost for growing fruits and vegetables that mature later in the year. Water loss is becoming a critical factor as the region becomes hotter and drier, the result of climate change. Belnap's group is working to reduce the impacts.

Working tirelessly, without fanfare, they are to be commended for their dedication.

The future is not just exciting it's breathtaking. The really cool idea is that it all makes sense. Our microbes are not just beneficial they are vital to our lives. The remarkable benefits microbes engender will remake and allow our civilization to sustainably produce the materials, energy, and by-products in ever greater demand. The versatility of microbes is downright stupefying.

Microbes do run the earth: run its biogeochemical cycles, remove all manner of waste, are responsible for clouds, rain and snow; provide a major portion of our food and beverages, protect our health and well being, and will surely be providing the fuel to run our vehicles, homes and offices.

Can we ever again think of microbes as anything but necessary, beneficial and collegial? It's time for these unsung heroic organisms to come out of the shadows, into the light of day, to receive the plaudits due them. That can only happen if we're ready to accept them as our collaborators FOR LIFE.

ABOUT

Melvin A. Benarde

Potential buyers are flipping through copies of *Germs Are Us* considering "Buy or no buy," wondering who is this Dr. Benarde who wants to turn our lives around and have us believe that microbes are not only beneficial, but crucial to our existence. From whence cometh his expertise? Is he to be relied upon? Good question. So, for what it's worth, Dr. Benarde began his scientific ascent with a B.Sc. degree in Biology/Psychology from St. John's University (NY). His service in the Air Force was followed by a M.Sc. degree from the University of Missouri medical school, (Columbia, MO). A Ph.D. in Microbiology/Public Health followed from Michigan State University (E. Lansing, MI).

Benarde's professional career included a six-year stint as Professor and Director of the University of Maryland's Seafood Laboratory. He then received dual appointments at Rutgers University's Departments of Microbiology, and Civil Engineering, (New Brunswick, NJ), where he introduced new courses in Public Health. While at Rutgers, he was awarded a World Health Organization (WHO) Fellowship that took him to the University of London's School of Hygiene and Tropical

Medicine, where he added Epidemiology to his armamentarium. Continuing to burnish his epidemiologic credentials, he spent a summer at the International Agency for Research on Cancer (IARC), a WHO/UN affiliate, (Lyons, France). This was followed by an interval at the Centers for Disease Control (CDC) in Atlanta, and an epidemiologic summer workshop at the University of Wisconsin's medical school, (Madison, WI). At Rutgers, he developed and presented *Environment and Health*, a weekly half-hour program on ABC-TV (NY); and wrote *Race Against Famine*, which was selected by the U.S. State Department for distribution to its worldwide libraries, and was translated into Arabic, Japanese, Portuguese, and other languages.

An outgrowth of his TV program was the first edition of his book, *Our Precarious Habitat* (WW Norton, NY). After Rutgers, he joined the newly created Department of Community Medicine at Hahnemann Medical School, (now Drexel College of Medicine) in Philadelphia. During his 16 years at Hahnemann, with a dual appointment in the Dept. of Microbiology, Benarde published *The Chemicals We Eat*, (McGraw-Hill), *Disinfection*, (Marcel Dekker, NY), and *The Food Additives Dictionary*, (Simon & Schuster, NY). He was then appointed Associate Director of Drexel University's Environmental Studies Institute with a dual appointment in the Dept. of Food Science & Nutrition. At Drexel, he was awarded and appointed Director of the USEPA's Region Three Asbestos Center, covering six states: Pennsylvania, New Jersey, Delaware, Maryland, Virginia, and West Virginia.

Dr. Benarde moved his Asbestos Center to Temple University where it expanded to become the Environmental Studies Center, dealing with Asbestos, Lead, and Mercury, among other environmental issues. At Temple University he published a second edition of *Our Precarious Habitat*: *Fifteen Years Later* (Wiley/ Interscience), as well as *Global Warning: Global Warming*, (Wiley/Interscience); *You've Been Had: How the Media and Environmentalists Turned America into a*

Nation of Hypochondriacs (Rutgers University Press); and *Asbestos: The Hazardous Fiber*, (CRC Press, Boca Raton, Fl.)

In his semiretirement, a completely new edition of *Our Precarious Habitat: It's in Your Hands* (Wiley/ Interscience, 2007) was published and also translated into Portuguese and published in Brazil.

During his career, Dr. Benarde has been elected a:

Fellow, World Health Organization

Fellow, Royal Society of Health (London)

Fellow, American Public Health Association

Full Member, Society of the Sigma Xi (The National honorary scientific society)

Surely with the credits, this background, experience and expertise he's reliable, someone we can trust. Bring him on! We'll buy this book.

.

GLOSSARY

AFFINAGE. The final or finishing process of cheese making that can take weeks or years, depending upon setting the optimal chemical environment for the cheese, at the outset, to bring cheese to its appropriate maturation. Affinage is used primarily for cheese with rinds, and the exacting work, ensuring control of temperature, humidity and acidity, is done by an Affineur, who brings the cheese to its ultimate ripeness. Affinage is a French word, from the verb Affiner, to refine, which comes from the Latin, ad finis, meaning, towards the limit, or end of the process.

AMINO ACID. A building block of proteins. There are 20 essential amino acids, each coded for by three adjacent nucleotides in a DNA sequence.

ANTIBODY. A protein produced by the immune system in response to infection by a foreign organism, or foreign protein.

ANTIGEN. A protein that stimulates the immune system to produce antibodies against it. Antigens include microbes, cells of transplanted organs, toxins, and foreign proteins generally.

ANAMMOX. The formation of nitrogen gas by the anaerobic oxidation of ammonia and nitrite.

BACILLUS. (plural, bacilli) a rod-shaped microbe

BIOFILM. A slime layer that develops when microbes congregate on surfaces, such as teeth, food, rocks and metal.

BIOMASS. The substance from living or recently living things, usually referring to plants, grasses, or plant-derived material often called lignocellulosic biomass. Wood is the largest, current source of biomass.

BIOREACTOR. A fermentation vessel for the controlled growth of microbes.

BIOREMEDIATION. The use of organisms, usually microbes, to degrade pollutants in soil or groundwater water.

BIOTECHNOLOGY. The industrial use of living organisms that is as diverse as removing unwanted chemicals, genetic engineering, or making wine, cheese or bread.

BUBO. The swelling of lymph nodes, most often in the groin, but also in arm pits, because of plague, syphilis, and tubercular infections.

COCCUS. (plural, cocci) a spherical-shaped microbe.

DENITRIFICATION. The reduction, anaerobically of nitrite to nitrate to nitrogen gas.

DNA. The abbreviation for deoxyribose nucleic acid, and the molecule containing the genetic code for all forms of life. It consists of two long, twisted chains of nucleotides. Each nucleotide contains one base, one phosphate molecule, and the sugar, ribose. The bases in all DNA nucleotides are adenine, thymine, guanine and cytosine.

ENZYME. A protein that speeds up, catalyzes, chemical reactions without being altered or consumed in the reaction.

FERMENTATION. A microbial process in which carbohydrates-most often-are metabolized, producing alcohol, acids, and gas.

FOMITES. An inanimate objects capable of transmitting infectious microbes from person to person.

GENE. A unit of hereditary information. Genes are sections of the DNA molecule that specify the production of specific proteins

GENETIC CODE. The 64 triplet codons used to specify all proteins.

GENETIC ENGINEERING. The removal, modification or addition of genes to a DNA molecule, thereby changing the information it contains. By changing this information, genetic engineering changes the type or amount of proteins an organism can now produce.

GENETICALLY MODIFIED ORGANISM. A plant, microbe or animal that has been modified or transformed, and is commonly referred to as a GMO: a genetically modified organism. (See Recombinant DNA)

GENOME. The totality of an organisms genes.

HORIZONTAL GENE TRANSFER. (HGT) The transfer of genetic material between microbes. Typically, only short fragments are exchanged, which allows them to easily adjust to new environments via acquisition of new genes.

LONGITUDINAL GENE TRANSFER. (LGT) See HGT.

MALTING. The stage in beer making in which grain is soaked in water to initiate germination and activate starch-digesting enzymes.

MASHING. The stage in beer making in which water soluble material is released from the grain in preparation for fermentation.

MICROBIOTA. The individual microbial communities that dwell in various body areas.

MICROBIOME. The totality of microbes, types and numbers, that dwell on, and in us.

MUTATION. A change in a DNA sequence.

PARENTERAL. Refers to a medication, a solution, given intravenously or intramuscularly.

PATHOGEN. A disease causing organism. Can be a bacterium, virus, fungus, yeast, or other microscopic organism.

pH. A measurement of the acidity or alkalinity of a solution. The pH scale runs from 1 to 14. One to six is acidic. 7 is neutral, and 8 to 14 is alkaline or basic. The lower the number, the more acidic. The higher the number the more alkaline and corrosive.

PHAGOCYTOSIS. The ingestion, digestion and elimination of foreign particles from our body by specific immune cells.

PHOTOSYNTHESIS. The process by which light energy is trapped by chlorophyll and converted to energy driving molecules for the synthesis of carbohydrates.

PRIMER. A short sequence of single-stranded DNA or RNA required by DNA polymerase as a starting point for DNA chain extension and amplification.

RECOMBINANT DNA. DNA that is formed by combining DNA from two different sources: a plant with a gene from microbe or animal; an animal with a gene from a plant or microbe; a microbe with a gene from an animal or plant. All that is being transferred are the four bases, and all selective breeding and genetic engineering are done by us humans.

RIBOSOME. The structure within a cell in which proteins are made. Most cells contain thousands of ribosomes.

SANITIZE. To make things, tables, counters, sinks, toilets, and other inanimate objects dirt-free, and partially free of microbes. Disinfection is synonymous with sanitization .

SEQUENCING. Often referred to as DNA sequencing is a means of determining the exact order of nucleotides of a specific fragment of DNA.

T-CELLS. Also known as T-lymphocytes, are a form of white blood cell that plays a central role in our immune system. There are T-helper cells, natural killer T-cells, and regulatory cells-Treg. cells, each with specific responsibilities during the battle against foreign invaders.

TESTACEANS. Testaceans are single-celled, amoeba-like organisms, living in freshwater and mossy soils. Many have finger-like projections used for locomotion, and are frequently encased in a shell. All appear to reproduce by budding.

VACCINATION. The procedure of inoculation or spray of a vaccine to provide protective immunity to specific diseases.

VACCINE. A preparqtion of dead or inactivated living pathogens, or their products, used to provide protective immunity.

ZOONOSES. A disease of animals transmissible to humans

REFERENCES

ONE

1. McCartney, E.S. Spontaneous Generation and kindred notions in antiquity. Trans. Amer. Philolog. Assoc. 51:101-115,1920. See also: Wilkins, J.S. Spontaneous generation and the origin of life. www.The talking origins archive. Posted April 26,2004.

2. van Helmont, Jan,B. Encyclopedia Britannica. www.britannica.com EBchecked/topic/260549/Jan-Baptiste-van-Helmont

3. Lechevalier, H., & Solotorovsky, M.Three Centuries of Microbiology. McGraw-Hill, New York, 1965. See also: Francesco Redi and Controlled Experiments. Scientus.org http://www.scientus.org/Redi-Galileo.html

4. The Spontaneous Generation Conflict, pgs. 2-8, Chap. One, History and Scope of Microbiology, in, Microbiology, 3rd. Ed. 1996. Prescott, L.M., Harley, J.P., & Klein, D. Wm. C. Brown, Publishers, Dubuque, Ia. See also: Who named it? Lazzaro Spallanzoni. http://www.who named it.com/doctor.cfm/2234.html

5. Galvez, A. The Role of the French Academy of Sciences in the Clarification of the Issues of Spontaneous Generation in the Mid-nineteenth century. Ann.Science. 45: 345-365, 1988. See also: Farley, J., et al. Science, Politics and Spontaneous Generation in nineteenth-century France: the Pasteur-Pouchet debate. Bull. Hist. Med.48:(2);161-198, 1974.

6. Brock, T.D. Milestones in Microbiology. ASM Press. Wash.D.C. 1975

7. Dubos, René. The Unseen World. The Rockefeller Institute Press. New York, 1962

8. Cullen, C.P. The Miracle of Bolsena. Amer. Soc. Microbiol.News.60:(4);187-191,1994

9. Merlino, C.P. Bartolomeo Bizio's Letter to the Most Eminent Priest, Angelo Bellani Concerning the phenomenon of the red colored polenta. J.Bacteriol. 9:(6); 527-543, 1924

10. Carter, C.K., & Carter, B.R. Childbed Fever: a scientific biography of Ignaz Semmelweis. Greenwood Press, Westport, Ct. 1994.

11. Nuland, S.B. The Doctor's Plague: Germs, Childbed Fever, and the Strange Story of Ignác Semmelweis. W.W.Norton & Co., New York, 2003. See also: Noakes, T.D.,et al, Semmelweis and the etiology of puerperal sepsis 160 years on. Epidem. & Infect. 136:(1); 1-9, 2008.

12. Woodham-Smith, C. The Great Hunger. Harper & Row, New York, 1962.

13. Snow, J. On the Mode of Communication of Cholera, in Cholera, Snow, J. Ed. The Commonwealth Fund, New York, 1936.

14. Cameron, D., & Jones, I.G. John Snow, The Broad Street Pump and Modern Epidemiology. Int'l. J. Epidem. 12:(4); 393-396, 1983.

15.   Whitehead, H. Remarks on the Outbreak of Cholera in Broad Street, Golden Square, London, in 1854. Trans. Epidemiol. Soc.(London) 3:97-104, 1867.

16.   Snow,J. On the Adulteration of Bread as a cause of Rickets. Int'l. J. Epidem. 32:336-337,2003. Reprinted from, The Lancet ii:4-5,1857.

17.   Dunnigan, M. Commentary: John Snow and Alum-induced rickets from adulterated London bread: an overlooked contribution to metabolic bone disease. Int'l. J. Epidem.32:(3); 340-341, 2003.

18.   Baldacci, G., Frontali, L., & Lattanzi, A. The Debate on Spontaneous Generation and the Birth of Microbiology. Fundamen.Scient. 2:(2); 123-136, 1981.

19.   Landis, H.R.M. The Reception of Koch's Discovery in the United States. Read before the Section on Medical History, College of Physicians, Phila. PA. Ann.Med.Hist. N. S, 4. Pgs. 531-537,1932.

20.   Allen, P. Etiological Theory in America Prior to the Civil war. J.Hist.Med. II: (4);489-520,1947.

21.   Richmond, P.A. American Attitudes Toward the Germ Theory of Disease. (1860-1880). J.Hist.Med. 9:(4); 428-454, 1954. See also: Richmond, P.A., Some Variant Theories in Opposition to the Germ Theory of Disease. J.Hist.Med.9:(3); 290-303, 1954.

TWO

1.   Lederberg, J. Infectious History. Science. 288:287-293, 2000.

2.   Lederberg, J. Of Men and Microbes. New Prospect. Quart. 21:92-96,2004

3.   The NIH Working Group. The NIH Microbiome Project. Genome Res. 19:2317-2323, 2009. See also: The NIH Common Fund. NIH Human Microbiome Project Completes Seminal Study of Microbial Diversity in Healthy Volunteers. June 13, 2012. http://copmmonfund.nih.gov/highlights/Index.aspx

4.   NIH. NIH News.Human Microbiome Project Awards Funds for Technology Development, Data analysis and ethical research. Oct. 7, 2008.

5.   Davies, J. In a Map for Human Life, Count the Microbes Too. Science. 291:2316, 2001

6.   Hulcr, J., Latimer, A.M., Henley, J.B., & 5 others. A Jungle in There: Bacteria in Belly Buttons are highly Diverse,but Predictable.PloS One. doi:10.1371/Journal.pone 0047712. Nov.7, 2002

7.   Avery, O.T., MacLeod, C.M., & McCartney, M. Studies of the chemical nature of the substance inducing transformation of pneumococcal types. J.Exptl.Med. 79:137-158,1944

8.   McCartney, M. Purification and properties of deoxyribose nuclease isolated from beef pancreas. J. Gen. Physiol. 29:123-139,1946. See also: McCartney, M. Discovering genes are made of DNA. Nature. 421:406, 2003.

9.   Griffith,F. The Significance of Pneumococcal Types. J.Hyg.27: 113-159, 1928

10. Downie, A.W. Pneumococcal Transformation-A Backward View. Fourth Griffith Memorial Lecture. J. Gen. Microbiol. 73:1-11,1972.

11. Crick, F.H.C. The structure of the Hereditary Material. Sci. Amer. 191:(4); 54-61, 1954

12. Henig, R.M. The Monk in the Garden: The lost and found genius of Gregor Mendel, the Father of Genetics. HoughtonMifflin, Co., Boston, 2000.

13. Dietz, H.C., Ramirez, F.,& Saki,L.Y. Marfans Syndrome and other microfibrillar diseases. Advan.Human Genet.22:Chap.4;153-186, 1994. See also: Ramirez, F., and Dietz, H.C. Extracellular microfibrils in Vertebrate Development and Disease Processes. J. Biol.Chem. 284:(22); 14677-14681,2007.

14. McLaren, R.E., Groppe, M., Barnard, A.L., & 11 others. Retinal gene therapy in patients with, choroideremia:Initial findings from a phase 1/2clinical trial. The Lancet. 383:1129-1137, 2014.

15. Mullis, K.B. The Unusual Origin of the polymerase Chain reaction. Sci. Amer. 262:(4); 56-65, 1990. See also: Arnheim, N., & Levensen, C.H. Polymerase Chain Reaction. Chem.Eng. News. 66:36-47, 1990.

16. Brenner, S. Frederick Sanger, 1918-2013. Science. 343:262,2014.

17. Kolbert, C., & Persing, D.H.Ribosomal DNA Sequencing as a tool for Identification of bacterial pathogens. Curr. Opin. Microbiol. 2:299-305, 1999.

18. The Human Microbiome Consortium. Structure, Function and Diversity of the healthy human microbiome. Nature. 486: 207-214, 2012.

19. The Human Microbiome Consortium. A Framework for Human Microbiome Research. Nature. 486: 215-221, 2012.

20. Kodaman, N., Pazos, A., Schneider, B., &13 others, including, Correa, P. Human and Helicobacter coevolution shapes the risk of gastric disease. PNAS. www.pnas.org/content/early/4/01/08/131809311

21. Bongers, G., Pacer, M.E., Geraldino, T.H., & 11 others, including Sergio A. Lira. Interplay of host mircobiota, genetic pertubations, and inflammation promotes local development of intestinal neoplasms in mice. J. Expt'l. Med.211:(3); 457-472, 2014.

22. Balter, M. Taking Stock of the human microbiome and disease. Science. 336: 1246-1247, 2012.

23. Hunt, K.M., Foster, J.A., Forney, L.J., & 7 others. Characterization of the diversity and temporal stability of bacterial communities in human milk. PLoS One6 (6); e21313.doi:10.1371/Journal.pone 0021313

24. Aagaard, K., Riehle, K., Ma, J, Sejata,N.,& 7others. A metagenomic approach to characterization of the vaginal microbiome signature in pregnancy. PLoS One 7(6): e36466. doi:10.1371/Journal.pone 0036466.

25. Lida, N., Dzutsev, A., Stewart, A.C.,& 18 others, including Trinchieri,G.,& Goldzmid, R. Gut commensal bacteria promote antitumor innate immune responses in distant tumors after immunotherapy and chemotherapy. Science. 342: 967-970, 2013.

26. Viaud, S., Saccheri,F., Mignot,G.,& 22 others including Zitvogel, L. The intestinal microbiota modulates the anticancer immune effects of cyclophosphoramide. Science. 342: 971-976, 2013.

27.   Smith, M.I.,Yatsunenko,T.,Nanary, M.J.,& 15 others. Gut microbiomes of Malawian twin pairs discordant for Kwashiorkor. Science.339: 548-554, 2013.

28.   Garrett, W.S. Kwashiorkor and the gut Microbiota. NEJM.368:(18); 1746-1747,2013

THREE

1.   Vance, E. Safe From Spiders. Sci.Amer. 308: 14, 2013

2.   Reddy, M.M., Wilson, R., Wilson, J, & 5 others. Identification of Candidate IgG biomarkers for Alzheimer's Disease via combinatorial library screenings. Cell. 144:(1);132-142, 2011.

3.   National Cancer Institute. Understanding cancer series: The immune system: Markers of self: Major Histocompatibility Complex. 2007. See also: Janeway's Immunobiology. Murphy, K.P. Garland Science, London & New York, 2012.

4.   Ahmed, R., & Gray, D. Immunological Memory and protective immunity: understanding their relation. Science. 272:54-59, 1996.

5.   The Rockefeller University Awards. Ralph M. Steinman. Henry G. Kunkel, Prof. 2011 Nobel Prize in Physiology or Medicine. See also: Steinhuysen,J.,& Nichols,M. Insight: Nobel Winners last big experiment:himself. Reuters. Oct.6, 2011. www.reuters.com/article/2011/10/06/us-nobel-medicine-experiment-idUSTRE7956CN2011006.

6.   Stadinski, B., Kappler,J., Eisenbarth,G.S. Molecular targeting of islet autoantigens. Immunity. 32:(4); 446-456, 2010.

7.   Rho, J.H., Zhang,W.,Mandakolathur,M.,& 2 others. Human proteins with affinity for Dermatan Sulfate have the propensity to become autoantigens. Amer.J.Path. 178:(5);2177-2190,2011.

8.   Lee, Y.K., Menenzes, J.S., Umesaki,Y.,& Mazmanian,S.K. Pro-inflammatory T-cell responses to gut microbiota promote experimental autoimmune encephalitis. PNAS.org/cig/doi:/10.1073/pnas.1000082107.2010. See also: Liston, A., & Gray, D.H.D. Homeostatic control of regulatory T cell diversity. Nat. Rev. Immun.14:154-165,2014.

9.   Strachan, D.P. Hay Fever, hygiene and household size. BMJ. 299:1259-1260, 1989.

10.   Strachan, D.P. Allergy and Family size: a riddle worth solving. Clin. Exp. Allergy.27:235-236,1997.

11.   Strachan, D.P., Taylor, E.M., Carpenter, R.G. Family Structure, neonatal infection and hay fever in adolescence. Arch. Dis. Child. 74: 422-426, 1996.

12.   Von Mutius, E., Fritzsch, C.,Welland, S.K.,& 2 others.Prevalence of Asthma and allergic disorders among children in the united Germany. BMJ. 305:1395-1399,1992.

13.   Von Mutius, E., & Vercelli, D. Farm Living: effects on childhood asthma and allergy. Nat. Rev. Immunol. 10:861-868, 2010.

14.   Gern, J.E. Barnyard Microbes and childhood asthma. NEJM. 364: 769-770, 2010.

15.	Bergroth, E., Remes, S., Pekkanen,J.,& 3 others. Respiratory tract illnesses during the first year of life: Effect of dog and cat contacts. Pediat.130: (2); 211-220, 2012.

16.	Ege, M.J., Mayer, M., Normand, A.C. & 7 others. Exposure to Environmental microorganisms and childhood asthma. NEJM. 364:(8); 701-709, 2011.

17.	Rook, G.W.W. A Darwinian View of the Hygiene or "old friends" hypothesis. Microbe.7:(4); 173-179-2012.

18.	Rook, G.W.W. Review series on helminths, immune modulation and the hygiene hypothesis. Immunol.126:(1); 3-11, 2012.

19.	Matthews, D. Dirt is good for the Brain. Mother NatureNetwork. 2010. http://www.takepart.com/article/2012/03/26/5-reasons-let-your

20.	Olszak, T., An, D.,Zessig, S, and 8 others including Blumberg,R.S. Microbial exposure during early life has persistent effects on natural killer T-cell function. Science. 336:489,493, 2012.

21.	Hepworth, M.R., Monticelli, L.A., Fung, T.C.& 14 others. Innate lymphoid cells regulate CD4 T-cell responses to intestinal commensal bacteria. Nature. 498: 113-117, 2012.

22.	Ding, T., and Schloss,P.D. Dynamics and associations of microbial community types across the human body. Nature. doi:10.1038/nature13178.April16, 2014.

23.	Wu, H-J.,Ivanov,I.I., Darce,J.,& 6 others. Gut residing segmented filamentous bacteria drive autoimmune arthritis via T-helper 17 cells. Immunity. 32: 6);815-827, 2010.

24.	Lee, Y.K., and Mazmanian,S.Has the microbiota played a critical role in the evolution of the adaptive immune system? Science.330: 1768-1773, 2010.

25.	Maslowski, K.M., & MacKay,C.R. Diet, gut microbiota and immune responses. Nat.Immun.12: 5-9, 2011.

26.	DeFilippo, C., Cavalieri, D., DiPaolo,M.,& 6 others. Impact of diet in shaping gut microbiota revealed by a comparative study in children from Europe and rural Africa. Proc. Nat'l. Acad. Sci. 107:14691-14696, 2010.

27.	Gomez, A., Luckey, D.,Yeomin,C.J.,& 5 others including Taneja,V. Loss of sex and age driven differences in the gut microbiome characterize arthritis - susceptible 0401 mice but not arthritis resistant 0402 mice. PloS One, 2012;7(4): e36095 doi:10.1371/Journal.pone0036095.Epub.2012 Apr.24.

28.	Scher, J., Sczesnak, A., Longman, R.S.,& 9 others including Littman, D.R. Expansion of intestinal Prevotella copri correlates with enhanced susceptibility to arthritis http://dx.doi.org/10.7554/eLife.01202.Nov.5.2013.

29.	Lady Mary Pierpont Wortley Montague: Letters from the Levant, during the embassy to Constantinople, 1716-1718. J.A.St.John,London, 1838. www.questra.com/pm qst?

30.	Mary Sydney, Lady Wroth,(pg.4). www.Ashgatebooks.google.com/books? isbn=075466532

31.   Edward Jenner and the discovery of vaccination. www.sciedu/library/spcoll/nathist/Jenner.htm_ See also: Morgan, A.J., Parker,S. Translational mini-review series on vaccination: the Edward Jenner Museum and the history of vaccination. Clin.Ept'l. Immun. 147:(3);389-394, 2007.

32.   Dufour, H.D.,& Carroll, S.B. History:Great Myths Die Hard. Nature.502: (7469);32-33,2013.

33.   Nobelprize.org: The Nobel Prize in Physiology or Medicine 1901Emil von Behring. Biography. http://www.nobel_prizes/medicine/laureate/190..

34.   Paul Ehrlich-Wikipedia, the free encyclopedia. http://en.wikipedia.orgwiki/PaulEhrlich

35.   Jonas Salk: Biography Academy of Achievement. www.achievement.org/autodoc/printmember/SalObio-1. See also: About Jonas Salk.Salk Institute of Biological Studies. www.Salk.edu/about/Jonas_Salk.html.

36.   Schmeck, H.M., Jr. On this Day. Albert Sabin, Polio Researcher, 86, Dies. http://www.NYtimes.com/learningt/general/on this day/0826.html. See also: The legacy of Albert B. Sabin. www.sabin.org/legacy-albert-b-sabin.

37.   Yusutzai, A. Health Workers Murdered as Pakistan Vaccinates. Canad. Med.Asso. J. News. April 22,2014. See also: Ahmed,J. Militant Ambush Kills 12 of Polio workers escort in Pakistan. Reuters, March 1, 2014. www.reuters.com/article/2014/03/01/us-pakistan-polio-attack

38.   Bill & Melinda Gates Foundation, Press Release: Bloomberg Philanthropies to donate 100 million to help end polio. Feb.28, 2013. www.gatesfoundation.org /media-center/Press-Releases/2013/02/Bloomberg-Philanthropies-to-Donate-100-million-to-help--end-polio.

39.   TAG Archives. Dr. Saad Omer. Flu shots help prevent preterm birth. Feb.27, 2013. http://marks loan.wordpress.com/tag/dr-saad-omer

40.   Wheeler, M. Study suggests link between untreated depression, response to shingles vaccine. UCLA Newsroom. Feb. 15, 2013. Newsroom.ucla.edu/releases/ucla-study-suggests-link between-243590.

41.   FDA. US Food & Drug Administration.Vaccines, Blood & Biologics. Flublok. Oct. 22,2013. Supporting Documents. www.fda.gov/biologicsbloodvaccines/approved products/

42.   Weise, E. USA Today. FDA Targets Flu Drug Claims. This Flu season has spawned a number of fraudulent products that claim to treat, prevent or shorten the duration of the flu, the FDA says. www.usatoday.com/story/news/health/2013.01/30/flu-drug-scam-germbullet/1875505

43.   Rowland, V. New Study Discovers Unique HIV features. University of the Witwatersrand, South Capetown, South Africa. Oct. 24, 2012. www.wits.ac.za/newsroom/news.tem/201210/8131 See also:McNeil, D.G.,Jr. A weak Spot in HIV's Armor Raises Hope for Vaccione. The New York Times. Oct. 30, 2012. D5.

44. Helleberg, M., Afzai, S., Kronborg, G. & 6 others. Mortality attributable to smoking among HIV-1 infected individuals:a nationwide population-base cohort study. Clin.Infect.Diseas. 56:(5);727-734, 2013.

45. Harris, G. As Dengue Fever Sweeps India,a Slow Response Stirs Expert's Fears. The New York Times. Nov.9, 2012, A6.

46. RTS,S, Malaria Candidate Vaccine Reduces Malaria by approximately one third in African infants. Results from on-going Phase III clinical trial announced Glaxo-SmithKline media archive. Nov. 9, 2012. US.gsk.com/html/media-news/pressrelease-2012/2012/pressrelease-1251217.htm. See also: Rathi, A. The Conversation: New Malaria vaccine the first to offer complete protection. The Conversation.com/new-malaria-vaccine-the-first-to-offer complete-protection16862.

47. The New York Times, Editorial. An HPV Myth Debunked. Oct.19, 2012. A30. See also: Mayhew, A., Mullins, K., Ding, L., & 5 others. Risk Perception and Subsequent Sexual Behaviors after HPV Vaccination in Adolescents. Pediat. 133:(3);404-411,2014.

48. Kotz, D. Throat cancer and Oral Sex. The Boston Globe. June 10, 2013.

49. Humphreys, K.A. Vaccine to Curb Addict's Highs. The Wall Street Journal, Nov. 24-25, 2013, C3.

50. Peterson, E.C., Gunnell, M., Che,Y,& 5 others including Dr. Owen. Using Hapten Design to Discover Monoclonal Antibodies for Treating Methamphetamine Abuse. J.Pharmacol.Expt'l.Thereapeut. 322: (1); 30-39, 2007.

51. Weil Cornell Newsroom. Cocaine Vaccine PassesKey Testing Hurdle: New Anticocaine Research Shows Drug Can't Reach the Brain. Human Clinical Trial on the horizon. May 10, 2013. http://Weil.Cornell.edu/news/

52. The Michael J. Fox Foundation. First-Ever Vaccine Approach to Treating Parkinson's Disease. May 15, 2012. http://www.michaelJFox.org/foundation/publication-detail.html?id=68

53. Grady, D. In Girl's Last Hope, Altered Immune cells Beat Leukemia. The New York Times. Dec.10, 2012. A1.

54. Ryan, K.A. Target the Super-Spreaders. Inoculating kids is the best way to protect everyone from the flu. Why don't we do it? Sci. Amer. Oct. 2012, pg.14.

55. McNeil, D.G., Jr. After Measles success, Rwanda to get Rubella Vaccine. The New York Times. Feb. 26, 2013. D7. See also: World Health Organization, Regional Office for Africa. Rwanda First Sub-Saharan African Country to Introduce measles-rubella vaccine Nationwide with GAVI support.

56. GAVI Support.March 18, 2013. www.afro.who.int/fr/rwanda/press-materials/item/5383. See also: Mehrotra, K. Measles Cases Spike to Highest Level Since 1994. The Wall Street Journal. May 30, 2014. A6.

57. Editorial, The New York Times. Aftermath of an Unfounded Vaccine Scare: May 22, 2013. A30. See also: Cheng.M. USA Today. Measles Surges in UK Years after Flawed Research. May 20, 2013.

58. Gerber, J.S. & Offit, P.A. Vaccines and Autism. A tale of shifting hypotheses. Infect. Dis.48: (4);456-461,2009. See also: Editorial, The New York Times. Journal Retracts 1998 paper Linking Autism to vaccines. Feb. 3, 2010, A9.

59. Kluger, J. Jenny McCarthy on Autism and Vaccines. www.time.com/time/health/article/0,8599,1888718,00.html. April, 2009. See also: Hollywood Life Staff. New Report Says: Jenny McMcarthy's Son may not have had autism after all. Feb. 26. 2010. http://hollywood life.com/2010/02/26/Jenny-mccarthy-says-her..

60. Bruni,F. Autism and the Agitator. The New York Times. April 22, 2014. A25

61. Doctors Without Borders Press Release. June18, 2013. Syria: Measles Epidemic Reveals Growing Humanitarian Needs. www.doctorswithoutborders.org/article/syrians-measles-epidemic-reveals-growing-humanitarian-needs.

FOUR

1. MacFarquhar, N., & Droubi,H. In Syria's Civil War, Doctors Find Themselves in Cross Hairs. The New York Times. March 24, 2013. A6.

2. Berriman, M., Aksoy S., Attardo, G.M.,& 143 others of the Int'l Glossina Genome Initiative. Genome Sequence of the Tetse Fly(Glossina morsitans):Vector of African Trypanosomiasis. Science. 344:380-386, 2014. (April 25)

3. Bingham, A.M., Graham, S.P., Burkett-Cadena,N.D.,& 3 others. Detection of EEE virus RNA in North American Snakes. Amer. J.Trop. Med. 87:1140-1144, 2012. See also: Armstrong, P.M.,& Andreadis,T.G. EEE virus-Old Enemy,New Threat. NEJM. 368:(18);1670-1673, 2013.

4. Vora, N.M., Sridhar, B.V., Feldman, K.A.,& 26 others. Raccoon Rabies Virus Variant Transmission Through Solid Organ Transplant.JAMA.310:94);398-407, 2013.

5. Hinshaw, D. Dozens Die as Ebola Outbreak Hits Guinea.The Wall Street Journal. March 25, 2014. A7. See also: Ebola Outbreak in West Africa Kills Over 140, UN Agency Says. Assoc. Press. April 22, 2014.

6. Winslow, R.,& Cohen,B. What Surgery Can do for Kevin Ware's Bad Break. Wall Street Journal. April 2, 2013, D1

7. Robertson, C.E., Baumgartner, L.K., Harris, J.K., & 4 others, including,Pace,N.R. Culture-Independent Analysis of Aerosol Microbiology in a Metropolitan Subway Station. Appl. Environ.Micro.79:(11);3485-3493,2012 (June)

8. Soper, G.A.The Curious Career of Typhoid Mary.Bull.New York Acad.Med.15:(10); 698-712,1939. See also: Leavitt, J.W. "Typhoid Mary" Strikes Back. Bacteriological Theory and Practice in Early twentieth-Century Public Health. ISIS. 83:608-629, 1992.

9. IDRI-Infections Disease Research Institute. Transforming Science into Global Health Solutions. IDRI & OrangeLife Register Rapid Diagnostic for Leprosy for use in Brazil. Seattle, Wash. Jan. 24, 2013. See also: McNeil, D.G. Fast New Test Could Find Leprosy Before Lasting Damage is Done. The New York Times. 2/20/13. A1

10.   Recent Theories Surrounding the Eruption of Mount Krakatoa. www.roman-empire.net/decline/krakatoa-535ad.html.

11.   Harbecks, M., Seifert, L.,Hansch,S.,& 8 others. Yersinia pestis DNA from skeletal remains from the 6th century reveals insights into Justinianic plague. PLoSPathog9(5):e1003349doi:10.1037/Journal.ppat.1003312.

12.   Barry,D. With Shovels and Science, a Grim story is Told.The New York Times, 3/25/13. A12. See also: O'Shea,K. Irish Central. Donegal Welcome Home Duffy's Cut Murder Victim-John-Ruddy After 180 Years. 2/28/13. www.irishcentral.com/news/donegal-residents-welcome-home-duffy's-cut-murder-victim-John-ruddy--193980811-237856876.html.

13.   History Channel.This Day in History.July 9,1850. President Taylor dies of Cholera.www.history.com/this-day-in-history/president-taylor-dies-of-cholera.

14.   Snow, J. On the Mode of Communication of Cholera. The Commonweath Foundation, New York, 1936.

15.   Chen-shan, C., Sorenson,J.,Harris, J.B.,& 14 others. The Origin of the Haitian Cholera Outbreak Strain. NEJM. 364:33-42, 2011. See also: Rosen,A. How the UN Caused Haiti's Cholera Crisis--and don't want to be held responsible. The Atlantic. Feb. 26, 2013.

16.   Barford,E. Parasite makes mice lose fear of cats permanently. Nature.Sept.18, 2013. doi:10.1038/nature.2013.13777. See also: Ingram, W.M., Goodrich, L.M., Robey, E.A.,& Eisen,M.B. Mice Infected with low-virulence strains of Toxoplasma lose innate aversion to cat urine even after extensive parasite clearance. PLoSOne Sept.18, 2013 Doi:10.1371/Journal.pone0075246

17.   Flegr, J. Influence of latent Toxoplasma infection on human personality, physiology and morphology: pros & cons of the toxoplasma-human model in studying the manipulation hypothesis. J Expt'l.Biol.216: 127-133, 2013.

18.   Soloman, C. How Kitty is Killing the Dolphins. Scient. Amer. 308:(5);72-77, 2013.

19.   FDA News Release. News & Events. Dec.31. 2012.On Dec. 28, 2012, the FDA approved Sirturo to treat multidrug resistant pulmonary tuberculosis. www.fda.gov/NewsEvents/Newsroom/Press announcements /ucm333695.htm. See also: Johnson & Johnson News Release 3/6/2014. Sirturo (Bedaquiline) receives Conditional approval in the European Union for the treatment of multidrug resistant tuberculosis.

20.   Schuch, R., Pelzek, A.J.,Raz, A.,& 11 others. Use of a Bacteriophage Lysin to identify a novel target for antimicrobial development. PLoSOne. April 10,2013. Doi:10.1371/Journal.pone0060754

21.   Hare, R. New Light on the History of Penicillin. Med.Hist. 20:(1);1-24, 1982.

22.   Mackie, B.The Almost Cure-all Urine of Albert Alexander. Posted Aug.10, 2012. bmackie.blogpost.com/2012/08/the-almost-cure-all-urine-of-Albert-html.

23.   Medawar, P., Sir. Howard Florey: The Making of a Great Scientist. Oxford Univ. Press. Reviewed by MacFarlane, G. The London Review of Books. V.1(5);3-14. Dec. 20, 1979.

24.   Darwin, C.R. On the Origin of Species by Means of Natural Selection;or the Preservation of Favored Races in the Struggle for Life. John Murray, Publisher, London, 1859.

25.   Kolter, R, & Maloy, S.R. Eds. Microbes and Evolution: The World That Darwin Never Saw. ASM Press. Wash.DC. 2012.

26.   Hughes, D. Antibiotic Resistance, Chap.7, in, Microbes and Evolution: The world Darwin Never Saw. ASM Press. Wash.DC., 2012.

27.   Misgav Companies, Medical Devices. The Flexicath Sterile Catheters. www.misgav-venture.com/companies-in,asp?num=4

28.   Sharklet Patterned Medical Devices. Sharklet technologies,inc.. www.sharklet.com/sharklet-products/sharklet-safetouch-f.

29.   EOS Surface. Large-Scale, Multi-site Test of Copper-Based Antimicrobial-Protected Materials. http://eos-surface.om/2013/01/sentara-healthcare-cupron-eos.

30.   Cupron/Purthread Technologies Reduces Bioburden on Soft Surfaces. www.purthread.com/About-us/contact-us/.

31.   MaKay, M. How to Stop Hospitals From Killing Us. Review Section.The Wall Street Journal. Sat/Sun. Sept.22/23, 2012, C1 & C2. See Also: Boyle, C. Study at Long Island's North Shore University Hospital Finds when CAM is on, med staff do keep hands really clean. NY Daily News. 11/30/2011. www.nydailynews.com/life-style/health/study-long-island-article-1.984723

32.   Landro, L.The Secret to Fighting Infections. Dr. Peter Pronovost says it isn't that hard. If only hospitals would do it. The Wall Street Journal. March 28, 2011.

33.   Duffy, J. Smallpox and the Indians in the American Colonies. Bull. Hist. Med. 25:324-347, 1951.

34.   Koenig, R. The Fourth Horseman:one man's mission to wage the Great War in America. Public Affairs Press, New York, 2007.

35.   Reidel,S. Biological Warfare & Bioterrorism:a historical review. Proc. Baylor Univ. Med. Center. 17:(4);400-406, 2004.

36.   Relman, D.A. "Inconvenient Truths", in the pursuit of scientific knowledge and public health. J.Infect.Dis. 209:170-172,2014. See also: Barash, J.S., & Arnon, S.S. A Novel Strain of Clostridium botulinum that Produces Type B and Type H Botulinus Toxins. J. Infect. Dis. 209:183-191,2014.

37.   Pollack, A. Traces of terror: The Science; Scientists create a Live Poliovirus. The New York Times. July 12, 2002. A16.

38.   Bioterrorism: A threat to agriculture and the food supply. General Accountability Office; GAO-04-259T, Wash.DC. Nov. 19, 2003.

39.   Dept. of Environment, Food & Rural Affairs, Great Britain. Archive:Foot and Mouth Disease, 2001 Outbreak; and the 2007 Outbreak. Archive:Defra.gov.uk/foodfarm/farmanimal/diseases/atoz/fmd/2007.

40.   US. Dept. of Homeland Security. Bioterrorism: Ready; Prepare; Stay Informed. www.dhs.gov/ready.

41.   Willson, R.C. Cullen College of Engineering, Dept. of Chemical & Biomolecular Engineering. Univ. of Houston, TX. Research: Molecular diagnostics & sensors; Genome based identification of microbes.

FIVE

1.   Bannerot,S.,& Bannerot,W. Health Underway: an unexpected intruder. Cruising World. 94-102, (Sept), 2001.

2.   Becker, K., Southwick,K.,Reardon,J.,& 3 others. Histamine poisoning associated with eating tuna burgers. JAMA. 285: (10);1327-1330, 2001.

3.   Deardorf, T.L., Kayes, S.G.,& Fukumura,T. Human Anisakiasis transmitted by marine food products. Hawaii Med. J. 50:(1);9-16, 1991. See also: Audicana, M.T., & Kennely,M.W. Anisakis simplex: from obscure infectious worm to inducer of immune hypersensitivity. Clin.Microbiol.Rev. 2:(12); 360-379, 2008.

4.   Torok,T.J.,Tauxe, R.V.,Wise,R.P.,& 8 others. A large community outbreak of Salmonellosis caused by intentional contamination of restaurant salad bars. JAMA. 278:(5);389-395,1997.

5.   Hennessey, T.W., Hedberg,C.W., Slutsker,L. & 8 others. A national outbreak of Salmonella enterididis infections from ice cream. NEJM.334:(2)1281-1286,1996.

6.   CDC. Morbidity and Mortality Weekly Report. 25:7; For the week ending, Feb. 21, 1976. Staphylococcal Foodborne Illness, Tennessee, North Carolina, South Carolina.

7.   Effersoe, P. and Kjerulf,K. Clinical aspects of Staphylococcal food poisoning during air travel. The Lancet. 306:(7935); 599-600, Sept. 27,1975.

8.   Layton, L. E.coli tainted beef infects 21 people in 16 states: ABC news:Health Highlights. Dec. 28, 2009.Beef recalled because of E.coli concern. ABC News.com/Health/Healthday/health-highlights-dec-28-2009/story?id=9436156

9.   U.S General Accountability Office. Food Irradiation Available Research Indicates that Benefits Outweigh Risks. GAO-RCED-00-217. Wash. DC.Aug. 24, 2000.

10.   Irradiation of Food, Report 4 (I-93) American Med. Asso. Council on Scientific Affairs. (Ref.Comm.E) Chicago, Adapted, 1992.

11.   Position Paper: Food Irradiation. J. Amer. Diet.Assoc. 100:(2);246-253, 2000.

SIX

1.   Davisdon, L. The Sun Chemist. Alfred A. Knopf. New York, 1976.

2.   Kaufman, G.B. Chaim Weizmann (1874-1952): Chemist, Biotechnologist, and Statesman. The Fateful Interweaving of Political Conviction and Scientific Talent. J.Chem. Edu. 71: (3); 209-214, 1994.

3.   Kessler, J.D., Valentine, D.L., Redmond, M.C., & 9 others. A Persistent Oxygen Anomaly Reveals the Fate of Spilled Methane in the Deep Gulf of Mexico. Science.331: 312-315, 2011. (Jan.21)

4.   Redmond, M.C., and Valentine, D.L., Natural Gas and Temperature Structured a Microbial Community Response to the Deep Water Horizon Oil spill. PNAS. Early Edition. Sept.7, 2011. www.pnas.org/cgi/doi:/10.1073/pnas.1108756108.

5.   Brigmon, R.L. Methanotrophic Bacteria: use in bioremediation. http://sti.srs.gov/fulltext/ms2001058/ms2001058.html

6.   Cologgi,D.L.,Lampa-Pastrick,Speers,M.A., Kelly,S.D.,Reguera,G. Extracellular reduction of uranium via Geobacter conductive pili as a protective cellular mechanism. PNAS. 108:(37);15248-15252, 2011.

7.   O'Malley, M., Theodorou, M.K., Kaiser, C.A. Evaluating expression and catalytic activity of anaerobic fungal fibrolytic enzymes native to Piromyces sp.E2 in Saccharomyces cerevisiae. Environmental Progress & Sustainable Energy, In Press. See also, Amer. Chjem. Soc: Enzymes from horse feces could hold secrets to streamlining biofuel production. April 11, 2013. http://phys.org/news/2013-04-enzymes-horse-feces-secrets-biofu

8.   Hargens, A., Bernie, F.,Schopp,S, Lin,J.,Cohen,M.F. Simultaneous biotic and biotic degradation of lignocelluloses under extreme alkaline conditions. Sonoma State University & Berkeley Labs, July 10, 2013. www.lbl.gov/publicinfo/newscenter/assets/docs/cohen-poster.pdf. See also: Preuss,P. A creature from an alkaline spring could improve biofuel processing. News Center Berkeley Lab. U.S.Dept. of Energy, June 10, 2013. lbl.gov/feature stories/2013/06/10/creature-fr.

9.   Wargacki, A.J., Leonard, E.,Win,M.N., & 12 others. An Engineered Microbial Platform for Direct Biofuel Production from Brown Macroalgae. Science. 335:308-313, 2012. (Jan.20)

10.   Takeda,H.,Yoneyama,F.,Kawai, S.,& 2 others. Bioethanol production from marine biomass alginate by metabolically engineered bacteria. Energy. Environ. Sci. 4:2575-2581-2011.

11.   PR NewsWire. Synthetic Genomics Inc. Purchases 81 acre site in South California for testing of innovative algae strains. www.prnews wire.com/news-releases/synthetic-genomics. May 24, 2012. See also: Hylton,W.S. God of Small Things. The New York Times Mag. pgs. 47-51, 64-65, 70-71, June 3,2012.

12.   Howard,T.P., Middlehaufe, S.,Moore,K.,& 8 others, including John Love. Synthesis of customized petroleum-replica fuel molecules by targeted modification of free fatty acid pools in Escherichia coli. PNAS. 110:(19);7636-7641, 2013.

13.   Cardwell, D.A. Side Trip on the Road to Clean Fuel. The New York Times. Sunday Business.June 23, 2013. Pgs. 1& 6.

14.   Strobel, G. Methods of discovery and techniques to study endophytic fungi producing fuel-related hydrocarbons. Natu'l. Prod. Rept. 31:(2); 259-2782, 2014.

15.   Metchnikoff, I, L.The Prolongation of Life! Optimistic Studies. (Engl.Trans., P. Chalmers Mitchell) Classics in Longevity and Aging (series) Int'l Longevity Center, New York, 2004.

16.   Ishiwata, S.On a severe softening of silkworms. (Sotto Disease). Dainihan Sanbishi Kaiho. 9:(114);1-5,1901.

17. Berliner, E. Uber die Schlastsucht der Mehlmottenraupe (Ephestia kuhneilla Zelli) und ihren Erreger Bacillus thuringiensis n.sp. Zeit. Angewan. Entomol. 2: 29-56, 1915.

18. Rauch, J. Will Frankenfood Save the Planet. Atlantic Monthly. Oct. 2003. pgs. 103-108.

19. Brand, S. Environmental heresies. Technol. Rev. May, 2005. Pgs. 60-63.

20. Hallman, W.K., Hebden, C.W., Cuite, C.L., Lang, J.T. Americans and GM Foods: Knowledge, Opinion and Interest in 2004. Publ. RR-1104-007, Food Policy Institute, Cook College, Rutgers University, New Brunswick, NJ. See also: Hallman, W.K., & Hebden, W.C. American Opinions of GM Foods: Awareness, Knowledge and Implications for Education. Choices. 20:(4); 239-242, 2005.

21. Harmon, A., and Pollack, A. Battle Brewing over Labeling of Genetically Modified Food. The New York Times, May 25, 2012, A1. See also: Miller, H.I. Activism vs. the Rule of Law. Hoover Institution, Stanford University, May 22, 2013. www.hoover.org/print/publications/defining-ideas/article.

22. Gibney, M. Something to chew On: Challenging controversies in food & health. University College Dublin Press, Ireland, July, 2012.

23. Anthes, E. Frankenstein's Cat: Cuddling up to biotech's brave new beasts. Sci.Amer/Farrar, Straus and Giroux, New York,2013.

24. Masip, G., Sabalza, M., Perez-Massot, E., and 5 others. Opinion: Don't Fear GM Crops, Europe! The Scientist, May 28, 2013. www.the-scientist.com/articles.view/articlesNO/35578/title/opinion.

25. Harmon.A. Golden Rice: Lifesaver? The New York Times: Sunday Review. Aug.25, 2013, pgs.1& 6. See also: Hvistendahl,M.,& Enserink,M. Charges Fly, Confusion Reigns over Golden Rice Study in Chinese Children. Science. 337:1281-,2012, (Sept.14)

26. Harmon, A. A Race to Save the Orange by Altering its DNA. The New York Times, Sunday, July 28, 2013. A1,16,17. See also: Burke, K.L. The Race to Stop a Citrus plague. Amer. Scient.102:(3);166-167, 2014 (May/June)

27. University of California, Berkeley-IPIRA. Amyris Biotechnologies: Harvesting Nature Through Biotechnology. www.amyrisbiotech.com/5/21/14.

28. Sullivan, M.Chemical Analysis confirms discovery of oldest wine-making equipment ever found. UCLA Scientists use new scientific method to verify vintage 4100 bce wine. Jan. 11, 2011. msullivan@support.ucla.edu.

29. Wilford, J.N.Wine cellar, well aged, is revealed in Israel. The New York Times. Nov.24, 2013. A6.

30. Wade, N. Microbes May Add Special Something to Wines. The New York Times. Nov. 26, 2013. A15.

31. Kaplan, S.L. The Rise of Nations. Review of, Bread: A Global History. The Wall Street Journal. Nov.26/27, 2011. C8.

32. Salque, M., Boguki, P.I., Pyzel,J.,& 4 more. Earliest Evidence of Cheese making in the sixth millennium bce in northern Europe. Nature. 493: 522-525, 2012 (Dec.12)

33.   Kawash, S. Sex and Candy. OP-Ed. The New York Times. Feb. 14, 2014. A31

34.   Stokstad, E. Down on the Shrimp Farm: Can Shrimp become the new chicken of the sea without damaging the ocean? Science. 328:1504-1505, 2010. (June 18) See also: Lawrence, A.Texas A & M.Agrilife Extension & Research. Commercial Superintensive Raceway Shrimp Farming. July 2013. ccag.tamu.edu/monoculture-port-aransas-race-way-shrimp-farming

35.   Molloy, D.P., Mayer, D.A., Gaylo, M.J., & 6 others. Mode of Action of Pseudamonas flourescens Strain CL 145A,a Lethal Control Agent of Dressenid Mussels. J. Invert. Pathol. 113:115-121, 2013. See also 104-114.

SEVEN

1.   Chisholm, S.W. Unveiling Prochlorococcus: The Life and Times of the Oceans Smallest Photosynthetic cell. Chap.23, in, Microbes and Evolution: The World that Darwin Never Saw. Roberto Kolter, & Stanley Maloy, Eds. ASM Press, Wash.D.C. 2012

2.   Kashtan, N., Roggensack,S.E., Rodrigue,S., & 10 others. Single-cell Genomics Reveals Hundreds of Coexisting Subpopulations in Wild Prochlorococcus. Science. 344:416-419, 2014 (APRIL 25)

3.   Falkowski,P.,Scholes, R.J., Boyle,E., & 14 others. The Global Carbon Cycle: A Test of our Knowledge of Earth as a System. Science.290:291-295, 2000. (Oct.11)

4.   Gillis, J. Climate Change Seen Posing Risk to Food Supplies. New York Times. Nov. 2, 2013 A1

5.   Christner, B. Cloudy With a Chance of Microbes. Microbe.7:(2); 70--75, 2012

6.   Lindow, S.E. Competitive Exclusion of Epiphytic bacteria by ice-minus Pseudamonas syringae mutants. Appl. Environ. Microbiol.53:2520-2527,1987. See also: Skirvin, R.M., Kohler, E., Steiner, H.,& 4 others. The use of genetically engineered bacteria to control frost on strawberries and potatoes: Whatever happened to all that research? Scientia Horticult. 84:179-189,2000.

7.   Morris, C.E., Georgakopoulos,D.G.,& Sands,D.C. Ice Nucleation active bacteria and their potential role in precipitation. J.Physics.IV. 121:87-103, 2004

8.   Poschl, U.,Martin, S.T., Sinha,B.,Chen,Q.,& 19 others. Rainforest Aerosols as Biogenic Nuclei of Clouds and Precipitation in the Amazon. Science. 329:(5998);1 513-1516, 2010.

9.   Smith, D.J.,T imonen,H.J.,Jaffee,D.A.,& 5 others. Intercontinental Dispersion of Bacteria and Archea by Transpacific Winds. Appl.Environ. Micrbiol. 79:(4); 11343-1139, 2013

10.   Vaitilingom, M., Deguillaume, L., Vinitier,V., & 4 others. Potential Impact of Microbial activity on the oxidant capacity and organic carbon budget in clouds. PNAS. 110:(2); 559-564, 2013. See also:Microbe.7:(3);119-122, 2012.

11.   Rodriguez, N.D., Latham, T.L., Rodriguez,L.M.,& 7others. Microbiome of the Upper troposphere:Species composition and prevalence,effects tropical storms, and atmospheric implications. PNAS.doi.10.1073/pnas.1212089110

12.   SantiTemkiv, T., Finster,K.,Hansen,B.M.,Neilson,N.W., Karlson,U.G. The Microbial Diversity of a Storm Cloud as Assessed by Hailstones. FEMS Microbiol.Ecol.81:(3);684-695,2012. See also: PloS One 8(1)e53550.2013

13.   Jackson, N., & Genki, R. Rio Tinto (Red River) Considered the Birthplace of the Copper Age and Bronze Age, the River is Tinted From 5,000 Years of Mining. AtlasObscura. Palos de la Frontera, Spain. www.AtlasObscura.com/places/rio-tinto.

14.   Brock, T. Life at High Temperatures. Science.158:(3804);1012-1019,1967.

15.   Fiala, G., and Stetter, K.O. Pyrococcus furiosus sp.nov.represents a novel genus of marine heterotrophic archeobcteria growing optimally at 100ºC. Arch.Microbiol.145:56-61,1986.

16.   Glud, R.N., Wenzhofer, F.,Middleboe,M.,& 4 others. High rates of microbial turnover in sediments in the deepest oceanic trench on earth. Nat.Geo. 6:284-288, 2013.

17.   Pfeffer, C., Larsen, S.,Song,J.,& 11 others, including Lars Peter Neilson. Filamentous bacteria transport electrons over centimetre distances. Nature. 491:218-221,2012 (Nov.8)

18.   Acevedo,F. The use of reactors in biomining processes. EJB Elect.J.Biotech. 3:(3);184-193,2000

19.   Reith, F., Fairbrother, L., Nolze,G.,& 5 others. Nanoparticle factories: Biofilms hold the key to gold dispersion and nugget dispersion. Geology.38: 843-846, 2010.

20.   Johnson, C.W., Wyatt, M.A., Li, X., & 4 others,including Magarvey, N.A. Gold biomineralization by a metallophore from a gold-associated microbe. Nat.Chem. Biol. 9: 241-243, 2013 (Jan.)

21.   Belnap, J. Biological Soil Crusts in Deserts: a short review of their role in soil fertility, stabilization, and water relations. Algolog.Stud.109:(1); 113-126, 2003

INDEX

49209562R00251

Made in the USA
Charleston, SC
19 November 2015